The Clinical Esthetician

£62.00

The Clinical Esthetician

An Insider's Guide to Succeeding in a Medical Office

Sallie S. Deitz

THOMSON

DELMAR LEARNING

Milady's The Clinical Esthetician
by Sallie Deitz

MILADY STAFF:

President:
Dawn Gerrain

Director of Editorial:
Sherry Gomoll

Acquisitions Editor:
Stephen G. Smith

Developmental Editor:
Judy Aubrey Roberts

Director of Production:
Wendy A. Troeger

Production Editor:
Eileen M. Clawson

Text Design and Composition:
Pre-Press Company, Inc.

Director of Marketing:
Donna Lewis

Cover Design:
essence of 7 / Suzanne Nelson

contact us by
Tel   (800) 730-2214
Fax   (800) 730-2215
www.thomsonrights.com

Library of Congress Cataloging-in-Publication Data
Deitz, Sallie S.
  The clinical aesthetician : an insiders guide to succeeding in a medical office / Sallie S. Deitz.
      p. ; cm.
Includes bibliographical references and index.
  ISBN-13: 978-1-4018-1788-6
  ISBN-10: 1-4018-1788-2 (alk. paper)
  1. Skin—Care and hygiene. 2. Beauty operators. 3. Allied health personnel.
  [DNLM: 1. Allied Health Personnel—organization & administration. 2. Skin Diseases—therapy. 3. Skin Manifestations. 4. Cosmetic Techniques. 5. Cosmetics. 6. Esthetics. 7. Interprofessional Relations. 8. Office Management. W 21.5 D324c 2003] I. Title.
  RL72.D44 2003
  616.5'0068—dc21
                                      2003013168

NOTICE TO THE READER

This book is dedicated to my mother,
Barbara Jean Strickler.
Her strength, courage, and wisdom have allowed
me to dream and to believe.

Contents

Foreword

by
R.E. Hecht, M.D.
Director, The Centre of Facial Plastic and Laser Surgery, Bellingham, Washington
Assistant Clinical Professor, University of Washington, School of Medicine

Man's concept of beauty has changed many times through the ages. Today beauty and preservation of youth are paramount in the minds of people from a wide spectrum of geography, genetics, and cultures. There is increasing awareness of the importance of wellness and self-preservation; we are all interested in skin care, prevention of problems, and good maintenance of our health and general appearance. Currently there is a surge in interest in cosmetic improvement; the aging of the "baby boomer" population is feeding the increasing demand for all types of rejuvenation surgery and medical care.

The clinical esthetician role is a recently established subspecialty and is often an integral component of a cosmetic plastic surgical/medical practice. Success with patients depends on exhaustive attention to detail, excellence in surgical technique, and a highly developed sense of perfection. This certainly includes patient screening and meticulous pre- and postoperative care. The esthetician has a role throughout this entire process.

There has been a paucity of current, meaningful material on this emerging specialty. Now this book strives to present a cogent outline and details of how to accomplish excellence in care through teamwork. This book expands our knowledge of techniques needed in the case of cosmetic and reconstructive patients. It provides an organized, easily understood, systematic approach to medical esthetics in practice today. The text fosters developing excellence in patient care. We all owe thanks to Sallie Deitz for taking on this project and developing this volume.

It has been the source of deep satisfaction and pleasure for me to be a small part of developing our comprehensive patient care protocols at the Centre for Facial Plastic and Laser Surgery in Bellingham, Washington. I have great pride in introducing Ms. Sallie Deitz, our clinical esthetician and my associate. She has labored to present this comprehensive volume so that it will be helpful to all striving to do the work of clinical esthetics.

We stand tall on the shoulders of those who have come before us, and I have been blessed throughout my life by close contact with fine teachers and wonderful patients, friends, and associates. Sallie Deitz arrived in our practice "from heaven" and has been a huge influence and help along the way. Sallie is an exceptionally talented, devoted, and intelligent young woman who has more than filled the gap as a medical esthetician in our busy practice. Her professionalism, compassion, and excellent judgment embody what a brilliant esthetician can bring to a cosmetic surgical practice. She, of course, had to learn and grow with us as we learned how to share patients in our practice—to the benefit of our patients and the satisfaction of ourselves. She has been patient, while ambitious to learn and practice new techniques, and has tirelessly educated herself and the rest of us. We are currently a good example of how well professionals can work together for mutual benefit. As a teacher, counselor, and compassionate human, Ms. Deitz continues to expand our horizons. This book is another step towards the goal of exceptional esthetic care.

Preface

As career opportunities in medical settings have become available, estheticians have expanded both their knowledge base and their responsibilities. Each setting determines the extent of the skills and training necessary to work in cooperation with the physician, nursing staff, and clinic administration. The esthetician's role in the clinical environment continues to develop, and recent rapid growth indicates that these professionals will persevere and obtain the necessary training to enhance this natural alliance.

There have been unfulfilled expectations on both sides of the union between physicians and estheticians, as well as many unfortunate misunderstandings. Physicians could gain greater understanding of the strengths, training, and vision for esthetic personnel if they would be supportive and nurture the gifts that the esthetician brings to a clinical setting. Conversely, estheticians need to improve their level of professionalism, team playing, and knowledge of the medical arts (language, procedures, chain of command), and, most of all, they need to develop greater confidence.

The Roles Played by the Clinical Esthetician

Many estheticians have found passion for their work in the medical milieu, and are increasing the value of their work. They are typically bright, thoughtful, compassionate, flexible, and eager to learn, and have an extraordinary aptitude toward service in working with clients and patients. Examples of existing liaisons and our roles within them are as follows:

- **Cosmetic and reconstructive surgery, otolaryngology (ear, nose, throat, and facial plastic surgery).** In cosmetic surgery the position may be more entrepreneurial than is the case with other settings. One may be responsible for an **ancillary profit center** (a separate department within the medical office that generates a profit). In addition to managing a retail center, performing routine and pre- and postoperative treatments, offering patient education, assisting medical staff with medical protocols, computer-imaging, and camouflage therapy, the esthetician may be involved in, or responsible for, marketing. This setting is excellent for one who is adaptive, has leadership skills, and is interested in business and teaching.
- **Dermatology.** In dermatology, the focus for the esthetician may be more analytical. For example, one may assist in research and clinical studies; many dermatologists conduct clinical trials. In addition, the esthetician may be working in tandem with the physician by cleansing or prepping the patient for a more advanced treatment or surgery that the physician administers. Other responsibilities may include performing routine facials, extractions, and microdermabrasion, and ordering supplies.

- **Outpatient clinic.**   The esthetician working in an outpatient surgery center will have responsibilities directed toward pre- and postoperative care. In addition the role may include being a patient educator, monitoring home-care compliance, developing protocols with nursing staff, coordinating patient care, computer-imaging, and/or fully managing the profit center.
- **Hospital.**   The function of the esthetician in a hospital setting may be team oriented. It might include assisting in research in clinical trials, providing pre- and postoperative care, and/or directing an ancillary profit center such as a medical spa.
- **Independent clinic.**   Estheticians working in an independent clinic located near a hospital or medical facility will provide services to clients and patients referred by physicians. One practicing in an independent clinic would need advanced knowledge of medical procedures, protocols, major malpractice insurance, and business acumen. The role may span from administrator to practitioner. In addition, it would require strong networking program within the medical community.
- **Laser centers.**   Laser centers offer unique opportunities for estheticians to act as coordinators for laser procedures such as spider vein therapy or laser hair reduction. Some states authorize physicians to supervise estheticians in performing laser treatments; in all cases, we can apply pre- and postlaser treatment.
- **Cosmetic dentistry.**   Estheticians providing comprehensive skin care in cosmetic dental offices may also manage a retail center to include facial products, makeup, and dental products.
- **Medical spa.**   The esthetician's role in a medical spa (**medi-Spa**) may include managing the spa, performing pre- and postoperative treatments, assisting nursing staff with protocols, and providing routine skin care to clients.

The Intention of This Book

This book is intended as support for the esthetician currently practicing in a medical office, or for those interested in working in a medical setting. In addition, it will inform nurses, medical and physicians' assistants, and physicians interested in supporting and benefiting from the skills, and talents of an esthetician.

It will also serve as a reference guide for cosmetologists including stylists, designers, colorists, aromatherapy specialists; estheticians working in skin-care salons and spas, massage therapists; and the department store beauty advisor. Statistics show that most clients will have some type of surgical procedure, as well as an alliance with a cosmetic surgeon, dermatologist, or clinical esthetician.

How This Book Came To Be

This book is a compilation of the author's 20 years of working in the skin-care industry, and 8 years of research while working in a medical office as a clinical esthetician. The result, *The Clinical Esthetician, An Insider's Guide to Succeeding in a Medical Office*, focuses on real work/life issues that come up while working in a doctor's office. Clinical estheticians have commented that they need specific information about how to work in a clinical setting. This book provides that information and more, and serves as a follow up to the Advanced Clinical section in the textbook *Milady's Standard Comprehensive Training for Estheticians,* 2003. The comments, questions, and answers have come from issues brought up at conferences, meetings, training seminars, and peer one-on-ones.

Here's How This Book Can Help

This client-patient–centered orientation reads easily for beginners, and can be a good review for veteran estheticians and for medical liaisons. This book will show how to:

- become a liaison for physician and client/patient
- resolve conflicts and office politics diplomatically and easily
- apply a code of ethics and learn boundaries
- treat clients who have special considerations or illnesses
- develop a method for interfacing with medical personnel
- chart legally and acquire risk management tools
- find appropriate forms of self-care and stress management
- avoid common pitfalls of burn-out
- build a booming retail business
- discover or revisit tried-and-true treatments, peels, and combinations
- build a major network/referral program
- create a BIZ Plan that really works
- improve your business acumen and bottom line

In general, you will learn how to create a thriving skin-care business in a clinical setting.

Who Can Benefit From This Book

- **student estheticians** interested in clinical work
- **clinical estheticians.** This book deals with real-life issues that face us working in a clinic every day.
- **nurses, physicians, administrators and other medical personnel**—all individuals working in a medical office wanting to make full use of the esthetician.
- **estheticians working in salons, spas and skin-care centers; massage therapists, cosmetologists, department store beauty advisors, and aromatherapists:** all practitioners dealing with clients having plastic surgery or appearance issues.

Overview

In the first half of the book you will find topics such as communication, referring to the doctor, consultations, both routine and preoperative, patient education and selection; computer imaging, business planning/marketing strategies; creating a code of ethics, dealing with office politics, OSHA standards made simple, risk management and insurance, medical documentation and treatment protocols for special needs patients.

In the second half of the book, subjects like pre- and postoperative care, skin-care conditions, tried-and-true treatments, and protocols are covered. In addition you'll find camouflage therapy, multicultural skin care, cases studies of acne, hirsutism, and dyschromias; handling challenging situations and patients, coping with the death of a favorite client, patient or co-worker, acknowledging and healing codependency issues; and unconventional methods to self-care for the esthetician.

The goal of the clinical esthetician across the disciplines is to provide support to the medical team and to give comprehensive care to the clients and patients. The expectations are that we are professional, ethical, and flexible. The medical setting is dynamic and ever changing. It will demand our best.

Sallie Deitz, clinical esthetician and patient educator

Acknowledgments

Very special thanks to my husband Gary Deitz for his love and support during the time that I spent writing this book. Thanks for the talks, walks on the beach, and the shoulder massages.

To Dr. Emil Hecht, thank you for your vision, creativity, patience and for taking a chance on me.

Thanks to Tannia Hecht, for paving the way so many years ago, and for exceptional help in research and development, and product acquisition.

To Drs. Robert Harris, Thomas Stackhouse, and Joost Knops: thanks for your continued support, and for allowing me to "run with it."

Thanks to all of our very special clients and patients at Bellingham ENT & Facial Plastic Surgery for allowing me to serve them.

Thanks to the following people and organizations who have contributed to this book through support, kind words, and input. The author appreciates all they have done in the creation of this book.

Pamela Lappies
Judy Roberts
Staff of Milady/Delmar Learning
R. Emil Hecht, M.D.
Robert Harris, M.D.
Thomas Stackhouse, M.D.
Joost Knops, M.D.
Tannia Hecht, M.A.
Staff of Bellingham Ear, Nose, Throat, and Facial Plastic Surgery
Margie Lykke
Katy Denooyer, CMA
Chris Hettick, CMA
Kelly Lequerrier
Susie Johnson
Karlene Caffel
Jean Hurlbert, LPN
Howard Gardner, Ph.D., Harvard University
Mark Rubin, M.D.
Albert Kligman, M.D.
Kathleen Young, Ph.D., Western Washington University
Annetta Vanandel, Ph.D.
Christa Hougan, L.A.
Small Business Development Center, WWU, Bellingham, WA
Tom Dorr

Angie Ellsperman
Mark Levinski, Ph.D.
Melanie Sachs
Megan Watt
Robin Gordon, Pre-Press Company
Christine Guiao
Bonnie Day, AAEA
Kathleen Driscoll, CIDESCO
Reviewers:
An Hinds, Catherine Hinds Institute
Beverly May, Redwood City, CA
Tena Northern, Academy of Hair Design
Keizer, OR
Margaret Groves, MA, Bellingham Technical College
David Scherrer, Photographer
Carolyn Alvis
Michael and Nancy Strickler, Lyte Speed Learning
Lynn Rosen, Steve Giordano
Barbara Forss
Jim Longman, Allstate Insurance
Suzanne Greene
Barbara and Mark Fuller, Our House Publishing
The Evergreen State College, Power in Perspective Program

Section I

Communication

1

Getting Started

- Introduction
- Building the Relationship
- Communication with a Purpose
- Building Trust
- Responsibility with Communication
- Summary
- Frequently Asked Questions

Introduction

Getting to know the client or patient is the key to the health of your practice. It will determine product choice, treatment, procedure plans and protocols, and it will serve as a guide to physician referral. Exceptional communication skills will be essential to your role as liaison between patient and physician and will establish a degree of professionalism, which leads to client and patient satisfaction. In this text, a person visiting an esthetician in the office for skin care and treatment shall be referred to as a *client*, and one meeting with a physician for medical care is a *patient*. When these roles overlap, they will be called patients, to avoid confusion.

Building the Relationship

In many ways, getting to know a client is like getting to know someone as a good friend. Especially because the evolving relationship can take many turns, it takes excellent communication skills to develop a healthy and committed liaison. The key elements in relationship building are universal: they are *respect*, *honesty*, and *compassion*.

In the client/patient-esthetician relationship, the focus always must be on the client. Therefore, we may say that the intention of our primary relationship in the office must be professional rather than private or personal. At times, it can become confusing and difficult because we develop feelings toward our clients and patients yet the distinction must be recognized. Figure 1–1 shows a consultation, which might develop into a long-standing professional relationship.

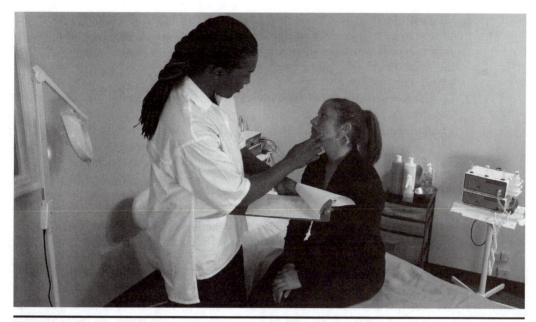

Figure 1–1   Clinical esthetician consults with a patient

Each esthetician has a unique way of fostering a sound relationship with a client. Some may share on a more personal level and know when to redirect conversation to the client; others may follow strict clinical protocol and feel uncomfortable sharing personal information. Whatever your particular method of interfacing with a client, there are three basic requirements that must be met. The client must always know and feel that you are taking the lead in the service, that your function is to assist them, and that you are practicing under the supervision of the physician.

Communication with a Purpose

Communication in a medical office is central to just about every task that needs to be accomplished. Since estheticians often serve as client and patient educators, it is natural that we want exceptional skills in this area. To learn about communication we want to look at our styles of communicating and, more importantly, the two-way transmission of information. In other words, it is essential that the information that we are sharing be properly understood.

People receive information based upon their own particular learning styles and intelligences. In 1983, Howard Gardner, Ph.D., psychologist and professor of education at Harvard University, developed a theory called **Multiple Intelligences**. He states that there are eight primary intelligences. They are defined as follows.

1. **Linguistic intelligence:** excellence in the use of words. Writers, teachers, politicians all tend to have linguistic intelligence. Such individuals like to express themselves in writing and will favor the use of words in communication. Poets Robert Frost and Maya Angelou could be considered examples of people possessing linguistic intelligence.

2. **Logical-mathematical analytical intelligence:** exceptional ability with numbers and logic. One is comfortable using statistics, graphs, numbers, and a logical sequence of events to apply to learning, understanding, and expression. Physicians, accountants, and engineers are examples of people possessing mathematical intelligence. Albert Einstein and Bill Gates are among those with logical and mathematical inclinations.

3. **Spatial/visual intelligence:** one is visually oriented and naturally adept at moving images around in space or visualizing images. This type of person will want to see and visualize something in the process of learning and creating. Artists, designers and visually oriented people will possess spatial intelligence. We could consider Michelangelo and Frank Lloyd Wright as examples of people with spatial intelligence.

4. **Body-kinesthetic intelligence:** excellence in physical movement; one may need to apply a "hands-on" approach to learning and doing. Michael Jordan and Lance Armstrong are superb examples of physical intelligence.

5. **Musical intelligence:** an above-average ability in music. The inclination toward musical intelligence will generate an interest in learning and expressing through rhythm and sound. Mozart and vocalist Ella Fitzgerald were endowed with musical intelligence.

6. **Interpersonal intelligence:** strength in dealing with people and emotional maturity. Individuals with this type of intelligence are understanding and compassionate and express those qualities in their learning and communication styles. One could say that Oprah Winfrey and Jimmy Carter possess emotional intelligence.

7. **Intrapersonal intelligence:** great self-knowledge and self-awareness. This type of individual will also exhibit confidence. Examples of people with this type of intelligence would be Abraham Lincoln and Gandhi.

8. **Naturalist intelligence:** strong ability with the natural world. People possesing this type of intelligence will communicate and work in the natural environment. Examples of those with naturalist intelligence, include Jane Goodall or Aldo Leopold, the writer and ecology pioneer.

Gardner's theory has been implemented in varied educational settings, to maximize learning potential. Typically, our culture uses linguistic and logical-mathematical intelligence to communicate information. However, our government documents, schools, businesses, churches, and other institutions often use media that may compromise some types of learning and communication styles. One example might be a visually oriented individual trying to comprehend a long written article detailing a logical-analytical approach to using a voters' booth, when a couple of diagrams might be more easily understood by that person.

For estheticians, this way of looking at learning styles has strong implications. Although many people possess multiple intelligences, estheticians often have **interpersonal intelligence** or **emotional intelligence** predominantly. This type of intelligence, useful in bonding our population, is clearly significant as an esthetician strives to enter a relationship with a client. When **emotional intelligence** is combined with **linguistic intelligence, spatial intelligence** and **kinesthetic intelligence** and are purposefully used in the office, it is easy to see that compassion (using interpersonal intelligence) expressed with words (using linguistic intelligence), that explained a hands-on treatment through the use of a sketch or other visual aid (using spatial intelligence) could be beneficial to preparing a patient for a procedure. Here are some examples of predominant intelligences and learning styles:

- A person showing the predominance of **spatial intelligence** or **visual intelligence** may make statements like, "May I see a picture or brochure of what you are describing?" This question is your first clue that the client or patient is visually oriented and would benefit from use of visual aids—the more colorful and esthetically pleasing, the better.
- A client asks, "How many of these procedures has the doctor performed?" Further, she comes fully prepared to write down everything you say in numbered sentences, is asking about percentages of eyelifts to facelifts that the doctor has performed, and has a copy of an article from *The New England Journal of Medicine*. You know that this individual has a very *logical-mathematical* type of orientation. Do not bother to give them fluffy or slick marketing materials when a good level-appropriate clinical study, with graphs, diagrams and solid definitions demonstrating a scientific approach, will give them what they need to absorb information.
- Patients with physical or *kinesthetic intelligence* may need to actually move their bodies or apply in a hands-on fashion in order to learn or communicate something. If you find someone using his hands to describe details, then you may want to actually *show*—not tell—that individual how to use something. As estheticians we often do this anyway, but applied demonstrations are the best way for people with kinesthetic intelligence to assimilate information.

Internet and Communication

One of the many reasons we find the Internet useful is that we can often assimilate information easily because of the various methods it uses to express material. We see graphs, diagrams, and statistics (logical-mathematical oriented); images and photographs (visual and spatially oriented); voice, music, or sound (musically or audio-logically oriented); and articles, books, prose, and poems (linguistically oriented); frequently the Internet provides a composite of two or more intelligences. This makes absorbing information even easier as most of us are in two or more of these orientations.

Building Trust

From the clients' perspective, we initiate work with them to offer products, services, and support in a medical setting. As questions arise during the consultation, most clients will be pleasantly surprised when we move to the position of educator. Depending upon your level of experience and knowledge, you can move from educating and sharing information to problem solving and acting as a resource specialist.

An example of problem solving might be that you are able to determine from your knowledge of cosmetic chemistry that an ingredient to which a client is allergic shows up in a product under a different name. For the client this insight begins to foster the idea that you have a much larger knowledge base than what was originally expected. From there, the client begins to feel understood. He or she will feel connected with the appropriate person, and perceive that there is hope for their particular situation. If you do not have the solution, it is important that you refer them to another health care professional or colleague. This way, every request or situation is an opportunity to serve. Clients always know when you have their interests as a main concern.

Four essential tips to building trust and creating a good consultation are:

- do your homework and continue to learn
- share what you learn in a comprehensible way
- be enthusiastic about their interests
- network with other practitioners and businesses

Once you have connected with clients in this way, they will listen to you and have confidence in what you are recommending. Without this vital bond, your services may seem unnecessary.

Responsibility with Communication

When you consider that people coming in for a consultation are sharing information to which not even a best friend, spouse, or co-worker may be privy, there is not only a legal responsibility created through the exchange, but a trust becomes sanctioned. We take into confidence the innermost personal grievances an individual is experiencing about his or her appearance issues. As estheticians, we need to remember that our role is to act as a liaison between the client and the physician, and to create a comfortable atmosphere for the subsequent visits.

Be prepared and know your boundaries.   We must be prepared to serve at the level of our purpose and function. Consulting with people in a friendly, professional, competent, compassionate manner is a necessary skill set for an esthetician—so, however, is observing a code of conduct while working with clients and patients.

We learn a tremendous amount about an individual as we consult and counsel, and it is necessary to keep this in perspective. You may find clients and patients wanting to share many details about their lives with you. Often estheticians can find themselves quite innocently in the middle of issues that are beyond their scope, and can encounter manifestations of both stress and depression unknowingly. Keep in mind: unless you have an advanced degree in mental health, it is unlawful to practice as a therapist. We are often interacting in a milieu with unclear boundaries, and this poses many problems for estheticians, their co-workers, and their patients.

Clients visit a clinical setting primarily because they are interested in results, and there is an assumption that products and treatments will be more aggressive than those found in a salon or spa. There is also a belief that an esthetician working in a medical office will have advanced degrees, training, and experience beyond what they may find elsewhere. This assumption may be erroneous and often includes unrealistic expectations, but it is often what is perceived. During the consultation, you will want to focus on realistic expectations and results from products, services, and procedures.

Summary

It takes time to get to understand and know your client, but cues received during your consultations can be helpful, and the way you present your material can be critical to a positive outcome. Structure your consults to yield maximum informational benefits to both of you. Make it clear that you are a liaison, a patient advocate, and a resource person, in addition to being a skin care professional. If you approach your consultations this way, you will create unions that will last long after they have left your office and you will be the first person that they think of when considering skin care or other services such as microdermabrasion peels or laser hair reduction that you have shared with them. In addition, if people sense that you are there to support them from the point of initial contact—through a treatment, procedure, and beyond—you will not need to *sell* them anything; they will trust you and see you as the consummate professional.

Frequently Asked Questions

1. **What does the esthetician do if a client begins to talk about all of her personal problems?**

   This is an issue for most of us working in the esthetics field. The difference in the *medical* setting is that there is an implicit belief that we may have more training because we are associated with a physician. When the client goes beyond the realm of skin care, or takes the conversation out of your scope, it is important to use a compassionate voice, and open, sympathetic, body language, to communicate that you want to be of help in the best way *possible*. Stand up and begin to pull out brochures, cards, or articles that are directed toward the topic and assure the client that your resource is a specialist in the subject of concern. Hand the information to them while you begin to sit back down, and as you are taking your chair say, "I am wondering if, for now, we can get back to the matters at hand, as this is your time for skin care." For most, this will send the message, and redirect the consultation. For a few, it will not.

   If someone is persistent, and continues to share personal stories, you will need to come right out and say, "I have really enjoyed meeting you today, but these issues cannot be solved here. Let us make a referral for you to speak with someone who can help you with these other matters." They may be terribly lonely and have many emotional problems. This is always challenging, and difficult to ignore, but you will not be able to help them if you are untrained in this area. It is necessary then for you to share this with the doctor, and make a chart note reflecting the referral.

2. What if during the consultation, the esthetician is asked by the client to perform a treatment or application that is beyond the level of experience or licensure?

If the request is made by the client or patient, tell them directly that you are unqualified to perform the treatment or procedure. Most people will appreciate your integrity, and you will not be in an uncomfortable—or potentially liable—situation if something fails.

If the request has been made by the physician, tell him or her that the procedure or application is beyond your scope. The physician may not know this. Conversely, if it is within guidelines and you are learning a new technique or peel, for instance, ask the physician to remain with you during the entire treatment. Physicians appreciate this type of disclosure, as they are ultimately responsible for all of your work.

CHAPTER 2

Consultation and Office Visits

- Introduction
- Prepare for the Consultation
- Seven Steps to a Good Consultation
- Record Maintenance
- Summary
- Frequently Asked Questions

Introduction

Depending on the type of physician with whom you are associated, and the policy or protocol of the office, you as esthetician may be the first representative in the office to visit with the client. The key to participating in a consultation is to be in attendance. That means participating with the client on many levels, listening and demonstrating that you are compassionate by using nonverbal cues such as head nodding, good eye contact, and a soft relaxed facial expression. All of these behaviors lead to good communication. Leave the intense "game face" for workouts in the gym.

Prepare for the Consultation

Clients and patients feel overly processed and managed today, with all of the changes in the medical field. Make certain that their visits with you are *about them*, and that your work is centered on their needs. Verbal response to questions, observing body language and—the least of all participation elements—becoming and remaining well organized will serve as a good foundation.

Two Key Elements to the Initial Consultation

During this initial consultation, you will discover whether the *client* is interested in becoming a *patient* and needs to be referred to the physician, or if their interest is skin care. It may be that they are interested in both. Herein lays an opportunity to visit expectations and to gain as much information as possible. It is important not to rush this process for two basic reasons:

PATIENT CONSULTATION Date _____

How did you hear about us? Newspaper Ad ❑ Yellow Pages ❑ Referring Physician ❑ Friend ❑

Please explain _____

Name _____ E-mail Address _____

Social Security _____ Birthdate _____

Home Address _____

City _____ State _____ Zip _____

Home Phone (_____) _____ Business Phone (_____) _____

Occupation _____ Employer _____

Employer's Address _____

Name of Spouse ❑ Parent ❑ Guardian ❑ _____

Address *(if different than above)* _____

Occupation _____ Employer _____

Employer's Address _____

Friend or Relative we may contact in an emergency:

Name _____ Phone _____

Please complete this health questionnaire

A. If you have had any of the following, check the appropriate box

❑ Anemia   ❑ Eye, Vision Problems
❑ Bleed Easily   ❑ Liver Disease, Hepatitis, Yellow Jaundice
❑ Cancer, Tumor   ❑ Phlebitis
❑ Diabetes   ❑ Stomach Ulcer
❑ Dark Skin Spots *(hyperpigmentation)*   ❑ Skin Lesions / Cancer / Moles
❑ Heavy Scarring   ❑ Anxiety

Lungs–   ❑ Cough or Pain
         ❑ Do you Smoke? _____   How much? _____
         ❑ Drugs / Alcohol? _____   How much? _____

Heart–   ❑ Angina
         ❑ Heart Attack
         ❑ Stroke
         ❑ High blood Pressure

Skin Problems (please list) _____

Have you ever tested for HIV? ❑ Yes ❑ No Result + –

Other _____

B. Operations and Approximate Year: _____

C. Medicines — List all medicines, birth control pills, aspirin or vitamins you currently take: _____
_____

D. Medicine Allergies — List all medicines you are allergic to or have had reactions to of any kind:
_____

If this visit is related to an ACCIDENT or INJURY, please fill out portion below:

How injured _____ Date injured _____

Job Related Accident/Injury ❑ Yes ❑ No

Describe Injuries: _____

Care Given _____ Where? _____

Figure 2–1 Patient Consultation Form

10

PATIENT CONSULTATION (*continued*)

My Appearance Concerns Are:

- ❏ Wrinkles
- ❏ Eyes — bags under / droopy eyelids
- ❏ Facial Scarring — uneven texture
- ❏ Thin Lips

- ❏ Nose
- ❏ Jowling / Neck
- ❏ Frown Lines
- ❏ Facial Hair
- ❏ Spider Veins

- ❏ Other _____

I Would Be Interested In Knowing More About:

- ❏ Laser Surgery
- ❏ Face Lift (Rhytidectomy)
- ❏ Nose (Rhinoplasty)
- ❏ Removal of Skin Lesions / Cancer
- ❏ Collagen / Botox

- ❏ Computer Imaging
- ❏ Eyelid Surgery (Blepharoplasty)
- ❏ Scar Revision
- ❏ Laser Hair Reduction
- ❏ Other _____

Esthetician Services:

- ❏ Skin Care Consultation
- ❏ Skin Health Products
- ❏ In Office Peels / Masks
- ❏ Microdermabrasion
- ❏ Camouflage Makeup
- ❏ Other _____

Figure 2–1 Patient Consultation Form (*continued*)

- **People do not always know what they want or need to achieve results.** It could be that a client coming to you may have erroneous information about clinical products for example, and may expect that a firming cream will eliminate a sagging jawline. Alternatively, a client may have seen an advertisement about **laser resurfacing**, and presents for information about the procedure, yet a **rhytidectomy** (face-lift) may be necessary to achieve the desired results.

- **The esthetician may not always know what the client truly desires.** A client may visit you ostensibly for skin care products, but may in fact be interested in having a procedure. This will often be the case in a medical office. You may experience a client visiting for several months prior to their disclosing that they are interested in having a more permanent result, as in a **blepharoplasty** (eyelift) or a **platysmaplasty** (necklift). Conversely, after a 15-minute consultation you may find that the client wants to meet with the doctor as soon as possible and you may facilitate that meeting by making introductions at the earliest opportunity.

CLIENT PROFILE FORM

Name _____ Phone _____ E-mail _____

Address _____

City _____ State _____ Zip _____

How did you find us? ❑ Advertising ❑ Friend ❑ Other_____

Is your skin dry? ❑ Normal ❑ Dry ❑ Oily ❑ Combination ❑ Sensitive ❑ Other_____

Have you seen a doctor in the past year for a skin disorder? ❑ Yes ❑ No

If yes, why? _____

Are you currently under a doctor's care? ❑ Yes ❑ No

If yes, why? _____

Are you taking any prescription drugs? ❑ Yes ❑ No ❑ Hormones ❑ Yes ❑ No

If yes, what kind? _____

Please complete this health questionnaire

Have you ever used:

❑ Retin-A®	❑ Scrubs
❑ Skin lighteners	❑ Salicylic Acid
❑ Accutane®	❑ Loofahs/sponges
❑ Benzoyl Peroxide	❑ Glycolic Acid

Do you exercise? _____ How often? _____ What kind? _____

Describe in detail what kinds of fluids you drink daily, and how much? _____

Are you pregnant? _____ Do you smoke? _____ If so, how much? _____

Have you ever had cosmetic surgery, a chemical peel or other treatment? _____ If yes, where and when _____

What products are you currently using? _____

SKIN CLASSIFICATION:

Skin Type	Notes	Rubin Photodamage Classification	Notes	Kligman Classification	Notes
Color		Level		Acne Grade	
I		I		I	
II		II		II	
III		III		III	
IV				IV	
V					
VI					

SKIN DISORDERS:

O None	O Sebaceous Hyperplasia	O Sebaceous Cysts	O Keloids
O Dermatitis	O Seborrheic Keratosis	O Miliam	O Scars
O Nevus	O Nodules	O Excoriations	O Hirsutisim

Location_____

_____

_____

Figure 2–2 Esthetician's Client Profile Form

Skin Thickness	Pore Size	Texture	Keratinization	Vascularity
❑ Thin	❑ Super fine	❑ Smooth	❑ Psoriasis	❑ Telangiectases
❑ Medium	❑ Fine	❑ Rough	❑ Eczema	❑ Erythema
❑ Thick	❑ Medium	❑ Granular	❑ Ichthyosis	❑ Rosacea
	❑ Large			❑ Rhinophyma

ACNEIC PATTERNS:

❑ Few   ❑ Many   ❑ Cyclical   ❑ Chronic

TYPES: LOCATION:

Medications _____
Frequency _____

- ❑ Comedones   _____
- ❑ Macules   _____
- ❑ Papules   _____
- ❑ Pustules   _____
- ❑ Nodules   _____
- ❑ *Propionibacterium* (*P. Acne*)   _____
- ❑ Rosacea   _____
- ❑ Vulgarus   _____

TREATMENT AND HOME CARE PLAN: ❑ Refer to Physician?

Date _____
Date _____
Date _____
Date _____
Date _____

PRODUCTS/PURCHASES:

Date _____
Date _____
Date _____
Date _____
Date _____

Figure 2–2   Client Profile Form *(continued)*

Seven Steps to a Good Consultation

By utilizing a methodical approach to a consultation, you will save time, energy and, most of all, misunderstandings. When enough experience has been acquired, the esthetician can abbreviate the consultation accordingly. However, if you find that it takes too long to determine what the client is requesting, or if this is often an awkward experience for you, try this method:

1. **Determine the subject of the visit.**   You may find within the first few minutes of a consultation that your client is not interested in basic skin care. Pay close attention here. There is nothing more uncomfortable for the client than feeling that no one is listening. If you find that the client really wants to discuss a surgical procedure, redirect all communication toward a consultation with the physician. Clinical estheticians today are well versed on procedures. They will often present the procedure to the client, briefly describing it, thus facilitating the meeting with the doctor by beginning the patient education process. Bring the nurse and doctor into the loop as soon as possible. This could be accomplished even just through a quick introduction if the doctor is busy with another patient. You want to finish your consultation with them so that they do not feel like you are saying, "Hey, here's a live one," but do not belabor the product orientation, or the long version of why we use glycolic acid in products. It is important to let the client assume the role of patient as quickly as possible.

2. **Begin your intake process.**   Once you have determined the subject of the client's interest, you may begin your intake process. By now you will have some information about the client from reading the required physician's standard **Patient Consultation Form** (Figure 2–1), and you will have access to their medical chart. Legally and ethically you must regard this information as highly confidential. In addition to the Patient Consultation Form, you will want to generate your own form for your records. This form is often called a **Client Profile Form** (Figure 2–2).

3. **Establish rapport while working through the Client Profile Form.**   This form is vital to your business. It will serve not only as a guide to remain organized during the consultation, but as a blueprint for setting up a treatment plan and home care program for the client. In addition to collecting information about your client for the purposes of being able to better assist them, you will be able to establish rapport through working your way through this form *together*.

Pertinent Background Information In the Patient Consultation Form and the Client Profile Form

The forms look straightforward, but let us consider the rationale for using some of this inquiry material. A few key questions will both garner information about a client and give a client an idea of your degree of interest and professionalism:

1. **How did you find us?**
   This question may seem of little significance to you now that the client is sitting before you, but the answer can give you three key pieces of information that are valuable to your practice:
   a. They are telling you how you are being perceived in the community.
   b. It shows you where to put your marketing dollars.
   c. It tells you whom to thank for the referral, and where to continue an alliance.

2. Medical history

- Note specifics like physician, dermatologist, or health care professional.
- Are there medical conditions such as allergies, headaches, and serious diseases such as HIV or hepatitis.
- Is the client pregnant or lactating?
- Is the client on **Accutane**?
- Note whether the client has had previous surgeries.
- Has the client had cancer? If so, where is she or he in treatment or recovery? (See Chapter 16.)
- Does the client have headaches? People suffering from migraines or allergies may not be candidates for your favorite aromatherapy treatment.

Patients with HIV or hepatitis will need special care given in the clinic and are not candidates for facial treatments. If your new client is pregnant, lactating, or on Accutane®, treatments or products containing **AHAs** (alpha hydroxy acids), retinoids, or bleaching aids with **hydroquinone** (skin lightener) should not be given.

3. Previous surgeries

Has the client had previous surgeries? If so, what were they? Who performed the procedures? Was the client satisfied with the results? If not, what is the nature of the dissatisfaction? The answer to these questions will give you insight as to whether or not expectations have been met. If the individual is unhappy with the results of previous surgeries, chances are he or she may not be happy with those performed in the future. Conversely, if a client seems reasonably satisfied and realistic, and recognizes that the benefits do not last forever, you may find a great patient in this client.

4. What is their primary concern or chief complaint (cc)?

Active listening skills are important here. Get to it. Again, if you spend time discussing products and services only to find out that this individual came in worried about a mole changing color, you will appear unknowledgeable and will probably create frustration for both of you. In addition, you need to know as quickly as possible if you are beyond your scope, so that you may make an appropriate referral.

4. Skin analysis.

A thorough skin analysis is not difficult to make since we do not get into diagnosis. A face diagram or graphic to present areas in question is helpful. Some clinicians use a narrative approach. Find what works best for you. It helps to have a list of potential disorders and conditions to check off, along with the head and neck region locators. Using terms such as *mental region* (chin), *orbital region* (eye), and *zygomatic region* (cheekbone) for charting purposes translates well to medical personnel. While looking at clean skin, use the following questions to direct your examination:

- Are the pores uniform? Where on the face are they the largest/smallest?
- Do you see **telangiectases** (spider veins)? Are they on the surface or deeper? Where are they located?
- How much photodamage is present? (Use **Glogau Classification** or **Rubin Classification** of photodamage in Chapter 14.)
- Does this skin present with blemishes? If so, where are they? Are the lesions open or closed? Do you see comedones, pustules, papules, or cysts? (Use **Kligman's Classification** in Chapter 14.)
- If there are scars, what types are present and where are they located?
- Do you see pigment changes?
- **Hyperpigmentation** (dark pigmented lesions)
- **Hypopigmentation** (void or loss of pigment)
- Write location on your CP form: Are there any other lesions such as:
  Hemangioma (red birthmark)
  Actinic keratosis (sun spots, can be dry flaky, red)
  Nevi or **lentigines** (moles or freckles)
- What is the skin type?
  Oily
  Dry
  Sensitive
  Normal
  Combination

- Are there distended or swollen areas such as the nose, chin, or forehead? How is the texture? Is it smooth, rough, uneven? (Glogau Classification) Is it wrinkled? Are there deep lines? Medium, or more on the surface? How does the neck and chest present? Is it crepy or photodamaged, or smooth and unlined? How do the hands look? Are they pigmented, lined, or rough—or are they smooth and hydrated?

Suspicious lesions
Here are a few words of caution about identifying suspicious lesions. While we do not make a diagnosis, with experience we can eventually recognize almost any type of disorder and disease with which we come in contact. It is vital that we refer the client to the physician as soon as possible, and always document suspicious lesions. Above all, regardless of what we think we see, allow the doctor to present the information to the patient. It helps to develop a professional response to the client such as, "We should have the doctor take a look at this area, we want to make sure that we are creating the best treatment plan for your skin." This is a precaution not to alarm prematurely (you may be wrong), or needlessly, and perhaps it may take a few days to get the client into the physician's schedule. Many of us have experienced firsthand what an unofficial diagnosis can be by well-meaning unqualified personnel. It can be nerve-wracking.

5. **Make recommendations.**   While making a skin analysis, you may ask what the client is using for home care. Once you examine the skin, you will begin to make some judgments about product recommendations and a treatment plan for your client. You will not be able to address every issue on this first visit, but you are building awareness about how best to proceed. Cues from your initial contact with the client will guide your recommendations. Remember what the chief complaints were and go from there.

Keep in mind that not every person you may see in a medical setting will want a full skin analysis. This service is often abbreviated. You may have several patients throughout the day as referred by the physician, and they may just want information, makeup, or an eye cream. You may ask them if they would like to come back at a later date for a full consultation; that way they will be prepared to focus on what you would like to share with them about how you may assist them with their skin care.

6. **Determine current home care and compliance.**   The answer to this question will give you a direction to follow in your own presentation. If you ascertain from your 50-year-old client that home care consists of soap and water, and moisturizing with a petroleum product, you will probably find that that person does not want an expensive, multiproduct regime. It will not be used. Keep it simple. Offer a cleanser that lathers like soap and a skin type and condition-appropriate, hydrating moisturizer with UVA and UVB protection. If you find however, that the client uses a cleanser, an AHA product, an eye cream, and a moisturizer with sunscreen during the day and a separate cream at night, chances are he or she will be willing to give a new product a fair try. Determine the missing item in the regime and augment the home care program piece by piece, rather than suggesting that the client throw it all out and start over. Even simply getting a sample of a new product in a client's hands is better than overselling and appearing like a *product pusher*.

   If clients tell you that they are dissatisfied with what they are using and want to replace everything, then by all means, share what you have. Nevertheless, keep in mind that it is better to have them come back in for something than to have them walk out feeling oversold and overspent.

7. **Detail protocol.**   Every client with a new product regime goes home with a written protocol on use and purpose of application. This avoids confusion, creates faster results, and is professional. It is worth the extra time to write them in clear order and add in medications as indicated. If you give out a computerized sheet with an entire product line listed, this can seem impersonal and creates uncertainty about products on the list which should actually be used. You can give them a product directory, with products that will be added in the future circled. Always make sure that they understand to look for products that are highlighted for their skin type.

Record Maintenance

Once you have made the transaction, be certain to maintain good records. Enter all purchases on the client profile form. As your client and database builds, it is very difficult to remember everything that you have sold to a client as you receive many calls for replacement items. In addition, as you build your product inventory, it is equally difficult to remember when you may have moved a certain client from one product line to another. It is unprofessional (not to mention embarrassing) if you put out the wrong product or introduce a product when you already spent 10 minutes describing the benefits and features of it during an earlier visit.

Summary

Today's consumers are well informed. By now, they have heard about AHAs, sunscreens, **antioxidants**, and laser surgery; however, often their main goal is to determine which office can best meet the complexities of their changing needs. You want to be that vehicle for them. By remaining committed to the health of their skin, and to continuing to learn about them as individuals, you will find they are returning to you and referring their friends to you.

Frequently Asked Questions

1. **What does the esthetician do if her client during the initial consultation reveals that she has tried every skin care product on the market, has been reading a book that says that all products are basically the same, and has found that nothing really works?**

   This happens frequently, when a client has been sold rather than educated. She feels she has been taken advantage of in the past, and needs to be empowered. Teach her about her needs, in a slow, methodical manner, and resist selling her anything without an extensive product-sampling program. In addition, she probably has some unrealistic expectations about products, which can happen with market hype and advertising. The features-benefit paradigm should be retired for this case. She will need honesty and possibly a more aggressive program, including a visit with the physician.

2. **What is the most appropriate way to handle someone who talks over your voice and is rude during a consultation?**

   It is often effective to stop speaking every time someone jumps in and speaks over your voice. Once a person catches on to what you are doing, he may feel comfortable enough to slow down and wait a turn. In addition, you can wait a few seconds before responding to a question. This will let the client know that you are aware of a tendency toward not allowing you to finish your statement, and you may put up one hand (if the client begins to interrupt again), almost as if you are saying, "Just a moment."

This communication flaw can be especially challenging when you are trying to help prepare a patient for surgery. It is another reason to have many forms of communication styles available, such as videos and images.

CHAPTER 3

Physician Referral, Patient Selection, and Computer Imaging

- Introduction
- When to Bring the Physician into the Skin-Care Consultation
- What Do People Look for in a Prospective Physician?
- Physician-Patient Match
- Patient Selection
- Computer Imaging
- Summary
- Frequently Asked Questions

Introduction

Since we estheticians are working on behalf of physicians, we want to keep all interactions with the client or patient extensions of the doctors' work. This will put everything into perspective for the patient or client, the esthetician, and for the physician. One of the problems that have frequently come to the attention of physicians is that the esthetic personnel sometimes behave as if the skin-care practice *belongs* to the esthetician. There is a difference between offering stewardship and guiding the practice—which is what we are hired to do—and owning the business—which clearly belongs to the doctor (unless you do in fact own your portion).

When to Bring the Physician into the Skin-Care Consultation

One thing is always clear. Whether we are seeing individuals for the first time as skin-care clients, or preparing them for a procedure, we must defer all questions that are out of our scope, decisions about surgery, and diagnoses to the physician.

Typically, a client or patient visiting a medical setting is coming to you because you are associated with a physician, and they will assume that you are sharing information about their skin health with the doctor. Clearly this is your obligation whenever a problem presents itself.

Legal issues arise if an erroneous account is made of a disorder or disease. As we know, the term *malpractice* means misconduct, mismanagement, and negligence. You may suspect or clearly know that you are viewing a particular disorder or disease, but it is essential that you let the physician make the determination. It is not because you do not have the experience, knowledge, or ability to recognize a problem, but the physician is the one who is legally qualified to make medical evaluations and diagnoses. Here is one account of a situation that went terribly wrong.

Case Study

A client told her clinical esthetician that she was interested in making an appointment for a consult with the doctor about some suspicious spots on her chest, and she wanted to know what else she could do to clear up some sun damage. The esthetician told the client that it really looked superficial, and that she recommended a light **hydroquinone** (bleaching cream), a **glycolic acid** cream for home care, and then a light **TCA** (trichloracetic acid) peel that she would perform in the office, in a couple of weeks. Standard protocol, seemingly.

One month later, the client called the esthetician and said that she had been to her dermatologist and had had two biopsies, one of which revealed a melanoma. She had been sent for **Mohs surgery** (a microscopic skin cancer removal technique), and further extensive surgery would be necessary.

At worst, this situation was life threatening and had some legal implications. At the very least, the esthetician lost a good client, by destroying her trust and confidence, as well as subsequent referrals in the process. It would have been morally, legally, and professionally appropriate to have referred the client to the physician, to allow the proper medical evaluation to take place. This lesson was learned the hard way, and the client has not held the esthetician responsible. She was lucky. Remember, no one will fault us for being cautious and professional.

What Do People Look for in a Prospective Physician?

Today personality often rules when people are considering a physician. Technically superior, highly skilled surgeons may lose patients after a consultation if they fail to relate or they intimidate or, worse, talk down to a person. People do not want to see themselves as patients; they want to feel empowered. Clients tend to behave in a variety of ways, in keeping with their generation.

Generation Y (1978–present)   This generation is still young, but not to be fooled. Its individuals are typically interested in having families and are starting earlier than their "boomer" parents in many cases. They will have some of the same demands, yet they are even more well informed when it comes to health issues; information gathering via the Internet comes as second nature to them. In addition, they appreciate a direct manner in a consultation and will often prefer a more traditional form of health care than their parents do. They will look for honesty and a forthright approach in a doctor.

Generation X (1964–1978)   The people of this generation are trying to balance it all—as are their big sisters and brothers (boomers), but they are slightly more realistic. Interested in preventative measures, they will begin taking care of their skin 10 years earlier, albeit they have seen their fair share of tanning beds. They are interested in small procedures such as lip augmentations, **Botox**, and **blepharoplasty**; they like peels, **microdermabrasion**, and personalized treatment packages. They do tend to be conservative in nature and like simple maintenance regimes, as they are raising families and usually do not have spare time. This group will want a doctor to be well versed in cosmetic procedures and be able to answer questions they have beyond the information that they can glean on-line.

Boomers   We know that Baby Boomers (1946–1964) have increasingly been having surgical procedures for some time now. Keep in mind that this is a generation of people with a certain sense of entitlement. They are as comfortable seeing a naturopath for basic health care as going to a medical doctor. We continue to see a growing number of boomers—and eventually their children (who have been raised with the knowledge of alternative or complementary medicine)—interested in skin care and procedures. This population will prove to be less tolerant of physicians indifferent to complementary forms of medicine, or to those who have not taken the time to learn about herbs, vitamins, and minerals.

In addition, this generation tends to share their innermost thoughts and feelings with their health-care providers in a sort of bare-all fashion. They tend to be professionals and are knowledgeable and self-evaluating about their health in general. With the help of their teenage and young adult children, they know that at a touch of a mouse, they have information available to them (even presentations of the very procedure that they are considering) on-line.

Physicians will need to be adroit at handling questions that come up in consultations such as: "Can I continue taking my **vitamin E** and primrose oil through surgery?" Or: "Are you familiar with cranial sacral treatments?" This **population** wants to know that we have done our homework and that the staff will be able to assist them through the entire process. They are looking for a health-care partner as well as a physician, and they will demand answers to questions, and attentiveness, or will they will go elsewhere.

Boomers' parents and the greatest generation   This group is a contrast to the boomers. This generation may wait for an hour or two in the waiting room, may take the doctor's word for the gospel, and may have a reverence for the physician as the final word. This may prove to be both positive and negative for them.

On the positive side, these patients may follow all home-care protocols, including follow-up appointments. This generation will want to know that the physician has performed many procedures and will trust that the doctor will know the best form of treatment. However, on the negative side, they may suffer needlessly with anxiety over an unforeseen or adverse outcome that could have been addressed if they felt that they were more in a partnership with their physician.

In general people look for a physician who is personable, energetic, well-rounded, experienced; has a good bedside manner, and is enthusiastic about performing the procedure the patient is requesting. The stuffy, all-knowing type that talks over the top of the patient's voice may have difficulty obtaining quality patients as information continues to become readily available to the public. Because people have so many treatment choices today, most physicians are retooling, cross-training, learning and implementing new ways of growing their practices, and improving their interpersonal skills.

Physician-Patient Match

It is important that the patient finds a match for his or her particular personality. If patients do not feel comfortable with their doctors, they may not follow instructions, and this may adversely affect the result. In addition, if a patient needs a warm, compassionate type of doctor, and the physician consulted is on the chilly side, the recovery may not go as smoothly, and the patient may require more office visits than normal. The interpersonal relationship is very important to the healing and well-being of the patient (Figure 3–1).

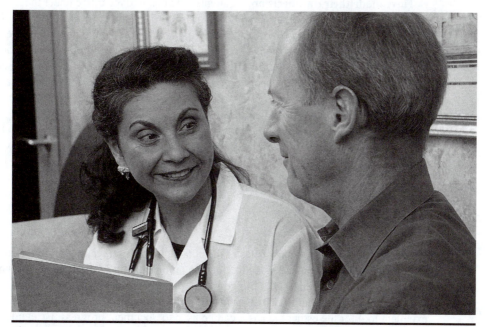

Figure 3–1   Dermatologist with patient

Patient satisfaction is highest when a partnership is created. Having surgery can bring up many unresolved issues for some people; sometimes these issues go undetected until the patient is under the stress of a surgical procedure. It is to the advantage of all concerned that the patient-physician relationship be a good one from the beginning.

Patient Selection

In today's litigious climate, physicians are wise to evaluate each patient carefully prior to entering into a relationship. It is no longer enough for doctors to consider a patient for a procedure just because they can perform a given surgery. Today, with malpractice lawsuits soaring, it is highly advisable to make an informed decision about a patient, and not rush the process of **patient selection**. It is better to spend more time up front in the *getting-to-know* phase in order to fully educate the patient, and to determine whether they will be compliant.

The patient-physician relationship can be vital to the outcome of a surgical procedure. If a doctor feels uncertain about performing a given elective procedure, it may be best to trust these intuitions. If it does not feel right at the outset, it will not improve later, after the fact. A candidate for a procedure must:

- **Have realistic expectations.**   Some patients may have unrealistic expectations for a medical procedure. A 50-year-old person will not suddenly appear 25, for example, or a patient with deep acne scarring will not have flawless skin after laser resurfacing.
- **Have made their own decision.**   Patients who come to the office under the direction of a spouse, friend, or another person for a procedure, do not do well. If there is difficulty postoperatively they may blame that other person for recommending the surgery. They could also experience a prolonged healing period if personal commitment was lacking.
- **Be physically and emotionally fit.**   Being physically capable of undergoing any type of surgery is essential; however being *emotionally* fit is equally important. The surgery may go well, but those not of sound mind may not have the ability to care for themselves or to receive the care that they need.
- **Be willing to become compliant.**   A patient must exhibit a rational desire to be compliant and follow all rules for the pre- and postoperative stages. Patients showing lack of interest in following orders may experience complications to their surgery or in the recovery phase.

Computer Imaging

Computer imaging plays many roles in the consultation. It serves as a rapport builder, as a tool in patient education and selection, and as an instrument in **medical documentation**. Many physicians routinely take images of all people who come in for consultations, for future reference, whether they plan to have a procedure or not (Figure 3–2). Imaging is an excellent tool for the esthetician as it can be used to document progress in treatment plans, product use, and to support the physician's medical documentation system.

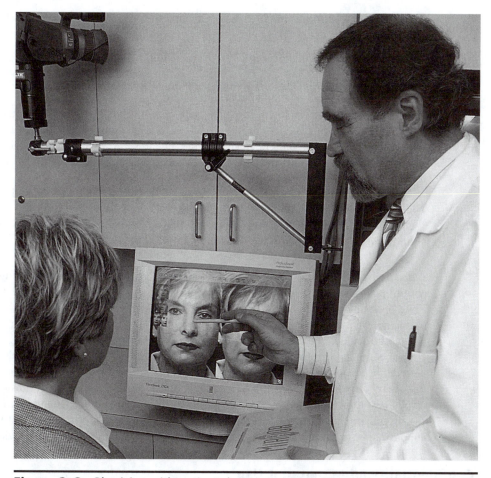

Figure 3–2   Physician with patient during computer imaging session

Because change may be viewed instantaneously on the imager, patients coming in for procedures are able to the see the future effects of treatment or surgery. Through use of the computer imager in a consultation, rapport is built between the patient and the doctor, nurse, patient care coordinator, or esthetician operating the computer. Do not rush this process. Patients like to see themselves on the monitor, and will be more open and receptive to the session if you relax and take it at their pace. This can be a very emotional experience for the patient, but usually it is a moment of elation as they see the transformation. The following points detail the logistics and use of computer imaging.

Operating the Imager

Depending upon the utility, staffing, and protocols set up in your office, some procedures currently being used might be applicable:

- The physician performs all functions of imaging the patient. Some doctors prefer to do all of their own picture taking and computer imaging, particularly if they have a small staff, or if they have a strong inclination toward this type of technology.
- All staff members learn how to perform all functions of the imager. Some offices expect that all staff members be trained in picture taking and in imaging, because appointments with patients may collide with staff days off.
- All staff members learn to take pictures, and then the physician does the actual imaging. This allows the patient to move through the consultation phase a little faster, and it frees up the physician, until he or she has the time to sit down and work on the imager. The patient would then come back for a second phase to the consultation, to view the changed image.
- A **patient care coordinator** (PCC) performs all functions of the imager, and consults with the physician to make certain that images are feasible. A PCC will work closely with the doctor to determine what procedure best suits a patient, and then fine-tunes the simulation when the doctor shares input.

Realistic expectations   As with all phases of the consultation, you are seeking information, but you are also *giving* information in a responsible and professional manner. While operating the computer, you need to place importance on creating a realistic image. You do not want to give the patient the impression that a change is possible when in fact it may not be doable. You may be able to make a client's scar go away on the imager, but it will not be ethical to allow them to think that this is what they can expect after a series of microdermabrasion peels.

There are parameters with all treatments and procedures. If you are unsure, it is always best to review the possibilities with the physician or other technician. In addition, if you are operating the imager for the client or patient, keep in mind that you are demonstrating, *not* recommending. The recommendations are made by the physician.

Confidentiality and Computer Use

If you are using the imager to show the benefit of a microdermabrasion series, or other peels that treat photodamage such as hyperpigmentation, make sure not only that the images are realistic but that the subject of your demonstration has agreed to be viewed. There are **informed consent** forms for this process (Figure 3–3). It is a great idea to check back with people who have agreed to have their images viewed for educational purposes, because over time they might change their minds. Repercussions can occur with patients who originally agreed to share images, while going through a procedure, and then later change their mind.

The Computer as Tool for Patient Selection and Education

The physician may use the imager for patient selection and **patient education.** While doctors are evaluating candidates for cosmetic surgery, or other surgical procedures, they are also making a determination as to whether a person would be a good patient. By demonstrating to the patient the possibilities for change, a clinician is able use the imager as an

INFORMED CONSENT

PATIENT COMPUTER IMAGING

In the course of consultations and discussion with certified medical professionals, I may have been shown or provided brochures and/or pictures of actual patients on an electronic computer imaging device._____Initial

I understand that pictures and/or alterations of said pictures seen are solely for the purpose of illustration and discussion, with the intent being to provide improved communication with medical professionals._____Initial

I also understand that the outcome of any type of surgical procedure is directly related to my individual characteristics and health._____Initial

I further understand and acknowledge that because of the obvious significant differences in how living tissues react to surgery, there may be no relationship between the electronic images created and the actual final surgical results._____Initial

The use of the computer imaging system offers an opportunity for me to discuss my interests and allows improved communication with the medical staff._____Initial

I hereby grant permission for the use of any illustrations, photographs, or imaging records created in my case, for use in scientific and professional journals and/or promotional presentations at any time during or after treatment, with complete confidentiality of my identity.

I certify my understanding that there is **NO WARRANTY,** expressed or suggested, as to my own final appearance after elective surgery by the use of these electronically altered images.

Signed_____   Date_____
(Patient)

Signed_____   Date_____
(Witness)

Signed_____   Date_____
(Physician)

Figure 3–3   Consent form for computer use

educational tool, and to incorporate into the session important details such as the necessity for following protocol to obtain desired results.

Summary

Once you have dealt with all types of patients with varying desires for change, you will learn whether a treatment or procedure is feasible for a given patient. Nevertheless, the physician makes the determination. As excited as you may become to have someone meet the doctor for a procedure, do not try to rush or force a partnership. In addition, if you notice a suspicious lesion during a skin analysis, always refer the client to the physician. Lastly, keep in mind that the computer imager is simply a tool used for simulation. It is not used in place of diligence by all practitioners to communicate effectively and to give the patient as much information as possible as they are making their heath-care decisions.

Frequently Asked Questions

1. **What does the esthetician do if while preparing to perform a routine peel/treatment on a client, they observe a suspicious lesion on the lip of a client?**

   Ask the client if they have a cold sore (herpetic breakout). If they do, let them know that having a cold sore precludes them from having a peel or clinical treatment, as the sore may spread. If they do not have a cold sore, tell them that they should have it looked at by the physician at the earliest opportunity. If the lesion is oozing, bleeding, or if the skin is broken, reschedule the treatment. If the lesion appears to be intact, perform the treatment avoiding the area, and reiterate the necessity for a visit with the physician.

2. **What does the esthetician do if a staff member is seen showing an unauthorized image on the imager to a new patient?**

   These situations can arise easily, and without any harm meant to the parties involved. Assuming that you are directly involved or in the room, suggest that the staff member go to an authorized image, or ask the staff member to step outside and tell them that the individual on the imager has not signed the appropriate consent form. This can be a legal nightmare with some liability issues, and can be embarrassing, especially if the image being shown is that of a community member with whom the new patient has contact or knowledge. Always think "Confidentiality."

The Business of the Practice

CHAPTER 4

The Business Plan

- ■ Introduction
- ■ Clinical Esthetics as a Business
- ■ The Business Plan
- ■ Sample Business Plan
- ■ Summary
- ■ Frequently Asked Questions

Introduction

Our primary focus as clinicians practicing in medical offices is to offer comprehensive, compassionate care. As we become absorbed in the daily rituals of seeing clients and patients, it is easy to become distracted from the business of managing the financial needs of our departments. It is important to make solid, educated decisions in all phases of our practice including product purchases, equipment, advertising, and even your salary, based on your merit and budget. This section will give you some ideas about how to address some of the questions about the business aspects of the practice, and offer some solutions toward achieving control.

Clinical Esthetics as a Business

One way to learn about your business from the ground up is to create a **business plan**. Even if you are walking into an existing skin-care practice, this will be one of the most effective ways to learn about what has been taking place and, more importantly, what you can do to grow the business and take it to new heights.

There is a major difference between dispensing service and handing out samples or selling products, and the processes of decision making, problem solving, growing a business, profit making, and creating financial goals that you can ultimately attain. Some questions that you may ask yourself along the way to success are:

- What does the esthetician need to do to make a business successful?
- What is a business plan?
- What is profit?
- How does the esthetician run a business and take care of patients?

This section has been written with the support of Megan Watt, Thomas Dorr, and staff of the Small Business Development Center at Western Washington University, in Bellingham, Washington.

- What happens if business drops off?
- How should products be priced?
- How do we educate the physician about the esthetic profit center?

Developing a business plan may seem a daunting task, but it can be a useful tool that will guide you along when you are at your highest points, and will help you get back on track if things are becoming more challenging than you would like. Statistics show that businesses are more successful when they have a plan. A business plan should be a fluid body of work, subject to change and updated every year as you create new goals. It also should include a mission statement, which is a simple sentence or representation that reflects your practice's primary goal and purpose.

The Business Plan

What is a business plan? A business plan is a description of your business, including your market, your personnel, and your financial needs. The purpose of creating a plan is to develop a blueprint for the management of your practice, to educate the physician about your practice and its needs, to provide a platform for patient education, and to facilitate opportunities of securing financial support at a lending institution should you require a loan.

Your plan should describe:

- your mission statement
- where we are now
- where we want to be
- how we are going to get there
- your practice/business and the industry
- your products, treatments/services
- the market and marketing approach you plan to use
- how the product and/or the treatments/services are acquired
- who is involved in the practice/business
- how much money the practice will need and what will you do with it

A business plan outline typically has the following sections.

Executive Summary

The summary is a condensed version of your business plan including your mission statement. Although this summary will appear first in the plan, it is often written last, after all other sections are completed.

Practice and Industry

This section provides you, the physicians, investors, and bankers with information about you and your practice and the nature and current condition of medical esthetics as an industry. This section should include:

The Practice

- start date and state of practice
- personnel, and the roles of each who played part in bringing the practice forward to where it is currently
- the business purpose of the practice and highlights of progress to date such as launching a new product line, or bringing in a new treatment such as the latest rejuvenating technique

The Industry

- your view of the current status and prospects for medical or clinical esthetics and the cosmeceutical industry
- the competition and how they are performing, including growth in sales, profits, and current market share
- the effect of major economic, social, technological, or regulatory trends of the industry

Product and Service

The objective of this section is to fully describe the products, services, special features, and future plans. It should include the following:

- **Description of your practice.**   Describe your practice's product and services in full detail, indicating what these products and services are and what function they serve. Include photographs, brochures, and other materials that may present this information clearly.
- **Research and development.**   Describe the extent of research, development, and planning that you must complete before you are ready to open. Record the costs and time required to set up your practice.
- **Special features and differentiation aspects.**   Describe any special features, exclusivity, or industry secrets that you may have. Present information about having authored articles on esthetics, worked with a famous physician, worked in product development, or taught esthetics. Announce anything that might show that you are in an advantageous position in the industry, and what makes you different from the competition.
- **Future development.**   Discuss plans for expansion of the present practice, such as bringing in new products, services, and personnel.

Market Conditions and SWOT

This section is designated to help you understand your market and to build a road map to achieve your sales target. Here is the information that can be helpful:

- **Market definition.**   Define the target market by describing potential customers, their locations, their interest in the products and services, and their potentiality of making such purchases. Here is an opportunity for you to discuss your past history, if you have one, and how well you have been received. In addition, discuss negative responses to such products or services (such as higher price points for example), and how you plan to overcome these responses or objections.

- **Market size.** Describe current market size. In addition, include new market opportunities, such as how to segment geographical factors and demographics for product lines, and synergies within the office. This needs to be supported with statistical data and discussions with potential distributors, sales representatives, and clients.

- **Market trends.** Describe the market's growth potential. Market projections should be created for 3 years. Clearly state the theory applied—including industry trends, new technology, and the developing interest in skin care by clients.

- **Competition.** One comprehensive approach to analyzing the competition is to use the *SWOT technique.* SWOT is an acronym for **S**trengths, **W**eaknesses, **O**pportunities, and **T**hreats (SWOT). We should all know our competition from the top down. Start by naming and discussing all major competitors. Then follow this outline:

  1. **Strengths.** Analyze the strengths of each of your competitors. Why do clients go to the competitor? Do they have more product lines? Better quality? Do they have better techniques in applying treatments? Are they better known or have they been around longer? Do they work with a well-known physician? Do they advertise more? What is their advantage? Target market? Obtain information about their practice, get brochures, marketing materials, and visit their Web site.

  2. **Weaknesses.** Analyze the weaknesses of your competition. What problems do you perceive them having? What is their history? High turnover in personnel? What do clients say about them? Are there markets they are not serving? Who are their vendors? What are their treatment/service prices? Product prices?

  3. **Opportunities.** Are there new opportunities that you could be seizing? Are there new products that the market needs now? Are there changes in the industry that could be creating new opportunities? You could be taking advantage of these opportunities. Follow up on requests that are being sought by your clients and those of your competitor.

  4. **Threats.** By analyzing your competition you will also learn about the threats to your practice/business. Is there new technology that may make some of your treatments obsolete? Are your competitors expanding or reducing? Are they going out of business? Why? What are potential problems that you could be facing? New government regulations for estheticians? Medical personnel? What are the economic conditions of the market?

Once you SWOT your competition, apply the same exercise to your own practice (Table 4–1). Discuss your own strengths and weakness. Ask co-workers, clients, vendors, and your partner or spouse for feedback. You will be able to not only find out what opportunities may be available for you; but also you will determine what your **differential advantage** is. In other words: why should someone come to you for products and service over someone else? Once you determine your differential advantage, it becomes the foundation of your sales and marketing message. This will help you position your practice against the competition and helps you target your market to those who need your products and services and are willing to pay for your differential advantage.

SWOT WORKSHEET

	Strengths	Weaknesses	Opportunities	Threats
Competitor 1				
Competitor 2				
Competitor 3				
Competitor 4				
Competitor 5				
Competitor 6				
Competitor 7				
Competitor 8				
Competitor 9				

Table 4–1   SWOT Worksheet

Marketing and Marketing Strategy

This section of your business plan is designed to provide projections of sales and market share and to show how you plan to achieve these projections. It should include:

Estimated sales and market share

- Provide an estimate of sales and market share that you plan to capture.
- Base this estimate on your assessment of your customers and their acceptance of your product and service, your market size, trends, and the competition.
- Identify any clients who have made or are willing to make purchase commitments. This could be a former client, new clients, or others who would be interested in supporting you in your practice.

Breakeven analysis

- Creating a breakeven analysis gives you a way to look at how much business you need to do in order to just break even. This affects your general operating decisions such as the buying and selling of products and services.

Strategy

- targeted clients (initial and later)
- methods of identifying and finding potential clients
- product and treatment features that will be emphasized

Pricing   Discuss the prices you will be charging for your products and services. Compare them to your competitor. Express how the prices that you set will enable you to:

- gain acceptance of your products and services
- maintain and increase your market share
- produce profits
- justify pricing that is above or below competitor

Sales   Describe how you plan to sell your products and services.

- Will you be the only one selling products in your office? If there are others, how will they be compensated? Salary and commission or will it be just commission?

Product and service guarantees   Discuss the importance of good customer service and how you plan to handle these problems.

Advertising, public relations, and events   Discuss your plans to bring your products and services to the attention of prospective clients. Include plans for:

- trade show participation, such as business shows, health-care events, women's conferences
- magazine advertisements
- promotional literature

Operations

This section provides a description of how and where you plan to practice. This includes the location, equipment, method of supplying service, and labor including training. Here are key points:

Location   Describe the location of the practice. Include both the advantages and disadvantages of the location and consider:

- proximity to clients, hospital, or surgery suite
- access to transportation and parking
- state and location
- area zoning—state and local laws
- utilities (including rates)

Plant and equipment   Describe the facilities and whether they will be leased or purchased. State costs and when the space will become available. In addition, comment on the future of the space and equipment needs, based on sales projections, including the acquisition of more space—the timing and its availability.

Product and services control   Describe the processes used to acquire products and control product and services. Consider:

- quality control, product and service control, and inventory control procedures
- organization and control of purchasing function
- breakdown of variable unit costs by product and service

Labor   Describe the local licensed esthetician pool (other than yourself) in terms of quality to supply you with sufficient product sales and treatments. Address any special training they may need to have and the costs that your practice may incur. In addition, detail any bonus programs and associated costs as well as:

- wage rate/commissions/percentages
- talent availability
- benefits offered

Management   The experience, talent, and integrity of your management team are of primary importance to the success of the business as a whole. Before agreeing to finance your practice, lenders will thoroughly review each member of your team. This section of the business plan should describe the following:

Organization

- what the key roles will be
- who will fill each position
- how the individuals' talents complement each other

Key Management

- duties and responsibilities of each individual
- career highlights of each (include a résumé)
- weaknesses of the team
- each individual's compensation

Professional Services

- state legal, accounting, public relations, advertising, banking, and other service organizations that you have selected for your practice; this will establish the credibility of the business component to your practice.

Financial Information

If you have been in practice, include your current financial statements. If not, your plan should describe the type and amount of funding you are requesting. In addition, you will need current information on the practice's present financial status and financial projections.

Funding needs   If you need funding, this section of your business plan should address the following:

- **Amount of financing.**   In general terms, state the amount of money that you need, and describe what you will do with it. Explain any other plans for acquiring capital.
- **Capitalization.**   Describe the impact that obtaining financing will have on the practice as a whole.
- **Use of funds.**   Explain how you plan to use the funds in a manner consistent with your financial projections. For example, if you need start-up money, express how the money will be used to purchase products and develop services along with developing your marketing plan.
- **Future financing.**   Explain the future need for financing. Mention key points along the way, such as when your practice grows and you need more space or personnel. Be clear and specific.

Current financial statements   If you have been in practice and have a record of accomplishment, provide financial statements from the last 3 years. In addition, include:

- detailed breakdown of income statement
- operating statistics and explanations of unusual fluctuations (such as September 11)

Financial projections   Create a 3-year profit and loss statement, **projected cash flow statement,** and balance sheet projections. If you have a record, the projections should be on a monthly basis for the first year, and annual projections for years 2 and 3.

Profit and loss forecast   Forecasted sales are the most important component of your financial projections since sales volume will dictate the necessary level of products and services. Start the financial projections with the sales forecast. This will help you define how much cash you will have coming from the business and when it will come in. This helps you to determine cash flow and how much debt capital and equity you will need until the practice generates a positive cash flow.

Your financial projections and your funding request must be aligned with your market expectations. The forecast should be consistent with your assessment of the market size, your competition, and your marketing strategy.

You may use unit or total dollar volume to project your sales, as well as assumptions about unit sales, price, and the percentage of unit or dollar volume increases in the future. In addition, product sales and treatment/services should be clearly defined.

Cost of goods sold (COGS)   The cost of goods sold is the cost of inventory that has been sold and the cost of actually performing a service or treatment. All costs must be considered. Overhead includes rent and utility, fringe benefits, and other incidental materials such as towels, laundry, and paper products. Fixed expenses of overhead that do not fluctuate with products and treatments/services should be identified. Changes or fluctuations in these fixed costs should be explained.

Selling, general and administrative expenses   These expenses should include marketing and sales, salaries, commissions, promotion, advertising, administrative expenses, legal expenses, and accounting costs.

Research and development   For physicians and estheticians developing their own products, research and development costs will depend upon the life cycle of your product and treatment/service and the need to bring in new or additional products and services to the market. Assumptions concerning the timing of a new product or treatment/service should be explained as well as the nature of these products and treatments/services.

Income taxes   Income taxes should be estimated using an annual effective tax rate applied to monthly or quarterly net income before taxes. The annual effective tax rate is an estimate of the income tax rate (both federal and state) for the entire forecasted year considering available tax credits and net operation loss carry-forwards.

Cash flow statements   A cash flow statement shows you what happens to your cash over a specific period of time. This allows us to know how much money we have in the bank to pay our bills. We may show a great profit yet not have capital for daily operations. This is just like looking at your checking account. Projected cash flow forecasts will assist you in determining the need and timing for additional financing.

Balance sheet forecast   A balance sheet is a document that shows your business/practice financial condition at a given point in time. It shows what you own (assets), what you owe (liabilities) and the difference between the two, which is called equity or net worth.

Overall Schedule

Create a time line for completion dates for major aspects of the business plan. This will show your practice and business as having an ability to manage the developments as you move forward.

Critical Risks and Problems

Discuss problems and risks inherent to all business ventures openly and directly with your professional service providers, lenders, and your team. Only through discussion will you be able to reveal potential problems and work to avoid the impact of negative developments in each risk area.

Sample Business Plan

An abbreviated sample business plan is shown. It will provide you with a context to develop your own plan, or give you some ideas about adjusting an existing one.

The figures described in this report, estimated costs, and all other materials are subject to change based on many factors including location, size, and type of practice. Use of this report is strictly for educational purposes and makes no actual or projected claims of profits/earnings or sales.

Business Plan
Financing Proposal

Wright Rogers
Clinical Skin Care Centre
Bay City, Washington

Prepared by
Suzanne Bergman
January 3, 2005

PART I

Executive Summary
Business and Industry
Product and Service
Market Conditions
Marketing/Marketing Strategy

PART II

Operations

PART III

Financial Information and Exhibits

1. Start-up Expenses
2. Sales Forecast
3. Monthly Expenses
4. Profit and Loss Statement year 1
5. Profit and Loss Statements years 2 and 3 Summary

PART IV

Personal Résumés

I

Executive Summary

Our goal is to provide comprehensive, compassionate care to our clients and patients, with the latest in technology rooted in sound science.

The Wright Rogers Clinical Skin Care Centre will offer comprehensive full-service benefits to clients seeking routine facial and body treatments, products, and cosmetic support and will retail higher-end clinically focused skin-care products which complement the treatments provided. In addition, the clinic will offer pre- and postoperative care for those patients undergoing plastic surgery procedures as provided by Drs. Greg Wright and Mia Rogers, and it will supply long-term follow-up care for patients until entering the client phase again.

Business and Industry

The skin-care industry is growing annually by 13 percent. The aging Baby Boomer has increased the market for plastic surgery in the last 10 years. According to the American Society of Plastic Surgery, cosmetic surgery procedures have tripled in 10 years.

Due to recent economic changes, we have seen a rise in less expensive or smaller procedures such as skin-care treatments (microdermabrasion, skin peels); product sales; injectibles such as Botox, **collagen**, or other fillers; and light laser treatments such as laser hair reduction and spider vein removal, which are more affordable. This all speaks well to our industry as a whole. People can afford the service and products that we are offering during a downturn in the economy; this indicates that when the prospects are better for the economy, we will realize even more business along with the more expensive procedures.

Product and Service

Wright Rogers Clinical Skin Care Centre will include products and services that will support three areas:

1. pre- and postoperative care
2. routine and general skin care
3. special conditions and considerations:
   - rosacea
   - acne—adult and teenage
   - age management
   - laser treatments (hair and vein)

Pre- and Postoperative

Pre- and postoperative care products and services are directed to those patients having facial and body procedures such as face-lift, eyelift, laser resurfacing, breast surgery, liposuction, and tummy tuck. Treatments and products that would support these procedures would be offered to reduce swelling and increase hydration and healing. The products may be offered in a kit formation (such as a cleanser, toner, moisturizer, exfoliant and sunscreen) or may be purchased separately. The in-office treatment packages would be purchased by the patient and applied to stimulate circulation and conditioning for proper healing. Pre- and postoperative services have been shown to increase patient compliance and recovery times and overall client satisfaction.

Routine and general skin care

Products and services for routine and general skin care sold in a medical office are vehicles for an ancillary profit center. They are considered highly desirable by clients and patients, as there is an assumption made that these products and services are more advanced because of the association with the medical milieu. These products would consist of products for all skin types such as:

- normal
- dry
- oily
- sensitive
- combination

Treatments for routine skin care would be determined by the skin type and condition, lifestyle, and commitment level desired by the client. They would consist of in-office treatments for normal, dry, oily, combination, acneic, and sensitive skin, as well as conditions of rosacea, cellulite, and stress, and would involve one or more of the following:

- peels
- microdermabrasion
- facials
- massage
- endermology

Special Considerations

Special considerations will include products and treatments for clients and patients with conditions that are beyond routine regimes. These products would include home-care preparations for rosacea, acne, and age management. The in-office treatments in the special consideration section would be targeting acne and age management with stronger peels and combinations of solutions, hair reduction, and spider vein removal.

Market Conditions

The Wright Rogers Clinical Skin Care Centre is well suited for the market in Bay City, Washington. Often consumers feel that they need to travel to larger cities and locations to find higher-end products and services, as the level of sophistication has not quite caught up with the level of customer moving into the area. By providing these products, treatments and procedures, the Centre will not only attract this clientele, but also encourage new upscale businesses to locate in the area of 125,000 population.

The medical practice has grown by 10 percent to 15 percent per year since its inception in 1997. The addition of the skin-care division will increase traffic and support the existing patient base. One of the problems of the practice has been that the doctors have not had enough time to spend in patient education due to the heavy surgery load. This can

Competition-SWOT Summary

	Strengths	Weaknesses	Opportunities	Threats
Derm 1	Location on main street	Bad reputation. High turnover, rude to patients	Could use more clinical approach in advertising	Dermatological technology, expansion in equipment
Derm 2	Well respected	No cosmetic savvy. Recommend bath soap routinely	Could work as partners—referral	Could expand and develop more cosmetic approach
Spa 1	Attractive presence	Not really a spa	Could do more spa-type treatments at some point	Their sales staff—good at selling business
Spa 2	Great spa	Untrained personnel	Clients appreciate well-trained, experienced personnel	They could get better at services and take more of market
Spa 3	Beautiful, new location, and clients trying out new facility	Could be considered sterile feeling, not friendly	Could create partnership referral/reciprocal agreement with them	Watch developing menu and product purchases
Independent 1	Well known	Works alone, can only take so many clients	Could send the "cosmetic police"-type clients to this practitioner as they use so-called natural products	Uses only "natural" product line—professes its value, downgrading all other lines
Independent 2	Very good esthetician, well liked and visited	Small practice area, cannot see more than five a day	This esthetician is a great resource, may send some clients our way if she cannot see them	Threat is minimal but only because of single-person business
Independent 3	Well trained and credentialed	Has not figured out how to maintain good customer service Owner not on premises	Run more as professional practice, focus on customer service	Speaks badly of others/gossips
Independent 4	High-traffic area	Has employee problem, no customer service	More opportunity to offer customer service, open Saturdays, evenings	Could "clean house" and become more successful

[Note: A true SWOT analysis should be expanded to include pricing, hours of business, number of employees, length of business, and key strategic partnerships.]

WRC SWOT

Competition	Strengths	Weaknesses	Opportunities	Threats
Wright Rogers Clinical Skin Centre	Full service, physician-directed skin-care clinic with history of successful cosmetic surgery practice	Some clients may not want to come to a medical setting for products and service	Unlimited—customer service, retail, treatment center, laser and cosmetic surgery procedures	Esthetician feeling overwhelmed with load and lack of personnel to support efforts

be remedied by having the clinical esthetician meet with those patients for additional educational support as directed by the physician.

Typically, clients and patients requesting cosmetic procedures have the income to support higher-end products and services; they have a personal income of $55,000 or above and are professional men and women with double-income households. Approximately 35,000 people that fit into this market in Bay City.

For those who may not be able to afford the higher-end products and treatments, we will have price-point items for the segment with income below $55k, and we will approach that market with a price/value concept. In today's product climate, there are products and treatments for both income levels.

Special Features and Competitive Differential Advantage Aspects

The primary competitive differential advantage is that each practitioner is a specialist with experience in creating comprehensive care in a private medical setting. Drs. Wright and Rogers and Suzanne Bergman are the only physician/esthetician consort in the area. As such, they will compete with two dermatological offices, three spas/salons, and four independent estheticians.

Drs. Wright and Rogers have received acclaim for their volunteer work in domestic violence cases, and in reconstructive surgery for accident survivors, and have been featured in various local magazines as pioneers in new techniques with respect to plastic surgery. Suzanne Bergman will be offering services such as pre- and postoperative counseling and treatments, which are currently unavailable in the area. The competitors are working in a more compartmentalized manner, offering medical care and then referring patients to the local department store. The Wright Rogers Clinic will see the patient through all phases of treatment and cosmetic support.

Future growth and development will be the inclusion of a second part-time clinical esthetician, expansion of products and treatments a PA-C (physician assistant), and additional nursing personnel.

Marketing/Marketing Strategy

In winter 2004, the Wright Rogers Clinical Skin Care Centre will execute an internal marketing plan by sending marketing materials to all regular and former patients informing them of this addition to the doctors' practice. In spring a marketing plan utilizing a combination of print and radio will be used to launch the new division and create awareness in the community that these services have been added to the doctors' practice.

II

Operations

The Wright Rogers Clinical Skin Care Centre will begin operations in spring 2005. Initially the practice will employ one licensed esthetician, Suzanne Bergman, and will add additional personnel as necessary. Greg Wright, M.D., and Mia Rogers, M.D., will provide space and physician support for the WR Clinical Skin Care Centre in their 8,000 square-foot plastic surgery suite located at 818 Sunset View Drive, in Bay City, Washington. The clinical administrator, Marian Black, MBA, will act as liaison between the WR Clinical Skin Care Centre and physicians, and will provide bookkeeping support to the clinic and to Suzanne Bergman, esthetician. Bergman will work closely with nursing staff as support to all clients and patients from initial consultation through to pre- and postoperative care, and then subsequently as a routine client.

III

Financial Information and Exhibits

Financial Information and Exhibits

1. Start-up expenses
2. Sales forecast
3. Monthly expenses
4. P&L year 1
5. P&L years 2 and 3

Start-up Expenses

Equipment List	$	18,000

1. facial bed
2. microdermabrasion machine
3. facial machines (a. steamer, b. galvanic, c. high frequency)

Inventory	$	10,000
Supplies	$	2,000
Brochures	$	1,000
Cards	$	500
Office Supplies	$	500
Leasehold Improvements	$	8000
Furniture	$	1000
License	$	60
Web Site Design	$	3,500
Working Capital (cash) Reserve	$	15,000
Total Operating Expenses	$	59,560

Sales Forecast

Instructions:

1. Identify the number of products you can sell per month and the average price per product.
   Multiply these two numbers to identify the projected monthly revenue from products.

2. Identify the number of treatments you will provide per month and the average price per treatment.
   Multiply these two numbers to identify the monthly projected revenue from treatments.

3. Identify the number of products returned per month and the average price per product.
   Multiply these two numbers to identify the monthly projected value of products returned.

Projected Revenue:	Month 1	Month 2	Month 3	Month 4	Month 5	Month 6	Month 7	Month 8	Month 9	Month 10	Month 11	Month 12
1. Products												
Avg. # of products sold per month	20	20	20	20	40	40	80	80	80	100	100	100
Avg. price per product	$ 50	$ 50	$ 50	$ 50	$ 50	$ 50	$ 50	$ 50	$ 50	$ 50	$ 50	$ 50
Total Revenue from Products	$ 1,000	$ 1,000	$ 1,000	$ 1,000	$ 2,000	$ 2,000	$ 4,000	$ 4,000	$ 4,000	$ 5,000	$ 5,000	$ 5,000
2. Treatments												
Avg. # treatments performed per month	20	20	40	40	40	60	60	80	80	80	80	100
Avg. price per treatment	$ 70	$ 70	$ 70	$ 70	$ 70	$ 70	$ 70	$ 70	$ 70	$ 70	$ 70	$ 70
Total Revenue from Treatments	$ 1,400	$ 1,400	$ 2,800	$ 2,800	$ 2,800	$ 4,200	$ 4,200	$ 5,600	$ 5,600	$ 5,600	$ 5,600	$ 7,000
3. Returns												
Avg. # products returned per month	1	1	1	1	1	1	1	1	1	1	1	1
Avg. price per product	$ 70	$ 70	$ 70	$ 70	$ 70	$ 70	$ 70	$ 70	$ 70	$ 70	$ 70	$ 70
Total Deduction from Returns	$ (70)	$ (70)	$ (70)	$ (70)	$ (70)	$ (70)	$ (70)	$ (70)	$ (70)	$ (70)	$ (70)	$ (70)
Total Net Revenue	$ 2,330	$ 2,330	$ 3,730	$ 3,730	$ 4,730	$ 6,130	$ 8,130	$ 9,530	$ 9,530	$ 10,530	$ 10,530	$ 11,930

Monthly Expenses

Insurance	$	85
Marketing	$	Varying 300–500
Phone	$	35
Utilities	$	50
Legal and Accounting	$	100
Wages	$	2500
Taxes	$	300
Travel	$	85
Education/Training	$	100
Internet Access/Web Site Host	$	100
Supplies	$	25
Office Supplies	$	35
Products Purchases	$	3000
Credit Card Fees (2% of credit card sales)	$	29
Bank Fees	$	71.50
Loan Interest	$	(yearly) 858

1rst Year Projected Profit and Loss Statement

	Month 1	Month 2	Month 3	Month 4	Month 5	Month 6	Month 7	Month 8	Month 9	Month 10	Month 11	Month 12	Total
Revenue													
Products	$ 1,000	$ 1,000	$ 1,000	$ 1,000	$ 2,000	$ 2,000	$ 4,000	$ 4,000	$ 4,000	$ 5,000	$ 5,000	$ 5,000	$ 35,000
Treatments	1,400	1,400	2,800	2,800	2,800	4,200	4,200	5,600	5,600	5,600	5,600	7,000	49,000
Returns and Allowances	(70)	(70)	(70)	(70)	(70)	(70)	(70)	(70)	(70)	(70)	(70)	(70)	(840)
Total Net Revenue	$ 2,330	$ 2,330	$ 3,730	$ 3,730	$ 4,730	$ 6,130	$ 8,130	$ 9,530	$ 9,530	$ 10,530	$ 10,530	$ 11,930	$ 83,160
Cost of Sales													
Products	$ 450	$ 450	$ 450	$ 450	$ 900	$ 900	$ 1,800	$ 1,800	$ 1,800	$ 2,250	$ 2,250	$ 2,250	$ 15,750
Treatments	140	140	280	280	280	420	420	560	560	560	560	700	4,900
Total Cost of Sales	$ 590	$ 590	$ 730	$ 730	$ 1,180	$ 1,320	$ 2,220	$ 2,360	$ 2,360	$ 2,810	$ 2,810	$ 2,950	$ 20,650
Gross Profit	$ 1,740	$ 1,740	$ 3,000	$ 3,000	$ 3,550	$ 4,810	$ 5,910	$ 7,170	$ 7,170	$ 7,720	$ 7,720	$ 8,980	$ 62,510
OPERATING EXPENSES													
Insurance	$ 85	$ 85	$ 85	$ 85	$ 85	$ 85	$ 85	$ 85	$ 85	$ 85	$ 85	$ 85	$ 1,020
Marketing	250	250	250	250	250	250	250	250	250	250	250	250	3,000
Phone	35	35	35	35	35	35	35	35	35	35	35	35	420
Utilities	50	50	50	50	50	50	50	50	50	50	50	50	600
Legal/Accounting	100	100	100	100	100	100	100	100	100	100	100	100	1,200
Wages	2,500	2,500	2,500	2,500	2,500	2,500	2,500	2,500	2,500	2,500	2,500	2,500	30,000
Commissions							1,230	1,440	1,440	1,590	1,590	1,800	9,090
Business Taxes	300	300	300	300	300	300	300	300	300	300	300	300	3,600
Travel	85	85	85	85	85	85	85	85	85	85	85	85	1,020
Education/Training	100	100	100	100	100	100	100	100	100	100	100	100	1,200
Internet Access/Web Site Host	100	100	100	100	100	100	100	100	100	100	100	100	1,200
Office Supplies	60	60	60	60	60	60	60	60	60	60	60	60	720
Credit Card Fees	29	29	29	29	29	29	29	29	29	29	29	29	348
Bank Fees	72	72	72	72	72	72	72	72	72	72	72	72	858
Total Operating Expenses	$ 3,766	$ 3,766	$ 3,766	$ 3,766	$ 3,766	$ 3,766	$ 4,996	$ 5,206	$ 5,206	$ 5,356	$ 5,356	$ 5,566	$ 54,276
Operating Profit	$ (2,026)	$ (2,026)	$ (766)	$ (766)	$ (216)	$ 1,045	$ 915	$ 1,965	$ 1,965	$ 2,365	$ 2,365	$ 3,415	$ 8,234
Interest Income (Expense)	$ (72)	$ (72)	$ (72)	$ (72)	$ (72)	$ (72)	$ (72)	$ (72)	$ (72)	$ (72)	$ (72)	$ (72)	$ (858)
Net Profit Before Income Tax	$ (2,097)	$ (2,097)	$ (837)	$ (837)	$ (287)	$ 973	$ 843	$ 1,893	$ 1,893	$ 2,293	$ 2,293	$ 3,343	$ 7,376
Income Tax						$ 195	$ 169	$ 379	$ 379	$ 459	$ 459	$ 669	$ 1,475
Net Profit After Income Tax	$ (2,097)	$ (2,097)	$ (837)	$ (837)	$ (287)	$ 778	$ 674	$ 1,514	$ 1,514	$ 1,834	$ 1,834	$ 2,674	$ 5,901

3 Year Projected Profit and Loss Summary

Revenue		Year 1		Year 2		Year 3
Products	$	35,000	$	40,250	$	46,288
Treatments	$	49,000	$	56,350	$	64,803
Returns and Allowances	$	(840)	$	(966)	$	(1,111)
Total Net Revenue	$	83,160	$	95,634	$	109,979
Cost of Sales						
Products	$	15,750	$	16,538	$	17,364
Treatments	$	4,900	$	5,145	$	5,402
Total Cost of Sales	$	20,650	$	21,683	$	22,767
Gross Profit	$	62,510	$	73,952	$	87,212
OPERATING EXPENSES						
Insurance	$	1,020	$	1,051	$	1,082
Marketing	$	3,000	$	3,090	$	3,183
Phone	$	420	$	433	$	446
Utilities	$	600	$	618	$	637
Legal/Accounting	$	1,200	$	1,236	$	1,273
Wages	$	30,000	$	33,000	$	36,300
Commissions	$	9,090	$	14,490	$	16,664
Business Taxes	$	3,600	$	3,708	$	3,819
Travel	$	1,020	$	1,051	$	1,082
Education/Training	$	1,200	$	1,236	$	1,273
Internet Access/Web Site Host	$	1,200	$	1,236	$	1,273
Office Supplies	$	720	$	742	$	764
Credit Card Fees	$	348	$	358	$	369
Bank Fees	$	858	$	884	$	910
Total Operating Expenses	$	54,276	$	63,132	$	69,074
Operating Profit	$	8,234	$	10,820	$	18,138
Interest Income (Expense)	$	(858)	$	(884)	$	(910)
Net Profit Before Income Tax	$	7,376	$	9,936	$	17,228
Income Tax (estimated at 20%)	$	1,475	$	1,987	$	3,446
Net Profit After Income Tax	$	5,901	$	7,949	$	13,782

IV

Greg Wright, M.D.

Curriculum Vitae

GRADUATE EDUCATION:	University of Washington
GENERAL SURGERY RESIDENCY:	Wright State University
PLASTIC SURGERY RESIDENCY:	Medical College of Ohio
BOARD CERTIFICATION:	American College of Surgeons
	American Board of Plastic Surgery
	National Board of Medical Examiners
ACADEMIC APPOINTMENTS:	University of Washington:
	Associate clinical professor of plastic and
	reconstructive surgery
NUMBER OF PUBLICATIONS:	20
SOCIETY MEMBERSHIPS:	American Society of Plastic Surgeons
	American Society of Esthetic Plastic Surgeons
	Washington Society of Plastic Surgeons
	6 additional societies
CLINICAL INTERESTS:	Esthetic plastic surgery
	Maxillofacial surgery

Mia Rogers, M.D.

Curriculum Vitae

UNDERGRADUATE:	Stanford University: B. A. in Art and Sciences and B. S. in Biology
GRADUATE:	University of Kentucky School of Engineering, Lexington, Kentucky
MEDICAL:	University of Kentucky School of Medicine, Lexington, Kentucky
RESIDENCY:	Plastic Surgery: Loyola University Medical Center, Maywood, Illinois
BOARD CERTIFICATION:	American Board of Surgery American Board of Plastic Surgery
MEDICAL LICENSES:	Tennessee, Illinois, Mississippi
SOCIETY MEMBERSHIPS:	Memphis and Shelby County Medical Society Tennessee Medical Association American Society of Plastic Surgeons Southeastern Society of Plastic and Reconstructive Surgeons The American Society for Esthetic Plastic Society
UNIVERSITY APPOINTMENTS:	Vanderbilt University, Nashville, Tennessee, July 1985

Suzanne Bergman, LE

Curriculum Vitae

UNDERGRADUATE:	Seattle University, Seattle, Washington— B.A. in Psychology
GRADUATE:	Simon Fraser University, BC, Canada— Adult Education, M.A.
ESTHETIC SCHOOL:	The Catherine Hinds Institute, Boston, Massachusetts
CONTINUING EDUCATION:	Advanced Institute of Clinical Esthetics, Seattle, Washington
	Euro Institute, Bellevue, Washington
	Medical Alliance, Laser Training, Seattle Washington
SOCIETY MEMBERSHIPS:	American Estheticians Education Association
	American Society of Plastic and Reconstructive Surgical Nurses
CLINICAL INTERESTS:	Esthetic Plastic Surgery Patient Education

Summary

Once the business plan has been completed, it is ready for implementation. If the plan is being used to secure funds from a bank or other source, it should include a balance sheet, cash flow statement and break-even analysis, and financial statements. Conventional accounting practices must be employed and may be sought by your administrator or CPA. Whether you are using it to secure funds from a bank or other nontraditional source, or as an educational tool for the esthetician, physician, and administrator, it will be important to keep it current. A business plan should be updated annually, and your financial projections will become the basis in creating a budget for your department.

Frequently Asked Questions

1. Can the esthetician really affect the bottom line or net profit?

Yes. Once you set up your budget, make some choices about the products that you purchase, and learn how to price products and treatments properly, you can manage the numbers much more efficiently. Conversely, this is certainly more difficult if you have no idea where your business stands. It takes time to learn, but you will be rewarded if you make the commitment to study, so you will be able to show the administration where you are projecting to go with the business side of your practice.

2. How does the esthetician know which marketing vehicle to use?

Depending upon the type of medical practice and the culture of your specific office, the marketing vehicle should support the direction that your marketing strategy dictates. If you want to attract upper-income, 35- to 55-year-old career women, do not use value coupons in a package in direct mail. Use vehicles such as networking at women's conferences and professionally designed print ads in a local business journal, and speak with the local newspaper about doing an editorial/article on your practice.

Make certain that the physician is in agreement with your strategy, and that the approach supports the vision of the medical practice. A team effort may move more slowly in the beginning but may prove to have more longevity. If you are feeling that you are in a constant battle with conflicting ideas, this may show in your advertising (see Chapter 5) and ultimately to the public viewing your marketing materials.

Marketing Strategy

- Introduction
- The Vehicles
- The Message
- Target Audience
- Summary
- Frequently Asked Questions

Introduction

Marketing strategy is defined as using a **vehicle** to communicate a message to a **target audience.** A vehicle is the actual method that you use to send the message, such as radio, print advertising, Internet/Web, or television commercials. The message relates your **differential advantage** that you determine through your **SWOT** (Strengths, Weaknesses, Opportunities, Threats) research. The target audience is the specific group that you determine is positioned to hear your message, through the appropriate vehicle, and is the one that best suits your practice.

The Vehicles

The form of advertising that you use to communicate your message must be an appropriate medium to affect the target audience enough to want to meet with you for a consultation. Often vehicles are combined for maximum benefit: you could use a networking opportunity at a conference, hand out your business card or brochure, and give a 1- or 2-minute introduction about who you are and what you do. The vehicles are varied, and some work better for us than others. Let us look more closely at each of them.

Word of Mouth

Many physicians feel that the best form of advertising is offered through personal recommendation, or word of mouth. Former patients may offer friends as well-screened, qualified potential patients, and these new patients may appreciate the doctor more than someone responding to an advertisement may. Some physicians feel that formal advertising may be deceptive or misleading to prospective patients. When the subject matter is surgical procedures, this can create legal problems later on if a patient felt misled by an advertisement.

The key to obtaining word-of-mouth referrals is to have consistent, continued, excellent customer service. Clients and patients will share both the positive and negative aspects of their experiences with friends and acquaintances; a beautifully created advertisement shows only the splendor and may not be viewed as accurate. Another nice thing about referrals is that there is no cost for this form of advertising.

Noncompeting Physician Referrals

Physicians such as family practitioners can also be great resources for referral. Offer to do a treatment on your physician, dentist, ophthalmologist, or other specialist, to build an alliance. Nurses are another example of a group to whom you may market. You might offer a special peel series to all nurses in your community. E-mail or fax specials addressed to nurses, and make them feel at home when they come to visit you. They tend to be very loyal, are low maintenance, and share information easily with other nurses, a built-in referral base. Once they trust your work, they will refer their patients and friends to you.

Complementary Health-Care Professionals

Chiropractors, acupuncturists, hypnotherapists, and massage therapists are all good examples of referral/networking opportunities for you. Remember, everyone is busy, so have your brochures, cards, and other marketing materials ready to give to them when you visit. Make your presence truly helpful, not just one more project for them to handle. Before you know it, most of your business will come from referring specialists.

Networking

One of the more obvious ways of networking is to join women's or coed business groups. If you like the support that you may receive from such a group, you will find that you have much to offer other women with appearance concerns. Working on a project together always inspires questions like "What do you do?" This will give you an opportunity to offer a complimentary service or product.

If you do not feel comfortable in these types of groups, or are not delighted with the prospect of weekly or even monthly meetings, put together baskets of products, or gift certificates with a complimentary consultation, and donate them to the group for auctions or Most Valuable Member type of events. These groups are always looking for ways to highlight members at meetings, so if you make this easy for them, before you know it, they will be coming back in to you for treatments or replacement products.

Newspaper

Newspaper advertising is certainly one of the oldest forms of advertising, and if you get in on one of their special discounted offers, you can purchase a package of ads for a good rate. Most ads are black and white, so they do not offer much in the way of esthetics; they are usually scanned by the reader who may or may not be in your target audience. This is important to factor into your marketing budget. If your newspaper is the only game in town, however, and is well read, you might do well with this medium.

Press Releases/Publicity

Press releases are a great way to receive free advertising and to keep your name out there. Upon launching a new service or product, returning from a conference or a training seminar, or creating a special event, send a professional-quality photo, along with a brief description that includes a defining characteristic which made this event unique, to the local newspaper, business magazine, or journal for publication. The public actually perceives these as more credible than conventional forms of advertising. Make certain, of course, that everything you say or write is accurate and can withstand public scrutiny.

Often reporters and columnists are looking for a good human-interest story, and particularly one in which people are helping other people. Estheticians are famous for doing good deeds like donating their services for a particular fund-raiser, or to a women's shelter for a day of beauty. Invite a writer along to the fund-raiser, or take pictures and submit them to the publication along with a few descriptive sentences about the event. A reporter usually likes to do the writing but may call you for an interview or a feature story.

Another approach is to invite columnists in for a complimentary service. They are often busy running around and would enjoy having a treatment. You want not only to take care to pamper them, but to be certain to compile a press packet including your brochure, profile, and some samples of basic products to try such as a cleanser, sunscreen, or hydrator.

Telephone Book/Yellow Pages

This is often overlooked as a viable form of advertising but proves to be great for new business. When you move to a new area, what do *you* do if you are looking for a service? Exactly, you go to the phone book. The phone book by nature is highly utilitarian, but you can also list your e-mail and Web site address on your ad so that people can visit you on-line.

As with ads for the newspaper or other print mediums, it is important to have a well-designed ad that conveys your differential advantage. This is one place where you will be viewed immediately next to your competitor. If you are comfortable using your image, do so, or find a model that reflects your taste. Most of us seeking services are visually oriented, so we often respond to good images in advertising.

Magazines

Magazines are extremely expensive forms of advertising, but in upscale areas they can be considered the premier form of presenting one's business. You have an opportunity to target specific audiences, and readers often share articles in magazines with family, friends, and co-workers. In addition, you may be of interest to an author or editor needing research material for a feature article in a particular issue on skin care or aging skin.

Another idea worth exploring: write and submit an article to a local or regional magazine. If you look in the front of most magazines, you will see a list of employees on every issue. One category title is Contributing Writers. This could include you with a little time, interest, research, and practice.

Radio and Television

Radio and television can be good exposure. You can determine whether a station caters to your demographics or audience through research of a given station. The downside may be that your audience is not typically listening on the day your commercial runs. Frequency is key in both mediums, and most of the responses to commercials occur within the first week of being aired.

As with all advertising, it is necessary that your choice of exposure reflect the image and integrity of your office. In addition, you want to portray an accurate message to the audience regarding treatment; you do not want to make a surgical procedure seem like a spa treatment. This can be a risk-management problem. A patient may have felt enticed by an ad that made a procedure sound so easy, with little or no downtime—only to find out that their recovery was really more like that of major surgery.

Commercials selling individual medical services are not always well received by the viewing public. Hospitals and health-care centers are, however, doing a notable job at putting together comprehensive advertisements for radio and television through demonstrating a teamwork approach. The viewer can imagine that there are many people supporting the patient and that the whole group is trained to care and help them through to recovery. If done well, this can be an effective form of introducing your practice.

Newsletters

Publishing a newsletter to keep busy clients in touch with your practice is by far one of the best marketing tools for an esthetician's practice. This is a soft sell, and if you are a closet writer, you may enjoy writing about new treatments and products, medical procedures, staff additions, or your delivery service. You could also have a guest visitor write a column for you. Collaborate with a massage therapist, dentist, or naturopath for your clients' education. People are interested in just about everything today concerning their health, and if you can formulate information in a succinct, easy-to-read manner, you will become their trusted resource.

It will be important to build a database for marketing to your clients. Taking their demographics from the client profile card, you may easily enter the information using a software program such as Access, and you will be able to make labels for direct mailings.

Your newsletter may be put on-line and accessed for a fee if you are interested in selling the information. Have respect for your time and energy. It may take many hours to research and put one of these together, so you do not want to just give them away without a purpose.

Some vendors will give you credit toward products for using their advertisements, images of products, or quotes in a newsletter. This can create a solid working relationship between you and your vendor. We will discuss cooperative advertising later in this chapter.

Brochures

Brochures are the foundation of a growing skin-care business. It is your menu. Clients need to know which services you provide, what these services will do for them, and how much you charge for your services. A features-benefits approach works well on brochures, and you may stress that the prices are given as a range, because after a full consultation you may determine that you need to apply two or three services to achieve the result.

You should place your brochures in all of the examination and consulting rooms, in addition to the waiting rooms. Take them to complementary physicians' offices, health clubs, business meetings, trade shows, your dentist, and anywhere else that you may develop business. Ask permission to display them.

Always place a brochure or menu of your services in the physician's packet, which is given to patients after cosmetic consultation. That way they can look at it at their leisure, and they see you and your services as an integral part of the support team if they choose this doctor to perform their surgery. Remember to put your Web site and e-mail addresses along with other logistical information such as street address with map, phone number with extension, or cell phone number if you use one for business.

Web Sites/Forums/Seminars/Chat Rooms

Web sites have the potential of giving your clients and patients a place to visit if they cannot get in to see you. Keep simplicity in mind when designing your site. People are overwhelmed with information today, so make your site easy to navigate. It's worth taking the time to update your site often. Make certain that you have a secured server if you sell products on-line.

Forums, seminars, and chat rooms are a great way to visit with busy people and to answer questions that potential clients may have about skin-care products and treatments. Often people have trouble making space in their lives for attending yet another event, but they may have a few minutes to log on and chat about issues that are important to them. One word of advice: this can be a time-consuming endeavor for the practitioner. Make certain that you can do the follow-through, before you sign up for on-line seminars and chat rooms.

Many estheticians have found their Web sites increase their income, but they are not without challenges. Make sure that you give the consumer plenty of information about products, because you do not want to be dealing with returns. We do not experience the returns in a medical office that one might in other venues, primarily due to our product knowledge, client/patient selection, and education. If you eliminate these important factors from your business, you become just another Web company to them.

Some set up a questionnaire for the on-line shopper, utilize passwords, and create some dialogue before sending products out the door. In addition, many vendors selling only to physicians do not want you to sell products over the Web without a live consultation first. This is in direct conflict with the original purpose for clinical skin care. Often these more advanced products contain higher levels of exfoliants, which may be contraindicated for various skin types. Providing this type of service eliminates the need for our expertise—and our existence, for that matter. Why should someone come to you, if he or she can get everything on the Web?

Open Houses/Sponsoring Public Events

Open houses are an integral part of a launch. In addition, this is an excellent way to show appreciation to clients who have been faithful to you, or to celebrate an anniversary date or something special. Hosting an afternoon tea or evening mixer where invitations are sent to select or targeted businesspeople in the community can be very pleasant. These are often most successful when people are invited to visit and just mill around on their own to look at displays, with you available to talk briefly about products and treatments in a casual way. No heavy selling or campaigning here; these events are for fun. You can put together packets and a few samples for them to take home. The idea here is not to overwhelm them with information or turn them off with a sales pitch, but to make an appointment for their return for a full consultation.

Seminars

Seminars are appealing to a certain sector of the public. If educational, these events can be great for introducing the doctor, the esthetician, as well as new products or procedures. Many physicians use PowerPoint presentations of before-and-after images for these events. These presentations can be followed with a talk given by the esthetician on skin care and product use.

However, what may prove even more useful could be an integrated approach where the physician and the esthetician present together, showing the procedure and what methods were used pre- and postoperatively to support the patient through the entire process. For example, the doctor could introduce the procedure, then the esthetician briefly describes what products and treatments were used to support the preoperative stage, such as a kit containing glycolic acid cream, lightening agents, retinoic acids, antioxidants, amino acids, and sunscreens to condition skin for laser surgery. A brief description could be given for the postoperative care as well.

A word of caution about seminars. You may find that you become a source for evenings out for the lonely-hearts club. When you find that the same people are showing up for each seminar, along with some of your competitors, you may want to rethink this format. This is not always negative, but do keep in mind that you are trying to promote your business and the clinic through this educational event. These can be labor-intensive. If you are spending a large amount of time trying to pull together 30 to 40 people, a well-advertised on-line seminar might prove to be more efficient and more effective.

In addition, some of us have found that would-be clients and patients are not willing to have others see them at such events. People still do prefer to maintain privacy about plastic surgery, especially in small or close-knit communities. Moreover, as with all marketing programs, these ideas work, work for a time, or do not work, depending upon your community. You will need to try various techniques, and then remember: be flexible. You will want to change the mix.

Keynote Speaker

Estheticians are often great public speakers. If you are inclined toward public speaking, this can be a rewarding experience, and one that can inspire others when you speak with authenticity, passion, and humor. Start small, and then build. Whether you are speaking to 5 or 500 you will be in demand if you have contagious enthusiasm about the topic on which you are speaking.

In most cases, your speech does not need to be a slick, professional piece. It just needs to be well organized, of interest to the audience, and clip along at a steady pace. Reading well while engaging the audience is better than fumbling without notes. Shorter speeches, leaving the audience wanting more, are better than longer talks, which may have attendees looking at their watches. Most of all, be yourself.

Cooperative Advertising

Companies from various industries offer cooperative advertising whereby the company will support your events or print, radio, and television ads if you use their product or logo in the ad. Some will allow you to bank dollars based on what you have spent on product with them, in turn receiving credit toward your next purchase of product. This is free money and a business generator. Use it.

Some companies will fund your newsletters and brochures, others have marketing materials prepackaged and ready to go; you just put your logo on them. Always ask whether the representative of the product line that you are interested in using has a cooperative advertising program.

The key to selecting a vehicle is to have your differential advantage in the forefront of your marketing strategy. Think about which tool will put you in front of the greatest portion of your target market, for a particular intended response. That tool might be an event, a new product orientation, or other efforts to attract new business.

The Message

The message that you will be sending through your chosen vehicle, in your marketing strategy, will incorporate your differential advantage. This advantage is the key item that makes you unique from everyone else and that will elicit a response from your target audience. Some examples of using an appropriate message for your target audience are as follows:

- 20 years as professional esthetician
- graduate of a prestigious esthetic program (name that program and how your education will benefit the client)
- affiliation with well-known, published, or celebrity physician (name that physician)
- clinical esthetic practice in a private setting (often people looking for help with appearance concerns do not like to be exposed in a public setting)
- exclusive product line targeting antiaging or acne, or a unique ethnic skin-care program (you must tell the potential client that you have what they are looking for and what they need)

The importance of sending an accurate, appropriate message is crucial to the initial communication that your audience receives about you, because it makes the statement: "We have what you need or want." Historically the business of esthetics has been considered a luxury. We need to move the messages from a luxury to a *maintenance*—or in some cases, a *necessity*—focus in the clinical setting.

Target Audience

Your target audience is the group or subgroup that you want to serve. Through the marketing research you do while developing your business plan, you will SWOT and sift through the competition, create your unique advantage, and thus determine your target audience or consumer. Some locations may support products and services that are higher end; others may serve more moderately priced products. Some areas may be flooded by day spas, skin care centers, and **medi-spas**, making it necessary for you to focus on your specific differences and abilities. Examples of your target audience may be:

- **Boomers.** Midpoint Baby Boomers (44–54) going through menopause, with an interest in small procedures such as Botox, or laser hair reduction. This population will want antiaging products and sunscreens and are typically interested in noninvasive procedures. They are typically working, so they do not have time to recover from major procedures. In addition, you will find many in this population to be transitioning in image presentation, often open to streamlining, classic styling, and an occasional whimsical trendy item. They are much less interested spending time in front of the mirror than they are in quality products and services.
- **Retirees.** Newly retired, which may include the 55- to 65-year-olds. Typically they have more time and money, are older, and may be interested in more invasive procedures along with quality skin-care products. They may be less interested in long dissertations on ingredient functions and features of products or treatments, but they really are focused on benefits. In addition, they may be traveling frequently. Like the boomer, they are busy and appreciate simplicity and ease in making scheduled appointments for treatments, in product purchases, and in surgery scheduling.
- **Students.** College towns may have a need for a skin-care business in acne treatments and products, along with makeup and trendy items. This group may benefit from appearance or image counseling, as they will be soon entering the workforce. They will need to know not only about proper skin care regimens, but how to present for interviews, networking, and general career success.
- **Men.** The male population is seeking antiaging methods. They are undergoing procedures, having treatments, and using products. This may be a target audience or a subgroup as they are the fastest growing users of **cosmeceuticals**. They appreciate the clinical approach, are not interested in standing in lines in a department store for products, and are perfect clients for the clinical esthetician.

Keep in mind that you do not want to waste your energy and marketing dollars, on a **demographic** group (population of individuals united by common income bracket, interests, living styles, or location) that is not going to be interested in your service, such as targeting the college student with a higher-end, antiaging product. This can build negative stereotype about estheticians and serve to be a misuse of valuable capital. Make certain that your marketing strategy, product or service, and location are in alignment.

If you are targeting employed, 45- to 55-year-old high-income clients, who are in need of stress relief, you want to market accordingly. One example of a message given through an appropriate vehicle to a target audience idea would be to use a full color print ad, in an upscale magazine, with an attractive male or female model receiving a treatment (Figure 5–1).

Most of us will have more than one target audience, but we will have a primary point of focus, and then two, three, or more subcategories. Start with your primary target audience, and then add subcategories when you want to create new business. Contrary to what we hear from some experts, we will need more than one audience, more than one product line, and more than one service.

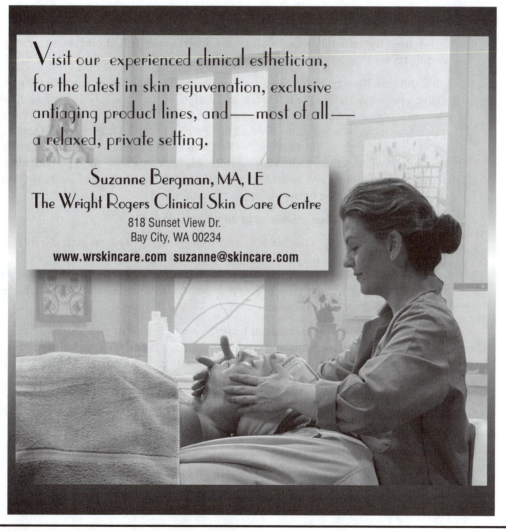

Figure 5–1 Print ad for clinical esthetician

Summary

Developing your marketing strategy can be a positive, enlightening experience, yet one with consequences. Create an image that best reflects the practice as a whole. Once your image is received by the market, it will set a tone for how you will be perceived by potential clients and patients. Select an appropriate vehicle for your target audience, and make certain that your message reflects your differential advantage. Continue to ask yourself, "Why should people come to us?" and then continue to remind them.

Frequently Asked Questions

1. **How does the esthetician and staff create a well-orchestrated marketing strategy while trying to meet the needs of the patients all day?**

   It is difficult. Most practices hire an advertising agency, practice management firm, or have a person designated to marketing and design work exclusively. If handled in the office, it is vital that this person have the experience, skills, and time to devote to marketing, as it can be a full-time job when there are two or more departments. There are press releases to write, ads to create, Web sites to update, media to contact, and a myriad of other duties that can be very exciting, yet too demanding for a practitioner to handle. Many estheticians have tried to be accommodating in this area and have found it taking too much time from building their practices.

2. **How much information should be in an advertisement?**

   Keep in mind your target market. If you are trying to bring in clients and patients from the 45- to 55-year-old range with an income of $100,000 and above, your message needs to reflect what your differential advantage is *over the other practices* in town. You will not need a laundry list of everything that you do, rather why you do it better. See Figure 5–2 for an example.

   From this ad, the prospective client learns many things about your office. They see that you perform Botox injections and are on the cutting edge, as this procedure has just recently become common practice. They will make an inference that there are many other treatments and procedures that this office does as well, and that you are obviously technologically savvy in having this seminar on-line. Incidentally, this is a great way to fill up an appointment schedule providing that you have a staff member poised to perform that function.

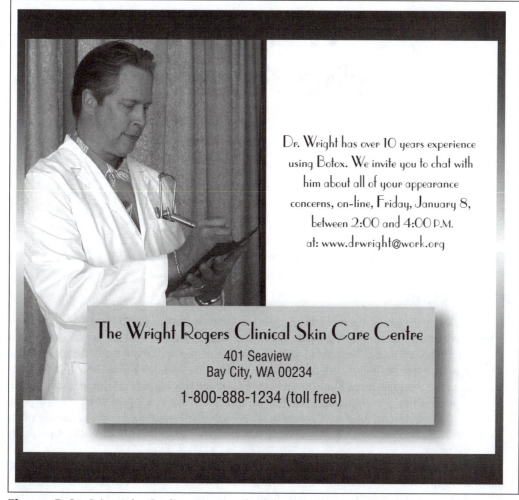

Dr. Wright has over 10 years experience using Botox. We invite you to chat with him about all of your appearance concerns, on-line, Friday, January 8, between 2:00 and 4:00 P.M. at: www.drwright@work.org

The Wright Rogers Clinical Skin Care Centre

401 Seaview
Bay City, WA 00234

1-800-888-1234 (toll free)

Figure 5–2   Print Ad—On-line Seminar for Physician

CHAPTER 6

Handling the Product

- Introduction
- The Pricing of Products
- The Pricing of Services
- Merchandising
- Summary
- Frequently Asked Questions

Introduction

Handling the product is a key function in our business, as our **profit**, paycheck, and client services depend upon it. We need to set prices based on the cost of the product (including all of the expenses), the **market value** (what the market will pay), the competition (what price are they selling it for), and your particular goal—whether in selling or dispensing (handing out) products. Some offices are less interested in profit advantages and may be against selling products altogether, thus having you to act as support by dispensing products in pre- and postoperative conditions. Yet others will want to take full advantage of the profit-making potential, and will want you to fairly and efficiently drive the retailing of the practice.

Retailing for profit requires that you know what you paid for a given product (including expenses). This is known as **cost of goods sold,** or COGS; from this point you know how to set your retail prices in order to make a profit.

The Pricing of Products

Pricing decisions are determined by several factors, and each must be carefully considered. We need to take into account our market, what our competition is offering and their pricing structure, and, the most important factor, what we paid for a product after all expenses have been taken out.

Cost of Goods Sold/Product

The cost of goods sold will dictate how much we will charge for the product. We would not remain in business if we sold products for less than we paid for them. The **profit margin** is the difference between the cost of the product and the price at which it is sold. In addition, we must factor in the all of the expenses such as shipping, compensation/wage/commission, and marketing. These must be covered by the sale of the product, or we are not truly looking at a profit. When we subtract all of these factors out of the sale, then we have what is called a **profit.** A profit is the difference between the cost of the product or service plus the *cost of doing business* (all expenses subtracted) and what is left over.

Compensation

Esthetician compensation is part of pricing a product as it is factored into the **cost-of-sale** forecast (Table 6–1). Depending upon the decisions negotiated by the esthetician and the physician, compensation packages are as follows:

- higher hourly wage, with a lower percentage in commission sales on products and treatments, health benefits, and training funded
- lower hourly wage with a higher percentage on product and treatment commissions (less risk to physician), health benefits, and training funded
- straight salary with no commission, health benefits, and training funded
- percentage of the surgery fee (as they close the surgical consult), in addition to hourly wage and commission on products and treatments, health benefits, and training funded

Markup

In retailing **cosmeceuticals** or skin health-care products, we typically obtain a two-time **markup.** This means if we pay $25.00 wholesale, including shipping costs, we sell it for the suggested retail price of $50.00. With volume package purchases or with generic or

Setting	Compensation
Cosmetic surgeon	12–30 hourly Plus commission 15%–30% on product and treatments
Dermatologist	12–15 hourly
Outpatient clinic	15–25 hourly Plus 15%–30% commission on product and treatments
Hospital	15–25 hourly
Independent clinic near physicians' office	15–50 hourly Plus commission on product and treatment
Laser center—physician or nurse directed	12–20 hourly
Cosmetic dentist	12–15 hourly Plus commission on product and treatment
Medical spa—physician directed	12–25 hourly Plus commission on product and treatment

Table 6–1 Compensation Chart

private label products, this formula may change. You may be able to price products at a three- or four-time markup in the case of generic brands, or, conversely, at a much lower markup on a well-known brand, if you are trying to increase business for a short period. An example of this would be holiday gift packages known as **value packages** in department store retailing. This technique would work in attracting clients by advertising a lower-priced item (also called the **loss leader**), to bring them in so that they also buy the more expensive, higher-quality items. Another example of discounting that is used is to close out slow-selling products.

Loss leaders and discounting products has a double-edged sword effect, however. Some clients become accustomed to value pricing, and will wait for it, so do not make your business about discounting; make it about good, quality service and stewardship.

Competition   The competition is another key factor in determining your markup on products. What are their prices compared to yours? To retain clients we need to have a very good reason to charge more for similar products. If the competition has a similar product or service, you may take a lower margin on those competitive products or services and make it up elsewhere, such as on generic products, an exclusive product line, or a service that no one else is performing.

Market supply and demand   Maybe there are several clinics using the same products or performing the same treatments, and the market is simply flooded with skin-care centers. Even in this climate however, pricing must be adequate to cover your costs, or remain above the **break-even point.** Your break-even point is a figure that is determined by knowing how many products and services that you need to sell each month to cover all of your expenses.

Corporate culture   Some physicians are not terribly concerned about the profit advantages of retailing, and feel that it is enough to have the esthetician assisting through the pre- and postoperative phases by offering support to the patient. They may look at the business of their practice from the perspective of a patient-care facility, and may want to offer products at the break-even point as a service, the cost of which is factored into the surgical fee.

The Pricing of Services

The pricing of services can be addressed as if the service is a product. The major difference, which may seem obvious, is that we can make more profit from our treatments and services. Once our start-up equipment and our treatment product supplies are paid for, it is just our time and expenses that are deducted.

Do keep in mind however, that we need to take out our wages/commissions, rent, marketing, and other expenses when looking at the profit from providing treatments. For example, if you charge $65.00 for a peel, which costs you $25.00 in commission or wages, and $20.00 in expenses, your profit may now be $20.00.

Merchandising

Merchandising is styling and displaying products in the clinic with the intention of increasing traffic and interest in point-of-sale purchases. It is important that you not only merchandise, but that you refer to it as such. Without making this profit-driving component of your business appealing, you have very little chance of moving it off the shelves. Here are a few pointers to keep in mind:

- **Keep all glass, étagères, cases, displays, props, and cupboards clean.**   This is not only important for OSHA standards (see Chapter 12); no one wants to purchase a bottle of cleanser from a dusty shelf.
- **Put all fast-moving products up front at eye level.**   Using a pyramid approach, start with tallest products in the center, and then move to smallest. If the eye has to go up and down across the case, it is not as easy to see all that it displays. Put all products that you want to move quickly at eye level, and make them easy to access (Figure 6–1).
- **Use a 3-month rate of sale to calculate purchase for stock.**   If you determine that you have sold 25 cleansers, give or take, per month for 3 months, at any given point—

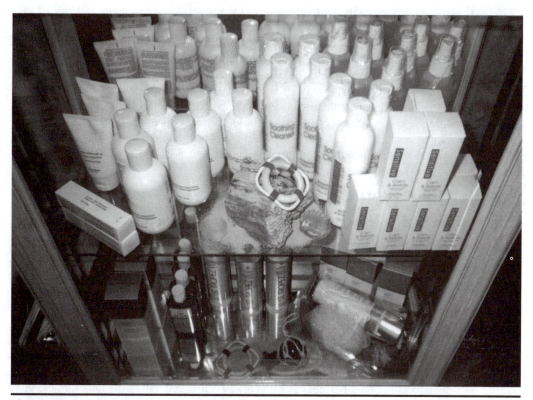

Figure 6–1   Merchandising your product lines

just to maintain that business—you should have at least six–seven pieces of that product on the shelf. If you increase sales by 10 percent, add 10 percent more in product and so on.

- **Perform an inventory at least every 3 months.**   This makes it easier for you to notice trends, order replacements, and keep stock balanced. If you notice that you are moving only cleansers, you are probably just servicing rather than educating, problem solving, advising, and ultimately selling. Use your inventory sheet as a research tool (Table 6–2).
- **Have style.**   Being a stylist is just that. It is using style to influence purchasing, not necessarily spending large amounts of money on displays. Depending upon area and demographics, for summer use sand and sunglasses around a sunscreen story. In winter use a snow look-alike with moisturizers and sunscreens, for spring use miniature birdhouses or nests for exfoliating products, and in fall use leaves or items in earth tones to promote environmental protectors and antioxidants. Use props that are unique or unexpected. They do not need to be expensive, large, elaborate, or ornate; just follow a simple, thematic approach.

Summary

Understanding the pricing structure of products and service seems complicated. Just keep in mind that you will need to consider every aspect of the cost of providing products and services—including your income, taxes, and benefits—before you can declare a profit. This department has been very difficult for many of us to comprehend if we work strictly as an employee. Administrators, owners, and managers have a very different perspective on business operations than we do, particularly if we are not made aware of how the consequences of our business decisions impact the practice as a whole. Becoming more educated on the general pricing and compensation packages is crucial when we decide that we want a raise. Chances are you can give it to yourself based on how you structure these pricing elements, your selling acuity, and your performance.

Frequently Asked Questions

1. How does the esthetician learn about business in general?

Attend all of the conferences, trade shows, and business expositions that you can, both those related to esthetics and those which are not. Many suppliers have business courses at trade shows, which are excellent for learning product knowledge, business plans, and simple accounting practices. Attend workshops on reading financial statements and balance statements. Work closely with your clinic administrator by setting up routine appointments for reviewing your department's profit and loss statements (P and Ls). This is one of the best ways to learn about your business practices.

Contact your local Small Business Development Center for upcoming seminars about business related topics, and join your local Chamber of Commerce. It takes time to learn about business and it is always changing, but in the long run, the more that you learn, the more opportunities you will create for yourself and for the team.

INVENTORY CONTROL SHEET

Supplier	Product ID	Product Description	Cost	Unit Price	On Hand	Rec'd	Sold	Current	Notes

Table 6-2 Inventory Control Sheet

2. **Is it possible to mark things up higher than two or three times the cost of the product?**

Yes, it is—depending upon the demand in your area for that item and your target audience's willingness to pay that price. Do keep in mind, however, that many products are sold on-line at a discounted rate and other estheticians in the area may sell products for less. In addition, if people learn that you are selling products at a great **markup**, they may go elsewhere in the future. Be fair in your pricing. This goes for treatments and procedures alike. It is important to remain competitive in prices, but providing excellent customer service will go a long way to determine client retention.

CHAPTER 7

Selling and Healthy Sales Practices

- Introduction
- Selling Products and Services in a Medical Setting
- Retaining the Client
- Simple Strategies for Successfully Running the Business of Your Practice
- The Best Policy
- Summary
- Frequently Asked Questions

Introduction

Visit with a successful, professional, sales executive, and you will often see a person with integrity, optimism, excellent communication skills, and interest in remaining an ardent student. Professional salespeople know that their future is based on their service to others, on retention of the client. They also know that they must remain current in general knowledge and be constantly researching specific information about their business to remain competitive and of continuing help to their clients. This is not unlike one of the goals of the professional esthetician, and this suggests what we need to do to build our business in the office. We need to keep abreast of trends, new products, treatments, and procedures in addition to learning how best to put skin-type/condition–appropriate products into the hands of the client or patient.

Selling Products and Services in a Medical Setting

Selling services and products in a medical office is a principled mission. Enthusiasm must be tempered by assessment of the client's clinical needs. As exciting as it can be, we must not be driven exclusively by our sales commission, a new product line, or by trying to increase the profit margin of the practice.

If the client is ultimately seeking a medical procedure, we do not want to sell them a product that they will not be able to use for 3 months as they are recovering from surgery. In addition, we do not want to apply treatments or products that may be contraindicated for a specific condition, such as selling a microdermabrasion series to someone with rosacea, or recommending high-level AHA products to a teenager who is on Accutane.

Presenting Treatments and Products to the Patient

Depending upon the plan set up by the physician and the esthetician, the consultation will often include a product and services presentation, generally offered by the esthetician (Figure 7–1). Many estheticians will have their brochures made up to reflect packages of products and services that the client can purchase in addition to the surgery price. Some physicians will prefer to have all of the products and treatments included in the surgery fee, so that there is a smooth transition and a one-time fee. Most offices operate somewhere in the middle.

One idea that combines the two approaches is, for example, to offer the prelaser resurfacing patient a preoperative kit that contains all of the products, medications, and written protocols for the procedure, along with two or three esthetic services, at no immediate charge. The charge for these products and services is factored into the surgeon's fee. The

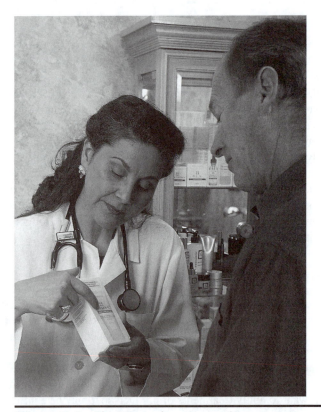

Figure 7–1   Physician educating patient on sunscreen use

patient is informed that subsequent products or treatments may be purchased by the patient at his or her choosing. Once patients experience the benefits of these products and services, they are often committed to long-term use.

Some physicians do not want to deal with factoring any other expenses into their surgical fee. If the decision has been made to offer these adjuncts separately, it is important to let the patient know that their products and treatments are not covered by insurance nor included in the surgical fee and must be purchased separately. This is a slightly more difficult presentation to make, and it can sound more like a sales pitch. But it can be done well. Show the patient that they may have a much better result if they follow a good skin-care regimen of certain products and treatments. You may want to take a leap of faith and offer a complimentary system such as a treatment and procedure-appropriate product to the patient, knowing that it will improve the outcome, and bring them back to you anyway.

Once you decide how to run this part of your business, be consistent. Trying to explain to the patient convoluted product or service prices that were assumed to be covered by the surgical fee has many pitfalls. In addition, a patient who feels as though they have to buy products and services above the surgical fee may see them as unnecessary.

Presenting Treatments and Products to the Client

Presenting and ultimately selling products and services to your clients will be exhilarating, affirming, and satisfying. When you see yearly repeat business you will realize these goals and know that all of the training and research is paying off.

Serving, educating, guiding, and caring are all part of presenting and promoting a comprehensive medical skin-care practice. Putting $400 worth of products in a glistening shopping bag, after performing a $300 treatment on a client is exciting. For some of us it is routine, for most others, a dream. Whether it is part of your daily schedule, or something that you are aspiring toward, keep in mind that in order for clients to come back to you, you must continue to serve them with all of the elements that made them trust and select you.

During your presentation, ask yourself:

1. What is the client looking for, wanting, asking?
2. What has she been using or doing about the current problem?
3. Can you improve upon what she has been doing/using, or should you send her to another professional?

To start, attend to the matters at hand. Try to address the immediate inquiry or problem, by defining or making an account of what is troubling the client. For example, "So your main concern, Jane, is that you have seen this mole change color and get larger?" or "You have noticed that you get these breakouts once a month?" Let the client describe to you what is happening, rather than guessing. Do not offer a solution too quickly; it may not be solvable, you do not want to suggest something that they are already using, and the problem may be beyond your scope or level of experience.

Also, do not give your recommendation until you have heard the complete story in the client's own words and you feel that you have established rapport and trust. You will appear as a real pro if you wait until all of the information is in. Moreover, you need to trust yourself enough to know that you can always add value, even if it means directing the client to another practitioner such as the physician.

Once you feel that you have enough information and the client seems to be waiting for suggestions from you, begin your presentation and keep these key items in mind:

1. **Be honest.**   While working in a medical office, you may be visited by clients with conditions or issues that are beyond your training. The person wanting to make a purchase for a product or treatment that is it not appropriate for their skin type, age, or need will find out later (often sooner) that the product or service was not good for them. In addition, people can feel a lack of knowledge or uncertainty from a professional; body language gives it away. It is better to be up-front about these matters. Keep in mind that if you don't have an answer or antidote, you will find someone who may be able to help. This will translate as professionalism.

2. **State clearly again for the client what you think that you have heard.**   Make certain that you both are addressing the same issue, and that it is the one in which they are the most interested. It is embarrassing to find that you are recommending a treatment or product that features benefits for a problem that the client does not see as an issue.

3. **Present a comprehensive plan to address issues.**   There are often many solutions to helping someone with skin care. As we know, there are many skin-care product lines and many treatments available. Rather than just focusing on selling your line, focus on a complete regimen for the client. Include a treatment plan, follow-up appointments, complimentary samples, or case studies or articles that have been written about the subject. All this will instill a sense of "I'm in the right place," or "This esthetician has really done the homework."

   This also shows that if one method does not work, there are other avenues to explore. Often if we present a solution as the *only* or *the best*, then you have nowhere to go if it does not work. Again, there is always another product, drug, procedure, treatment, or practitioner to try.

4. **Once you have given your presentation . . . BE QUIET!**   Do not go on about the product, treatment, doctor, colleague, or whatever. Let the client make the next move. Often you will find that if you apply this technique, the client will take you seriously. He or she will realize that you are waiting for an answer, assume that you have recommended the best plan at that point, and purchase the package that you have recommended.

   If a client comes back with objections such as, "Well, I have so many products at home," or "Let me think about it," then do so. High pressure has no place here. Send clients off with samples along with written, detailed method for use, and they will come back to buy when they are ready.

   A small percentage of the population—often logical/analytical types—will often need to think it over, look at their budget, talk to the spouse or partner, or just not want to make a decision on the spot. For these mathematical/logical personality types, it is wise to have a cost analysis on the products for them to take home along with their articles, samples, and treatment plan. This would be a breakdown of the product expense per month. It does not need to be formal. You may just write it down on the spot, as every program is different:

Cleanser	$25
AHA Cream	$50
Antioxidant Lotion	$45
Sunscreen	$35
Total	$155 ÷ 5 (months) = $31 per month

5. **After the client has made a decision to purchase, provide written home-care instructions.**   Make certain that clients leave with written instructions on how to use and apply the product program and employ the "Tell Them" approach:
   - **Tell them what you are going to tell them:** "I am going to tell you about . . ."
   - **Tell and show them what you want them to know:** "I am telling you and showing you . . ."
   - **Ask them to tell you what you told them:** "I am asking you to tell me what I have said . . ."
   - **Tell them what you told them:** "I am reiterating everything that I have told you . . ."

6. **Always give a client a sample, or a suggestion for next time.**   Plant the seed for the next visit or product purchase. When a client gets ready to leave, say, "Next time, let's look at masking. Here is a sample of a hydrating mask that I want you to try meanwhile." There is always a next time.

7. **Always schedule a follow-up appointment.**   Even during the busiest seasons of the year, people need products and services. Keep them on track by making an actual appointment to return to enforce the service-selling continuum.

Retaining the Client

Some of us are adept at bringing in new clients, planning promotional events, and creating excitement about new products and treatments, but maintaining a client base is what really drives the profit-making business over time. We need to think about all of the marketing strategies and new product and treatment acquisitions as nourishment for our existing client and patient base. If we do not look at our business this way and are just focusing on new clients, clients may come and go, thus creating an unstable practice. Long-term, satisfied clients and patients are the keys to a profitable business.

Research and share your findings with your clients. Think in terms of adding value during every opportunity that you have with them. Let the client and patients know that you are constantly searching for new technology in products and treatments through your quarterly newsletter, or on your Web site. Make certain, however, that new technology has been well tested prior to treating them, and charge a lower introductory fee. The concept of short-term profit in an expensive *not tried, nor true* treatment or procedure can eventually erode your client base. If clients feel that they have been overcharged in the name of new technology, they will go to a practitioner who is less apt to jump on a new bandwagon but who is consistent, fair with pricing, and waits until a treatment or product is proven.

Simple Strategies for Successfully Running the Business of Your Practice

We do not have to go very far to learn how to create a successful business. The application of that learning can be supplied with the guidance and support of others who have been through what we are trying to do. In addition, always remember how you like to be treated, and emulate that in all of your business dealings. Here are a few reminders.

- **Return calls immediately.**   When a client calls, put that person at the top of your to-do list. If colleagues call or e-mail, respond as soon as possible; they may have a client for you. We cannot assume the luxury of thinking that we are too busy to handle our business. It may seem like we are too busy now, but things always change.
- **Work with your pharmacist.**   Some compounding pharmacists have a manufacturing designation and can create products containing antioxidants, **retinoic acid**, hydroquinone, sunscreens, amino acids, lower-level alpha and beta hydroxy acids, and various other types preparations for the face and body. They have access to product containers, labels, and other items necessary for retailing. Products containing drugs dispensed through the office must have been prescribed by the physician and have the appropriate documentation, signed by the doctor and placed in the patient's chart. In addition, continual evaluations must be made by the physician for reorders, and documentations follow accordingly.

  Take a field trip to your local pharmacist. Call them and find out how much actual compounding work they do on-site, and offer to spend a day with them. Not only is it exciting to see how this is done, but also you can gain knowledge about ingredients, bases, chemistry, and compounding.

- **Buy generic product lines.**   With a little research, you can find excellent generic products, at lower entry-level prices, create your own label, and thus gain a greater markup. To make a profit on a generic line, you must:

  have creditability with the client
  have excellent ingredients and packaging
  buy it at a nominal price
  have excellent supporting materials and collateral (safety and guarantees)
  research your market to make certain that other practitioners are not carrying the product with their logo applied to the same bottle

- **Create a private label.**   It is extremely expensive to hire a chemist and formulate your own line. Moreover, for the record, some of these companies use chemists who are formulating products for many companies, which means that they are not as exclusive as they appear. A quick trip through a department store stockroom will show you that 75 percent of the lines are owned by the same company using the same chemists and formulation processes, under a different label. You may however find that once you are established, private labeling may be the best answer for your practice. Expenses for logo design and applications are becoming more affordable, and we are finding that we do not need to make the exorbitant quantity purchases that we have in the past.

- **Compete with large companies.** Large companies through well-researched focused groups creatively demand our attention with large-scale elaborate marketing plans. An average advertisement in a popular magazine can run as much as $60,000 to $70,000 per page. We can make an educated guess that the amount of actual product that goes into a hundred-dollar cream may well only cost $8–$10, or less, hence the balance of the profit may be in large part sent to the advertising budget for the company. We can compete for market share with these companies because we do not have these large advertising budgets to deal with, we can create our own brand, or buy from smaller manufacturers, and we can change product inventory instantly.
- **Dispel notions, myths, and marketing hype.** Dispelling myths and marketing hype, is part of our responsibility to educate our clients. If we train our clients to know what they are looking at, they will be empowered to make good buying decisions. Some notions and myths that consumers unknowingly buy into are:

    Brand recognition: These products must work because XYZ is promoting them.
    Natural is the best: The ingredients are *all natural* according to the ad, and they must be better than those chemical-laden products.
    Implied guarantee: The photo of a woman showed her appearing 10 years younger after using the product . . . it must work.
    Monkey see, monkey do: Everyone else is using it, so there must be something to it.
    Esthetically pleasing: These advertisements are so beautiful, I'm framing them.

Now if we are to examine this information in a useful and mindful manner, we will find that these myths are embedded in each of us. Every time something new reaches the marketplace, we trip over a colleague to obtain our sample. After having tried the new product, we once again become satisfied and committed to remaining professional estheticians. We know that this is just another product just like ones we are familiar with, packaged to look different. Further, ours is better than . . . because it contains . . . has clinical studies . . . and is available to them at half of the price. (Albeit, the package may not be as alluring.)

The Best Policy

So, how do we impart this information to our client who visits us for treatments, and yet rushes off to purchase that new cream which holds great promise? Be direct.

- **Be honest.** Tell the truth. Share with them information that will help in decision making such as explaining that some of the ingredients in a lower-priced product are the same as those found in a different product. (However, because of smaller marketing budgets we can purchase these products for a fraction of the price, hence we can charge less in some cases.) In cases where products are more expensive, you can tell them that clinical products can be more expensive as there have been more clinical studies performed to assure their efficacy, or they have used expensive ingredients and more advanced technology to manufacture them. In addition, because ingredients in clinical products can be more aggressive, communicate that you will need to monitor the client's progress.

- **Know up-front that some of your time will be wasted.**   Regardless of what you do, some will go from line to line ingesting the latest fragrance sample, asking the poor salesperson for a tissue to wipe off the lipstick tester (germs and all). Others will attend meetings that feature pyramid schemes where the focus is on enlisting family members to sign up as sales associates, in order to build an inordinate amount of wealth by selling products including skin care, of which they know nothing about. They will then ask you to join. Another type of consumer will come rushing back to you after a consult wanting you to evaluate their latest purchase, without giving one thought to the time that you spent presenting information on free radical proliferation, amino acids, and antioxidants in full detail, diagrams and all. They are convinced that the beautiful jar, the neighbor's opinion, or the infomercial is gospel. Again, let go.

- **Since some clients are well informed and may know more than you do, help where you can.**   Some clients have a fair amount of cosmetic savvy, possess basic to intermediate skin-care knowledge, and purchase products from all over the world. Be delighted that they consider you part of their team. Guide and direct where you can, pay attention to cues about how you may help them. Some travelers like products sent to their homes abroad, and will appreciate your making the effort to think outside of the typical service model. Keep them abreast of all new products and treatments by sending them a newsletter, or a brief note card. Take recommendations that they may provide seriously. Some of our best business ventures come from people traveling, or from other countries and cultures.

- **Be accountable.**   Recognize that on some level, you are doing the same thing—selling—as the major advertiser or competitor. Let's face it: we want the consumer to become our client. We are convinced that our products and services are better than what they could find elsewhere, and most importantly, WE KNOW WHAT THEY NEED.

- **Remember you are the licensed professional.**   We are credentialed. Our training is extensive; we have attended numerous courses on cosmetic chemistry, product application, sanitation, and bacteriology as well as advanced courses in dermatology, physiology, anatomy, treatment protocols, client services, and lymphatic drainage massage. Clinical estheticians interface daily with nurses, doctors, patients, clients, clinic administrators and staff members, and vendors and therefore often have higher levels of exposure to current information.

Summary

If you bring your clients along with honesty, enthusiasm, quality products and treatments, outstanding customer/client services, research, and continuing education that can be shared in a comprehensible fashion, they will be able to look beyond the advertising and marketing of major lines. When you are able to show clients that your unique clinical or medical lines have much to offer specific skin-care issues, and that you are taking the time to tailor your treatments and product lines to their individual needs, you will find that you are a good match.

Frequently Asked Questions

1. **Exhibitors at trade shows recommend offering only one skin-care line. How does the esthetician know which one to buy?**

This is an ongoing battle that affects both new and veteran estheticians. No one line will fill all of your needs indefinitely. In the clinic, you will find that drugs will be added to home-care program preparation for surgical procedures, some super-hydrating products will be too rich for patients on Accutane, and not everyone will be a candidate for aggressive AHA or retinol products.

Look back through your marketing plan and assess your target market. Build your skin-care program around the market that you are going after, by looking at all phases of their needs from the inside out. Start with what you will need for supporting the physician's procedures, both for in-office and patient home-care needs. Then go to the next largest target market and find a product line that best suits that group, and so on. Some lines may overlap, so it is important to study your chemistry and make certain that ingredients are compatible.

Several product lines are exclusively sold to physicians due to the active agents that are used in the formulas. They will always have support products that are companion pieces to the active products, along with sunscreens. These products are a great place to start, and from there you can venture out as experience and need dictate.

2. **What does the esthetician do if a product just does not sell?**

This will happen on occasion, despite the fact that the product may be popular in another market. Most vendors are willing to work with clients on slow or nonmoving merchandise. Ask if you can exchange it for something else in the line that sells for you. If this does not work, build a basket or two for the local women's shelter; they can always use these new products, and you can take it out as a tax deduction.

Territories and Office Relations

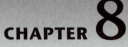

CHAPTER 8

Acknowledging Office Politics

- Introduction
- Office Politics
- Learn Office or Corporate Culture Before Accepting a Position
- Nepotism in the Medical Practice
- Know and Report to Your Immediate Supervisor
- Conflicts about Commission
- Summary
- Frequently Asked Questions

Introduction

This section contains material that is not politically correct. The subject matter is uncomfortable to discuss and could have managers and staff running for the door if you bring up any of the contents. The focus of this chapter is to identify some of the key issues that arise for estheticians during the process of integrating the esthetician into the medical practice.

Office Politics

Office politics has existed for years. It has been accepted and addressed with varying degrees of effectiveness. Visualize a huge invisible Bengal tiger pouncing through the office, bumping into desks and walls, bounding through the exam rooms, the operating room, the reception area, and even in the lunchroom. It toys with its victim by sweetly lying in wait, thus allowing everyone to let their guard down before the attack. During the attack, you are not exactly sure of what is taking place, but you sense an injustice somewhere. Then, when you least expect it, you can see the tiger over in the corner licking its chops after devouring the unsuspecting prey. This tiger's name is *office politics*.

Politics and power struggles exist in any work setting, and like it or not, we all have people around us with personalities that we do not like. There are duties and details that we find superfluous; limitations on our education, personalities, and comprehension; and, at times, a work life that can be oppressive. In addition, we may find that certain systems and organizations do not support our work style, philosophical beliefs, or career goals. It is important to identify basic truths about ourselves so that we may improve, in order to create a more satisfactory environment for ourselves as practitioners and for those co-workers and clients with whom we serve. We all have an opportunity to set the bar higher.

If you address sensitive problems head-on with a visit to the manager's office every time something comes up, the manager will become desensitized to your plight and will run from you. If you continually talk to other clinical workers about your fears, problems, or perceived slights, they will begin to see you as unprofessional and wonder what you are doing there.

People expect to live with a certain amount of gossip, one-upmanship, or other irritating factors in the workplace. However, if you feel that you continually need to keep your résumé buffed up and are one moment away from walking out the door, this can affect your productivity, interest, and the morale in the office.

Learn Office or Corporate Culture Before Accepting a Position

The first step to succeeding in a medical office is learning something about the culture in an office before your start date. Find out who the players are. It may seem that the manager makes all of the decisions, but with a little inquiry you may find a very different story.

If you are entrepreneurial, and you determine that you are entering a real *top-down* office (all decisions come from the doctors or manager, with no room for independent decisions), you may find that you will not function well in this type of environment. If you like to make your own decisions about product purchases or treatments that you will perform, and implement your own marketing ideas, it will be unbearable to work in an environment where you must ask for permission to make a move.

Conversely, if you are new in your profession or need a fair amount of direction to feel comfortable at work, working for a laissez-faire type of office with a lack of structure, may create some anxiety for you. It will be important for you to find an office with a staff that has an interest in educating you every step. Many physicians, nurses, and administrators are interested in teaching. It is important for you to connect with a group that supports your needs (Figure 8–1). In addition, if the office you are interviewing with is very formal, and you have a more informal type of personality, do not fight it. There are plenty of offices that like to have fun with the staff and patients; you will feel out of step all of the time if you try to fit into a more austere environment. Keep looking.

Expand the Interviewing Process

Take time in the interviewing process. Request additional interview components and ask to spend a morning in the office, to engage in the culture firsthand. Physicians and nurses do this activity, known as *shadowing*. With the consent of the physician and patients, following the doctor and nurses into consultations, appropriate-level meetings, and having lunch together are all good ways to find out how the health-care professionals relate to the patients and staff members. This is important.

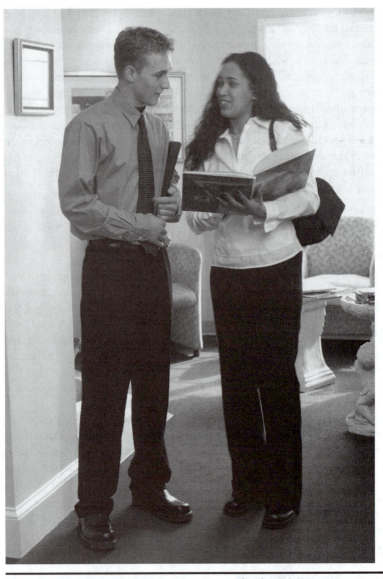

Figure 8–1   Esthetician interviewing with physician

If you are considering a long-term position with an office, a possibility beyond shadowing is creating an internship. This would be established by the esthetician, the clinic administrator, and the physician, to provide a brief status as an *esthetician in training*. You would go into an office at no charge to them, with a predetermined time allotment, goals, and objectives to experience yourself working in that environment.

This is a much-needed adjunct to esthetic education. It could improve office relations by establishing a context for the esthetician *before* the actual start date. The staff has an opportunity to experience the quality, interests, and construct of the esthetician's work; moreover, the esthetician can learn the office culture and politics, visit expectations, and determine if a specific office offers a good match. If this request is agreeable to the doctor, then you can discover if this could be a good opportunity for you. If not, you have lost nothing. Once you are in place shadowing or interning, trust your instincts. If you feel slightly intimidated by it all, this is normal. If you feel uncomfortable, you will grow. If you feel humiliated, put down, and as if you are waiting for the hours to pass, thank the supervisor for the experience, and move on.

Nepotism in the Medical Practice

Office politics can be exacerbated by conditions that are intrinsically difficult—seniority, hierarchy-patriarchy, and levels of education—and which are naturally occurring and operating in any office. There are additionally unique conditions that can be brought about by having relatives and friends working within the framework of an office. However, because medical offices are often small, private enterprises, family members may make up a part of the staff. This can make it difficult for staff members to take the lead roles that they need to make good business decisions.

If staff members feel that they are being negatively monitored by a close friend or family member of the doctor (or other authoritative personnel), creativity and production may suffer. If you find that a family practice means just that, bear in mind, it may be difficult for someone outside of that group to fit in. A husband, wife, son or daughter, or in-law may have a built-in blind spot to the problems that the family member possesses. This can create an uphill battle. Moreover, if you report to a family member who does not have the expertise or training to handle routine issues, this gap may become wider as you gain more knowledge about your position. It might be worth your time, energy, and peace of mind to look elsewhere to build your practice.

This is not to say that nepotism never allows smooth running of the practice. In some offices having a family member or close friend as a co-worker can be a contribution to the whole, and in general become a positive addition. When the family member has made a commitment to continuing education, is objective about each employee, and does not resort to favoritism, that enlightened individual may have insights about how to work with the relative that others cannot seem to find. It highly depends upon the *team* and its ability to assess, evaluate, and implement necessary elements in the office.

Know and Report to Your Immediate Supervisor

An esthetician should not be in the position of having to answer to five or six people on a daily basis. Moreover, physicians, nurses, and medical personnel should not be placed in the position of making management decisions for the esthetician during the workday.

Once you determine who your supervisor is, work directly with that person. This can eliminate the awkwardness of having too many bosses, or feeling torn trying to please everyone. Once again, a supervisor should have management training and possess the hard (office machines, equipment, etc.) and soft (human resources) skills necessary to be an effective leader and to act as an impartial liaison (Figure 8–2).

Conflicts about Commission

Conflicts often arise from a lack of defined roles or job descriptions in the office. They are sometimes financially motivated as well. Co-workers may become resentful or want to reap benefits when they find out that an esthetician is making a commission for sales and treatments rendered. It is important to keep this and all similar information confidential between the administrator and the employee, but sometimes information leaks. This may set up a chain of events that initially can be frustrating to everyone in the office. One way to resolve this is for the management to offer a bonus to all staff members when appropriate. Employees respond positively to financial rewards, and offices that engage in giving bonuses routinely, have diligent and loyal staff members. Lunches, dinners, and picnics are fine, but these can become obligatory. If a choice is to be made, staff members typically would enjoy having the extra money.

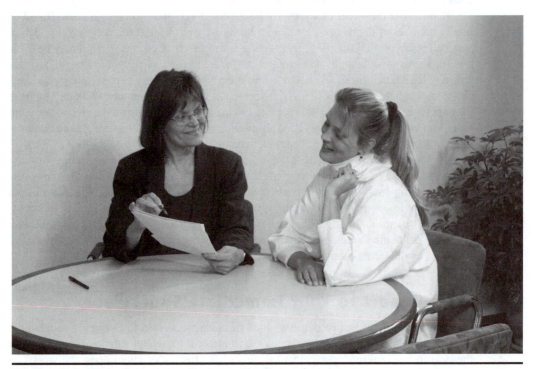

Figure 8–2   Esthetician interviewing with clinic administrator

Summary

Office politics will continue to plague employees whenever there are two or more people involved in a business or practice. The esthetician needs to pay close attention to detail when selecting an office in which to work. If unsuitable issues show up immediately, they do not go away later. As with all health-care service positions, we experience high stress, and often there is not enough time to communicate well with people having unresolved personal problems. Learn as much as you can about yourself, your needs, and create a wish list that indicates what type of office for which you are best suited.

It is necessary to designate at least one person to handle the details of the skin-care business; this lowers the stress level for everyone in the office. If the esthetician does not yet have the experience or interest in creating a growing business, then another staff member may provide this service. However, estheticians have received this training as a rudiment in their initial esthetic education. It is natural that most of us will be positioned as a lead or we will assume stewardship of the skin-care center. With time, maturity, and a bonus package given to all staff members, the commission conflict dissolves quickly when the complexity of the estheticians' work becomes apparent.

Frequently Asked Questions

1. **How does the esthetician go about setting up a day in the office shadowing or an internship?**

   Once you determine that the initial interviews have been successful, and the office is interested in hiring you, express your interest in coming in to shadow for a few hours or a day at no charge to them (remember, this is research for you). Explain that you would like to learn how you could best prepare for your role with them, and that you are interested in allowing them to view the quality of your work.

   If you are interested in an internship, create a proposal complete with objectives, goals, and plans for how you would like to spend your educational experience with the office. This can be developed with the support of an instructor, an experienced clinical esthetician, and a cooperating physician. This can be sent to the office along with your résumé or curriculum vitae, to be followed up by a phone call for an interview.

2. **What type of questions should the esthetician ask during an interview that may reveal something about the office culture?**

   Follow conventional wisdom at the onset of the interview. You want to appear graceful and collected under pressure. Allow the interview to be led by the interviewer(s) until asked if you have any questions. At that point, pull out a few well-constructed questions (it is fine to read) such as:

   - "What personal and professional characteristics are you looking for in an esthetician?" Alternatively, "What type of person do you envision in this position?" This will tell you what they are hoping to find.

- "How long have you been in practice? How long have you had the skin-care component to the practice?" This will tell you whether they are a start-up, expanding and adding a new department, or if you would be filling the shoes of a former esthetician.
- "Where do you see the skin-care department going?" This will tell you what their expectations are, and you will need to assess your skills. (What do you need to add, maintain, delete?)
- "Who does the buying?" The answer to this question will tell you how much control that you may have in the position. If the clinic administrator does all of the buying, and will continue to do so, then you will have less control. For some this may be great, for others it could be stifling. Think about what *you* need and what *you* will be bringing to the practice. If your skills, talents, and vision do not fit in one practice, do not despair. They will somewhere else.

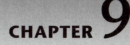

CHAPTER 9

Territories and Roles Defined

- Introduction
- The Roles and Legal Consequences
- Summary
- Frequently Asked Questions

Introduction

Many issues and conflicts in a practice can be resolved by looking at the territories, the roles that accompany them, and how they play out in the clinical setting. By acknowledging the differences in training and experiences, we can learn to complement and support each other, rather than allowing these differences to divide and polarize the team.

The Roles and Legal Consequences

By looking at the few key roles that members of a medical team fill, we can see that the nursing staff, the physicians' assistants, administrators, estheticians, and surgical staff all have very different functions and areas of responsibility. Should we move from our area of expertise, certification, and training there may be legal consequences. It is imperative that we find ways to support and enable each other to perform our tasks and yet follow the parameters as dictated by the laws of our state licensing.

The Nurse-Esthetician Relationship

Nurses and estheticians have a natural alliance. If you have been blessed with a nursing staff able to recognize your talents and skills in the treatment of clients and patients, be grateful. Estheticians can spend more time with the patient, freeing up the nurse to assist the physician in all phases of clinical work. The esthetician can supply the nurse with detailed information about **home-care compliance** and act as a liaison for the patient on behalf of the patient. The nurse and the esthetician can work together in organizing special clinics such as Botox or laser hair reduction, and may share in treatment applications. In addition they may co-create pre- and postoperative protocols, office flowcharts, and patient education materials.

Developing a good working relationship with the nursing staff is a priority. Here are a few ideas for generating goodwill:

- **Do not make outrageous claims.**   Don't tell them: "This product is a miracle," or "This product is all natural; it does not have chemicals in it." Nurses and physicians know that everything has chemicals in it and hope that there is a good preservative in a product to fight bacteria. While your new product may have some great benefits, it is better to talk function with them, rather than using marketing tools.
- **Offer nurses simple skin-care programs.**   They are in artificially air-controlled rooms for hours at a time, wearing masks, hair caps, scrubs, gloves, and other personal protection items. Their skin can often be dry, parched, and in need of nourishing hydrators, with an uncomplicated regimen for work.
- **Give them your time and services.**   Even the crustiest veteran nurses will respond to a hand massage or a lymphatic massage (Figure 9–1). Do not use a heavy aromatherapeutic treatment. Many have allergies and do not like fragrances.
- **Watch your timing.**   There is not always time for long, involved explanations or responses. Keep responses short and prioritized. (This works well with physicians, too.) Always approach them at an appropriate time.

The Physician-Nurse (RN, LPN, CMA) Relationship

Examine the role that the nurse or medical assistant plays in the work life of a physician. The nurse's role is that of primary support to the physician (Figure 9–2). Every movement is directed toward assisting, connected to the physician's actions. Their clinical work consists of having knowledge of and performing duties which are requested by the physician: administering medications or performing injections, patient education, scheduling, assisting in pre- and postoperative procedures, assisting in surgical procedures; and cleaning instruments as well as the OR (operating room) and all exam rooms. Moreover, they follow and direct all orders as given by the physician. Some Certified Medical Assistants are trained to perform administrative duties as well. Physician Assistant-certified staff members are more independent, as they are licensed to practice medicine under the auspices of the physician, but typically they do not manage a department.

The Physician-Esthetician Relationship

The physician-esthetician relationship is unique in that it is new, and from the perspective of the client or patient, their roles are parallel in nature. If you are an esthetician working for a physician, the physician obviously retains full responsibility and ultimately directs the work provided by esthetic personnel; however, the nature of the work of the esthetician is independent of the physician to a greater degree than that of a nurse. We are providing skin analysis/problem solving, conducting empirical research, managing a profit center, merchandising, researching and buying products and treatments, applying hands-on treatments, presenting product orientations, procuring clients and selling treatments and products, and managing client retention and marketing.

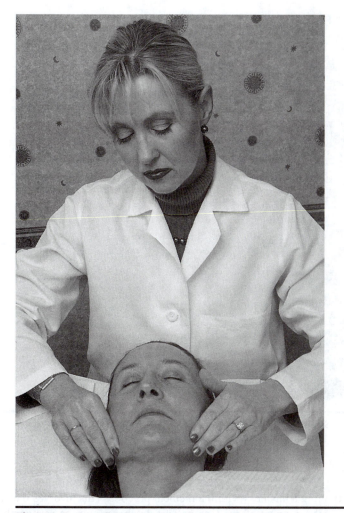

Figure 9–1   Client receives treatment by clinical esthetician

If you are a nurse *and* are a licensed esthetician, a different situation exists. If you are not responsible for a profit center unto its own, you are really operating as medical support. If your primary role is in assisting the physician in surgery, supplying an immediate response to gather instruments, cleaning rooms after office visits and/or scheduling, your role is different from that of the estheticians. The distinction is necessary to make when considering the business elements of a full-service esthetic practice in a physician's office (Figure 9–3). You will have a different perspective and focus and will make different decisions. Depending upon size and need, this configuration works well in some offices.

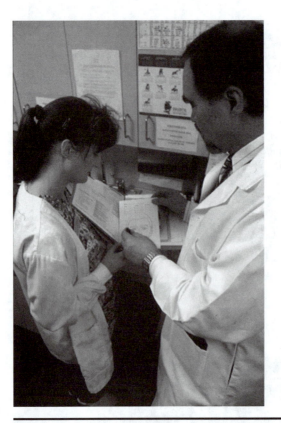

Figure 9–2   Nurse and physician

Summary

An esthetician is running a business within a medical practice. This involves the procurement of a clientele, the support of existing patient database, and the responsibility of creating a profit from both. That is, as an esthetician you are recommending and selling products and treatments for profit, in addition to seeing patients pre- and postoperatively. Estheticians are responsible for consultations, all treatments they perform, product knowledge orientation, retailing (including buying and selling of product and accepting payment for treatments and products). They take charge of marketing; they clean and maintain esthetic instruments, space, and machines; and in many cases they schedule their own appointments. They assist in creating protocols and are patient educators. They are interconnected with the physician but clearly operate duties that are independent from both physician and nursing staff.

If you are licensed as both a medical assistant and an esthetician, it is important to pick a primary role for yourself. It will be difficult to wear both hats such as in serving

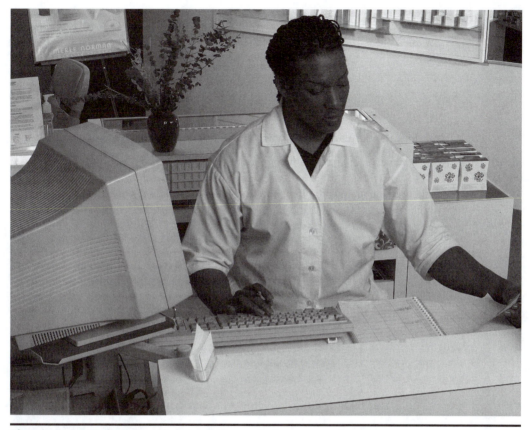

Figure 9–3   Esthetician planning a busy week

the doctor by taking patients in and out of rooms, and trying to present skin-care products and treatments for purchase in a consultation. This can be frustrating to the patient. Patients will have an easier time relating to one person who is selling them skin care, and then to the physician and nurse who are working on their behalf in procedures or surgery.

If you are working for a small office and you have been hired to fill the position of scheduler, receptionist, marketing personnel, certified or licensed medical support (i.e., nurse, medical assistant, etc.), and esthetician, you will need to be flexible. Many offices try to economize by having one person cross-train to work in multiple capacities and for the short term this may work, however, ultimately all roles will be diluted, and possibly your effectiveness as well. Eventually you will need to turn over some of the responsibility to other professionals so that you can concentrate on the goals of serving as the esthetician in the office if this is part of the vision for the clinic. As always, be respectful and mindful of the physician with whom you are connected.

Frequently Asked Questions

1. **How does the esthetician keep from feeling that they cannot seem to get anything done?**

   Often the esthetician's effectiveness is diluted by trying to perform too many tasks. Eliminate something from the job description, and focus on practice building. That would include caring for the patients and building your clientele.

2. **How does the esthetician deal with feeling left out?**

   Estheticians do spend more time on their own when compared with other medical personnel. It will be important to connect often with the doctor and nursing staff to make certain that you are aware of changes in scheduling, patient status, and office administrative changes. Doing this will lessen the exile status. Many estheticians actually appreciate the separate entity of their department.

CHAPTER 10

Survive Office Politics and Hierarchy—and Learn to Thrive

- ■ Introduction
- ■ Strategies for Thriving in a Medical Office
- ■ Ten Most Commonly Asked Questions by Estheticians

Introduction

Work in a medical setting requires a chain of command. This is typically quite different from salon, spa, or an independent skin-care center where the esthetician is acting on his or her own behalf. The hierarchy that exists can be difficult for some to adapt to if one feels a resistance to authority. It is important to find strategies that will assist you in coping with the existing power structure and office politics and learn to really thrive. Thriving is a necessary part of feeling successful, competent, relaxed, and creative.

Strategies for Thriving in a Medical Office

Here are strategies for creating success while working as an esthetician in a physician's office or medical setting:

Always treat your clients and the patients with respect. Do not ever complain to them about issues that may be coming up for you at the office. They may know the other person involved, and it puts them in an awkward situation. Be professional. Even unprofessional co-workers can identify respect. If for some reason you need to leave your current situation in the future, satisfied clients will have good thoughts of you, and may follow you to your next location.

Do not play the Pollyanna or Goody Two-Shoes role. This is always a bore. If you find yourself behaving in an overly exacting manner, or have a tone of *Everything I do is* *always perfect*, this will bring about aggravation from co-workers. No one is perfect, and you cannot possibly know everything.

Be enthusiastic!   Be excited and optimistic about things that come up for co-workers. Let them know that you feel that they are important. If you do not care for a particular person, find a way to honor them anyway; such as saying "Good job!" if you observe it. (People can also sense that we do not like them.) If a staff member is going through a challenging time, tell them that you are holding good thoughts for them. It does not need to be a grand gesture.

Build your knowledge bank.   Do everything you can to learn about new products, treatments, and procedures. Take advanced classes in other disciplines to round out your knowledge. Find ways of sharing that information with others in the office, such as copying an article about something of interest for a co-worker, or posting a seminar schedule on an interesting topic (gardening, fly-fishing, exercise, etc.) in the employee lounge.

Admit mistakes immediately.   Let the administrator or doctor know when you have discovered a mistake. This way they may gain time on correcting it. You will look more competent to others if you readily admit to making errors, and then resolve the issue, so that it does not happen repeatedly.

Do not engage in gossip.   When conversations switch to unkind words being said about co-workers, doctors, patients, or clients, know that it is just a matter of time before you are a subject of such activity.

Leave your personal problems at home.   We all have personal lives that can be loaded with issues that are not appropriate to share with co-workers. We see many clients and patients with problems, so it is necessary that we are healthy in this department.

Learn to de-stress in a situation.   It is important to take a mental time-out when you can see that you are responding negatively to a work situation. If you find that you are compulsively responding to everything a co-worker may say or do during in the day, you may need a break to process your response.

Follow all laws, rules, and regulations.   Following rules and regulations in a medical office will have legal consequences; so will endangering the lives of others by ignoring them. A lack of trust is created when co-workers cannot depend upon each other. This can bring up many feelings of irritation in co-workers, and can inspire conflicts in a heartbeat.

Become self-evaluating.   One of the most critical aspects of being a good business associate, employee, and co-worker is developing a method to evaluate one's own work. We cannot wait for that 5 to 15 minutes in a one-on-one with your supervisor once a year. Get ahead of the game. Find out what you are doing well, what areas of opportunity are laying before you, and how you can best go about implementing improvements. Then document everything that you put into practice. It is easy if you are observing yourself on a daily basis.

Keep a daily journal.   This simple exercise eliminates a backlog of ideas and unfinished projects that can cloud an otherwise clear day. It does not need to be formal, for anyone else's eyes, and does not even need to written in a known language. The important points are that you date your entries and that you understand what you have written.

Ask yourself, "Am I making my goals?"   Goal setting is akin to pulse taking in your clinic life. Achieving goals are not only about making your sales quota for the week, but also looking around for opportunities to improve upon patient care, treatment application, product orientation, volunteer opportunities, and education in general.

Take charge of your business.   Maybe you set a goal to connect with five new people a week to talk about skin care for example. Develop a method for tracking that activity along with the other items on your to-do list. Perhaps you decide to e-mail or mail cards to these people. Note this activity in your daily journal, as well as on their client or patient profile form/chart, along with the response that you receive from the client. This creates a template in which you will be able to evaluate the practices that you apply. In turn you will be able to determine how you can increase your performance effectiveness and define areas in which you contribute to the office. If duties are not documented, this can lead to a problem for administrators during employee evaluations. You cannot receive credit for something if no one knows that you have done it.

Become or remain a low-maintenance employee.   Do as much as you can to create opportunity on your own. If everything that you do requires a confirmation or buy-in from someone else, it will not only become tiring for others in the office, but off-putting. Remember other employees have completely different orientations, job details, and performance issues that are unique to their experience. For some, discussing promotional activity when they are trying to analyze a data control sheet, or perform other more logical/mathematical material could be a source of interference or, put bluntly, frustration. Check in to see the time is appropriate, before you decide to present an idea.

Avoid getting into schisms with co-workers.   If you find that you always get into a rift with a particular individual because of their ego, know that nothing that you will say or do will change the situation for them. These people may exist at the lowest level of the hierarchy, through the middle, and all the way to the top. Here are some ways to disarm the egomania in all of us:

- **Do not feed the fuel.**   If you find that the egomaniac is confronting you, remain calm and respond in an even-toned voice. Let them know that you can see that they are upset, and that it is disconcerting. Remember, *you* are not what they are concerned about . . . it is *they*. They are afraid. Give them that right. Think about what might be behind the ego, arrogance, or anger. What do they have to lose?

- **Be professional.** Do your homework. Make sure that you do the best job that you can, so that you are not the subject of debate.
- **Ask for a *sandwich*.** A sandwich is a liaison or a person between you and the egomaniac. Find a trustworthy person to act on your behalf rather than going directly to the egomaniac. Because of the fear that the egomaniac may be experiencing, a confrontation may be too direct. Remember others are living their lives, going through divorces, in debt, dealing with health issues, and experiencing an entire host of other problems that may inspire a person to act out.
- **If a person is abusive, take the problem to the administrator.** Some people are professional miserables, and nothing will ever be good enough, correct, or even marginal in their eyes, so bless the situation and move on.

Ten Most Commonly Asked Questions by Estheticians

These questions have been asked by estheticians. They have been taken from a compilation of conferences, meetings, small groups, and peer one-on-ones.

1. **It seems like no one takes the time to thank the estheticians for what they do in the office.** This can happen. Staff members become accustomed to being able to come in for treatment whenever there is extra time during the day. Some offices charge staff members a low fee for treatments, just to cover costs, but it reminds employees that this is a service for which clients and patients are paying. It could also be a kind of barter situation. Keep in mind that there are many items that other staff members help you with including those intangibles that you may not have knowledge of, such as referral by association. Research and development in your department also benefits by your being able to try out new products and treatments on staff members. For every treatment that you perform, you should be trying a new method, product, or treatment on a staff member to further your knowledge. In addition, they can be your consumer-loyalty advocate partners as well. For example, if a client has defected, you may have a built-in resource that can easily find out, in a nonthreatening manner, why this has happened.

   If you truly feel taken advantage of, look at how this situation has been created. Examine the part you played in it, so that this is not repeated. Perhaps when you start with the next new staff member, you can make an agreement about how you want to be compensated, so that you feel validated. Maybe they have a subscription to a magazine that they could turn over to you when they are through with it. Or, tell them that you would be happy to help them with their treatments if they help you with purchasing the color selection next time you order makeup. Make sure it is something valuable to you, so that it works for both of you. If we work as a team, there are countless ways that we can benefit one another.

2. **Can an esthetician make more money out in a freestanding clinical operation or as an independent contractor?** When we start looking at this option it is important to look back at the business plan in Chapter 4 to recall what you will need to create your own business. It is possible that you will make more money in a solo prac-

tice. However, keep in mind that you will need space, a receptionist (patients referred by doctors or other practitioners will expect that you have someone to greet them), participating physicians, marketing, equipment, products for retailing, and various other items that you will need to maintain a clinic.

Another concern about a solo clinical practice is that the stakes are higher. Clients or patients will need a more experienced esthetician; you do not have the doctor handy if something does not go well. In addition, there are treatments that should not be performed if you are in a solo practice, whereas if you were practicing with a doctor you could apply them with supervision depending upon the laws of your clinic and state regulations.

Make sure that the issues that are driving you to want your own practice are not ones that can be recreated elsewhere. For example if you have trouble with a co-worker, you may have the same type of problem in your own practice, with someone else. Always work through your issues, they are likely to come up again for you.

Issues for an independent contractor   The idea of working as an independent contractor is appealing when estheticians first become interested in working with physicians. On the surface, this seems like a great idea. You either rent your space in their office, or nearby. You do not have to follow office protocol or become involved in office politics and power struggles. In general, it may seem that you will be your own boss.

However, there is a downside. Your insurance coverage needs will be more extensive: you will need disability, liability (theft and damage), and business liability insurance or malpractice. Each physician that you provide services for will have their own ideas about how their patients are treated. In addition, each physician will:

- have a fixed protocol that you will be expected to learn and use while caring for their patient
- feel that they have less control over your methods and actions with their patients if you are not located in their office
- expect that you will enter into a legal contract, which may involve prohibiting you from working with other facilities for a certain length of time (even after you are no longer partnering)
- expect that you can obtain your own benefits, pay for your own products, have an accountant and legal counsel, and the list goes on

Once your research this type of agreement, you may find that it is not as beneficial to the esthetician as thought. It is typically less lucrative.

3. **The physician seems to be the only one benefiting from the marketing provided by the esthetician.**   Typically, when the doctor wins, you will. When he or she gains a new patient you will benefit in some way, even if it is a long time after the surgery. If the doctor does not take the time to bring the esthetician into the loop with a patient, the patient is the one losing out. Sometimes a physician will simply forget about the esthetician while consulting with a person about a surgical procedure. There are a few foolproof steps to take to tell the patient about your services:

- Make sure that you have your brochure in the doctor's patient packet that is created for home compliance.
- Look at the physician's schedule ahead of time for cosmetic consultations so that you may introduce yourself when the patient comes in the office for their appointment.
- Set up a separate appointment for the patient to see you for a tour and to show them how you may be of help to them during recovery and beyond when they go back to routine skin care.
- Make certain that you are not a hard-sell type of professional. Sometimes physicians may be reluctant to bring an esthetician into the scenario because they may feel that the patient will feel overwhelmed by product "must haves," and this could dilute the effectiveness of the consultation.

4. **The doctor seems to be resentful when we advertise for the esthetics department, yet it is benefiting his name and practice. How do we resolve this?** Make sure that the doctor wants his or her name used this way. Many doctors do not like advertising. It could be that they have unresolved issues concerning seeing their name being used when they do not feel that the business is coming their direction. Revenue coming from the esthetic department can be quite nominal at times, and there may not be a large enough trade-off for the expense. That said, many a patient has made a consultation for cosmetic surgery, and 3 years later, (after having spent monthly trips to the esthetician in the office), has scheduled a procedure.

   In addition, some physicians do not want the esthetician to appear more important than they. This is fair. If it is their practice, they should have top billing. However, many physicians will look favorably on promotional activities, and will honor good and fair practices by diligent estheticians who are in good faith trying to bring business to the office.

5. **The patient does not come back to the esthetician once the doctor sees them.** Even under the best of circumstances, this can happen. Sometimes a doctor may be in disagreement with something that you have recommended for a patient. Alternatively, maybe they have forgotten what you have to offer the patients. Doctors cannot possibly remember every detail of what is available from the esthetics department. Develop a method for introducing yourself to every person that walks in the front door, and remind the physician about you, your products, and your services routinely. When a patient walks in, let them know:

- who you are
- what you do
- what you can do for them

6. **What should an esthetician do about a rude relative of a staff member that comes to the office free of charge?** This is always challenging, and unfortunately this happens more often than we would like. It could be that this person comes to you because you are not charging them. It is always best to create value on the work that you do. Sad, but true, people will take advantage, challenge you with what the local hairstylist told them about skin care, or better yet, throw in some of the newest multi-

level marketing hype that they have heard at a friend's home party. You may even find staff members doing this. It is frustrating, but remember: *You are the professional.*

7. **It seems that a co-worker is always in competition for sales and clients, and will even take clients. What can be done?**   Competition, in small degrees, can be healthy. It can be a driving force for some, and for others it can be debilitating. If you find that your co-worker is taking a healthy competitive spirit to an extreme, find out what is motivating this person to do this. Could it be that she is a single mom needing money to support her family? Maybe this person sees things that could be improved upon but is uncomfortable about bringing it up to you in fear that you may see it as criticism. Perhaps this person is more aggressive or advancement oriented than you, and is interested in growing the business at a fast clip. Conversely, it could be that the individual is not even aware of being overly competitive, but is just trying to do a good job.

That said, however, there are some people for whom competition exists in all areas of their lives. Whether they are on the freeway, in the grocery store, or in a class-room, they will compete for whatever they perceive as the prize. They thrive on it, creating a great deal of chaos in the process. Building a business is not always calm or relaxed and selling products and treatments can be a real motivator (adrenaline, en-dorphins flowing, excitement building). These people can be important allies if they do not erode the integrity or natural flow of the office.

If *you* are the aggressive salesperson, and you find yourself having to apologize for employing techniques that you have learned to build a business, realize that not everyone has had this training, or is interested in approaching their work from a sales perspective. Some people work best by spending time analyzing and coordinating tasks, building protocols, and talking with patients about various details. They are not interested in selling products. This style of operating is a great complement to a per-son who is maybe less detail oriented but likes sales and direct business building. Work with it. Offer to share a percentage of your product sales with them. This idea sounds like you are giving up something, but in the end you will be able to see more patients this way, and your co-workers will not feel that you are pushing them out of the way to get to the sale.

Start fresh by determining what each of you likes to do and set some goals.

- **Maintain a professional, friendly atmosphere.**   We want the client to feel com-fortable about coming to the office, regardless of whom they see. This is difficult, but it must be genuinely expressed. In addition, if they were truly your client they would wait for you.
- **Acknowledge that you have different working styles, and that it is important that you each attend to work at your own pace and level.**   Let your co-worker know that you are there to support them, and that you would like them to do the same for you. Tell them that it is clear that you approach things differently and that this can be strength. Find a common ground. Where are you alike? What is the vision? Work from that perspective.

- **Divide the menial tasks.**   Make certain that you are sharing the workload. It is not enough to be the star; one must be able to perform all of the other tasks such as cleaning, calling clients, putting away inventory, and other jobs that take time and are not as ego gratifying.
- **If you are the sales aggressor in the office, share the wealth.**   If you are able to easily make your commission and have a supportive environment, acknowledge those who have helped you with monetary means. Do not be stingy, because this will come back to haunt you. Always let others know how much you have appreciated the extra time they have spent on helping you. This goes for the receptionist, medical records associate, medical assistants, nurses, and even the doctors. Pick up a pair of baseball or concert tickets, give extra product testers to well-meaning staff members, or send flowers to someone who has really gone out of his or her way. Have style.

8. **The other esthetician in the office always gets credit for what has been done. She does not realize that it is a team effort. How do we make this fair?**   This is part two of question number 7. We must ask ourselves: What are our goals? Sometimes it is enough just to see that a job has been completed and has been done well. We often need to fire our "recognition machine" in order to work in the real world. Having confidence in your talents and abilities is one part of the equation, but we must understand ourselves well in order to meet even our own expectations.

   If we are always noticing what the other person is doing, perhaps we need to do some soul-searching and discover where and why we are not creating a healthy situation for ourselves. Then, we need to be ready and willing to act upon these findings. Here are some ideas to get you started:

   - **What is your Plan for Success?**   Make one up. A good solid Plan for Success is necessary for achievement. Your plan can be a written list, a huge poster, a video, or an audiotape that you create which describes success to you. Your plan may contain ideas such as becoming a good listener, asking for help when you need it, or to having the goal of empowering others to achieve, in addition to other more conventional ideas about being successful, such as financial rewards. If we do not know what we deem as success, we will not understand what we need for acknowledgment or recognition. We will be constantly frustrated and feeling at a loss. You may discover that the credit that a co-worker received on a project was well deserved. Conversely, it may have been given for other political reasons, such as to reward that individual for doing a job that an administrator does not want to do. One never knows exactly what is at stake. By creating your own Plan for Success you may find that some of the accolades another is receiving are for deeds very low on your priority list or in your plan.
   - **Identify your strengths and weaknesses.**   List the attributes that *you personally* bring to the office. Think about things that the staff does not know about. Remember the time that you talked a frightened woman off the ski lift, or stopped to help someone in need after they had received some bad news. That is strength; think

about how to use what you have. Look at your weaknesses. What do you need to do to increase your visibility in the office, and yet be prepared to address the challenging issues that becoming more visible will bring? Becoming more visible brings expectations, criticism, and rivalry as well.

- **What are your goals with this job?**   Are you planning to stay long term, or is this position just something to get you started? *Get real with yourself* about your work. If you want to stay, learn, grow, and become a permanent fixture with this office, then you will need to make a plan to learn everything you can about how to develop your role and take it to a new level. Maybe you unconsciously want to become an administrator, or need to go back to school to get an advanced degree. Do not stand on the sidelines and wait for something to happen. It will not.
- **Observe the co-workers getting the credit.**   What do they do well? Not so well? What is it about these co-workers that people tend to give credit so easily? Do they work late or start early? Do they speak with confidence, or are they beautiful? If your co-worker is being given credit unduly, this will change when it becomes obvious to others. Let it unfold naturally. You will always appear envious or jealous if you point your dismay in their direction.
- **What can you do to get what you want in this situation?**   Through determining your Plan for Success, you will be able to create an appropriate approach, tailored for your needs alone. Learn what you can if you are there for just a short time. If you are planning to stay, continue to observe, collect data, and build your practice. When you are clear about your strengths and a method for presenting them, you will be receiving more of everything—including credit.

9. **A co-worker constantly shares long, drawn-out stories about his life, even in front of the patient, what do we do?**   The charm and comfort of hearing a well-placed short story, shared at an appropriate time, is immeasurable, especially in a medical office where things can be quite serious and sterile at times. Patients do like to know that they are not alone in their thoughts and feelings while receiving care from you and the doctor. This is a major judgment call . . . and not everyone has good judgment.

There is nothing more awkward and uncomfortable than going to the dentist, doctor, or any other professional, to be captive and forced to listen about the inner workings of a personal life. That patient may be struggling in their life, and it is insensitive to go on about your own, even if it is all very exciting to you.

It may be important to redirect the conversation to the patient or client such as: "Susan (patient) is doing well and has a new baby." Usually a colleague will notice your attempt at redirecting the focus to the patient. If the co-worker does not make the shift, tell them later that you thought that the patient was trying to share something, which is often the case.

We all get into this bad habit. We become acquainted with people, share stories, and the next time that you see them, some will ask you about a previous conversation. It starts innocently enough. Just know where to stop. We do not use patients, clients, or co-workers for that matter as the audience or sounding boards. Observe the "one-minute relief rule." If your story goes on longer than one minute, it should be left to share with family members, friends, or, if emotionally charged, a good counselor.

10. **What if the doctor prescribes a method of treatment that the esthetician finds contrary?**   Most doctors with whom you have earned trust and have a good working relationship will welcome a challenge. It is important however, to know when and how to ask about your conflicting thoughts. It is extremely intimidating to challenge a physician, but also rewarding and respect-igniting if you find something that they have missed. This is professional and can be a real learning experience for both of you.

    That said, there are some important aspects of handling a situation such as this, and it demands a respectful, mindful approach. We *never* want to try to gain an advantage over the doctor in front of the patient. This is unprofessional and you will find it will not be tolerated. Here are some guidelines to help you in this situation:

- **Develop a good communication system relationship with your doctor.**   Establish as soon as possible a protocol for sharing information or your assessment of a patient complaint or inquiry. Determine how open the doctor may be to your input, and in what form (in their office after the patient has left, in front of the patient, written communication) you should share this information.

- *Do not find fault with a physician's diagnosis in front of the patient.*   The appropriate way to handle this is confidentially. Wait until you have a few minutes, at an appropriate time for the doctor, to ask about your conflict. Remember your input is valuable, and as a team member you will be respected if you act professionally. In addition, you may be incorrect, and it is always good to approach these situations with humility and a sense of curiosity.

    However, do not discount your skills. Many estheticians referred patients to physicians through recognizing thyroid, diabetes, and melanoma and other types of cancer through visual observation or by hearing a patient speak of symptoms they were experiencing. If you are able to have an open dialogue with the doctor about your findings, your input will be respected, and you will be encouraged to increase your knowledge. Again, many physicians are teachers, and hold learning experiences in high regard.

- **Once you have done your homework, relax, and in plain terms share your thought with the doctor.**   Remember this is not a graduate thesis you are trying to defend. This is simply a sharing of information you are willing to do on behalf of a patient. When you each have a few minutes (make sure the time is appropriate), present your findings such as:

    Patient Smith had a slightly distended area across nose and cheeks, which accompanied telangiectases. She said that it becomes redder when she exercises, or if she has a glass of wine. It looks like rosacea, and I'm wondering if you could have a look.

- **If the doctor says that they disagree with you,** *let it go.*   If you are incorrect with your findings, accept it and let it go. If the doctor feels that you are wrong, and you still disagree, do not get into a battle over it. This is the practice of someone with 4 years of medical school and probably several years of experience ahead of you. If you feel emphatic about an issue and the patient continues to ask again about the specific unresolved problem, recommend a second opinion. This is the responsible thing to do, and the doctor would agree. Do not put yourself in the middle of these situations. Remember to facilitate as an impartial liaison, with the goal as the best outcome for the patient. This is also the goal of the physician.

Rules and Regulations—Legal and Mandatory Systems

CHAPTER 11

Ethics, Risk Management, and Insurance

- Introduction
- Ethics
- Risk Management
- Liability Insurance
- Summary
- Frequently Asked Questions

Introduction

As we look at an esthetician's code of ethics we can see how keeping a few golden rules in place can remind us all of the privilege that we each have of serving in this capacity. While doing so, it is necessary to employ some preventative measures and objectives to protect this honor, and to keep our work safe for the patients, co-workers, and the public.

Prevention is our chief objective in managing risk while working for the physician on behalf of the client or patient. Having the appropriate insurance products and legal counsel in place is necessary for all concerned.

Ethics

In a medical environment, strong boundaries serve as the construct, with the physician at the helm. In order to become licensed to practice medicine, the physician will make a pledge called the **Hippocratic Oath**. This name comes from the ancient Greek physician, **Hippocrates** (ca. 450 B.C.; see Figure 11–1). His teachings have influenced medicine through time, and although some say he may not actually have written the original oath, all subsequent works have been submitted with his name on his behalf. One of Hippocrates' famous quotes puts our work in a medical office in perspective:

Life is short, and the Art long: the occasion fleeting; experience fallacious, and judgment difficult. The physician must not only do what is right himself, but also to make the patient, the attendants, and externals cooperate (Collier 1910).

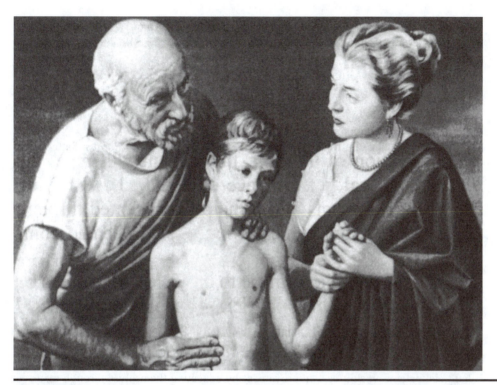

Figure 11–1   Hippocrates' teachings have influenced medicine through time.

Today, each medical school in the United States has adapted the Hippocratic Oath to suit its particular situation, and thus these codes have been brought into the twenty-first century. However, it is useful to consider a few phrases from one of the original versions (Collier 1910).

Hippocratic Oath

I swear in the presence of the Almighty and before my family, my teachers and my peers that according to my ability and judgment I will keep the oath and stipulation:

- To reckon, all who have taught me this art equally dear to me as my parents in the same spirit and dedication to impart knowledge of the art of medicine to others.
- I will continue with diligence to keep abreast of advances in medicine.
- I will treat without exception all who seek my ministrations, so long as the treatments of others is not compromised thereby.
- I will seek the counsel of particularly skilled physicians where indicated for the benefit of my patient.

- I will follow the methods of treatment, which according to my ability and judgment I consider for the benefit of my patient and abstain from whatever is harmful or mischievous.
- I will not divulge information that should be kept in confidence.

Hippocrates states in his preamble that an *attendant* or *personnel* should follow the direction of the physician. In our work with the physician, it is vital that we observe, respect, and follow such direction or not work in this capacity.

Perhaps we can additionally propose an *Esthetician's Code of Ethics* that could be used whether we work for a doctor, or are independent.

Esthetician's Code of Ethics

In creating an Esthetician's Code of Ethics, we first want to look at our duties, our intentions to serve, and rules of conduct to support those objectives. Here is one idea for creating such a document:

Preamble

Clinical estheticians work to develop a valid and dependable body of knowledge based on clinical studies, physician partnership, and empirical research. In doing this work they act in many roles to provide appropriate, competent support in areas such as patient educator, liaison to patient and medical personnel, skin-care clinic manager, practitioner (applies skincare treatments), product sales and adviser, and skin analyst. They strive to educate the client and patient on skin-care improvement by educating themselves through recurrent training. They follow the regulations set forth by the clinic administration and the physician.

This code is intended to serve as a general guideline to maintain the highest possible standard for estheticians working in a medical setting. And, to apply knowledge to clinical skin-care practices in a variety of contexts in any given day with the best possible outcome to serve as a goal for clients, patients, and co-workers.

Rules of Conduct for Working in a Medical Office

1. Do no harm knowingly, and when in doubt, do not use or perform a treatment.
2. Adhere to all laws and regulations.
3. Use accurate representation of your education, training, and experience.
4. Support, practice, and promote this Code of Ethics.
5. Maintain high standards of competence in your work. Stay abreast of new techniques and innovations in the field, and make a concerted effort to continuing education.
6. Promote integrity: be honest, fair, and respectful of others, both inside and outside of the office. Do not degrade fellow estheticians regardless of how egregious their practices may prove. Let the proper authorities handle these cases. Do not make exaggerated or misleading statements to others for personal gain verbally or in print.
7. Maintain accurate records: follow all office protocols with respect to **charting** and documentation.
8. Work within licensure and scope. Refer to physician for all diagnostic measures.

9. Maintain confidentiality and privacy at all junctures. Do not share information about a client or patient with anyone other than medical personnel at an appropriate time and place on a need-to-know basis.

10. Estheticians will obtain appropriate informed consent (signed agreement) from the client prior to treatment or procedure, after significant information has been given and accepted.

11. Disclosure: estheticians will disclose information to the physician if such information would deem important to the health of that individual, such as in pre- or postoperative stages.

12. Consultations
    • All consults with the client or patient are directed toward assisting them with their goals, whether the esthetician performs or offers a referral to another practitioner.
    • Strive to make all communications about matters at hand.

13. Honor commitments. Follow through on all promises made to clients, patients, and co-workers.

14. All products and services shall be truthfully presented as to price, grade, and availability.

15. Warranties and guarantees: the seller will fully and promptly offer all guarantees and warranties on products according to terms that conform to office policy.

16. Responsibilities and duties: if a client is dissatisfied with a product or service, the esthetician will attend to the matter promptly and fairly according to office protocol and policy.

17. Conduct outside the office: estheticians will not behave outside of the office in a manner that is inappropriate or that would bring undue ridicule or hardship to the practice.

18. Contract with employer: if a contract is created between the esthetician and the physician, the esthetician will fulfill obligations and agreed-upon matters consistent with office policy.

19. Service to community: always give something back to the community whether it is through volunteer, publishing, or of other service.

20. Maintain own health of body, mind, and spirit.

Having a code and plan in place helps to navigate through some of these difficult passages with clients, patients, and co-workers. If we maintain honorable intention, and preserve the ethical integrity of all relationships, we will create a healthy, thriving atmosphere in the office.

Risk Management

As we explore the concerns facing the clinical esthetician, safeguarding your career is as sound a practice as having one. The field of esthetics tends to attract an independent type of individual who is responsible and has multitask capabilities. The area of a practice known as **risk management** is just one more aspect of serving in a medical facility. Most offices will have some type of risk management protocol to follow, but here are a few ideas toward building a program for you.

Health History Questionnaire

Having clients and patients fill out an ever-evolving health history questionnaire is important to the health of any practice. Health conditions are constantly changing in the lives of our clients therefore we want to improve patient care and avoid any chance of liability. A questionnaire should address at a minimum the following:

- Questions regarding the family history of the client or patient, current and preexisting illnesses, diseases, injuries, operations, allergies, prescription and nonprescription medications. You might also ask specifically what type of facial treatments that they have been having including peels (AHA/Beta hydroxys), microdermabrasion (crystal/salt/diamond wand—no particles), and enzymes (papaya, pineapple, pumpkin).
- Avoid using jargon. Some of the medical terminology may be second nature to you but will seem isolating to the client.
- In our multicultural society, we must be sensitive to those for whom English is a second or third language. Always allow more time and patience with these patients. Offer the help that they require and treat them with compassion. Always remember to ask yourself, "How would you feel in a country where the people did not speak your language?"
- Take the time to review the form with them. This can be a great rapport builder. While reviewing their history however, *avoid commenting* on prior care. Do not suggest that you would have done something differently, or criticize the former practitioner because they may do things differently, and remember that you do not have all of the facts. Statements like "How did this happen?" or "Why did Dr. Good do this to you?" could unknowingly pull you into a developing legal case.

Client-Patient Selection

Observing and employing good patient selection practices (a patient being one who is mentally, emotionally, physically healthy and able) is key here. You may not always be able to select the patient, as this falls into the realm of the physician's jurisdiction, although in time, with experience, you will work as a team in this activity. You may however, become keen on what you will or will not take on. One must really consider risks with respect to a client coming to you for treatments. If a client is constantly complaining about the last bad experience that they had with an esthetician, do not jump right in. Chances are you will be next on their list.

Client-Patient Satisfaction

It can be difficult at times, but part of your job is to make certain that patients and clients are not only compliant but reasonably satisfied with their care. As we know, some patients are far more high maintenance than others, and when you encounter such an individual, *anticipate* problems. Find and employ easy solutions. If they will not use a preoperative home-care kit because there are too many things to do, find or make one product that does fit all their needs. If the patient is often angry, hostile, and downgrades the doctor when they are not in the room, tell the physician. This is risk management.

Avoid Office Payment Plans or Large Discounts

Patients able to finance their surgeries are not apt to sit around looking for loopholes and trying to get out of paying for their treatments. Those who do can get you into big trouble in any business. It is a version of *buyer's remorse*. A disgruntled patient may unconsciously blame you or the doctor for having spent money that they really could not afford to spend, which may inadvertently drive them further into financial problems.

Informed Consent

When the physician agrees to take on a patient for a procedure, the patient must agree both verbally and in writing that they understand both the risks and the benefits. This is true with the esthetician as well. If you are going to use a treatment, it is necessary that the client understand that there may be some risk involved, and by signing the agreement, they are allowing you to perform this application. Even if something unforeseen arises, they will not hold you liable.

Documentation

Documentation, a legal matter, also proves to be helpful in many kinds of problem solving. If a client complains at a later date that a treatment that you have applied has created a problem for them, you can go back into your chart notes and see exactly what has occurred, and offer the appropriate counseling and the antidote. Sometimes this may involve bringing the doctor into the loop. Sounds simple, but it happens. Documentation is visual as well as written.

- **Photographs** before surgery are mandatory for risk management; some say before-and-after photos declare good faith by the patient in showing their involvement. It is a good idea for the esthetician to invest in a good camera and take pre and post images to demonstrate patient willingness to have a given treatment or application.
- **Computer imaging** stored on the computer for pre- and postoperative sessions can be used for medical documentation. Make certain that there is simulation (corrected version) noted on the image that has had the artwork applied.

Follow-up/Follow-through

Dissatisfied patients typically point to one or more of three areas that are potential risk management issues. First, patients claim that they did not receive care that was promised to them during early visits. Secondly, they were not given a follow-up appointment schedule beyond the first 2 weeks. The third complaint is that the doctor was not interested in supplying a revision or second surgery if the initial surgery did not correct the perceived problem.

It is vital that we as a team have a good support system in place for the patient and client. There is nothing more frustrating or irritating than being forgotten, which is compounded if a patient is anxious about having, or having had, a medical procedure. Here are four key risk management rules to follow:

1. Make sure that patients have products, treatments, and written instructions for their use and a copy goes into their chart.
2. Make certain that all of the pre- and postoperative treatment appointments with the esthetician coincide with the doctor visits.
3. Make sure that all pre- and postoperative appointments are scheduled. In addition, give them a written document that tells them that it is their responsibility to set up follow-up appointments, which are to take place at 1 month, 3 months, 6 months, and 1 year, per office protocol. A copy of this document also goes into their chart.
4. Do not have patients waiting for product on back order. If you are out of a product, give them one that is just as effective, send them to the pharmacy, or contact a colleague to obtain a similar one.

Liability Insurance

Having good insurance is necessary for practicing as an esthetician in any capacity. In today's business environment, it is a good decision to examine all of your potential risks and areas of exposure. When shopping for insurance always look at the risk that you may be exposed to versus the loss you may incur.

Many questions you may have can be handled by a qualified insurance broker or insurance agent. They can analyze your coverage and point out the areas where you may have risk exposure; they will be familiar with the laws of your state.

State regulations set the standards for our licensure, in addition to those of the facility or clinic. As an employee practicing under the direction and supervision of a physician, you will be registered as a clinician acting on the physician's behalf. You will be covered under the doctor's malpractice insurance. The physician may pay $100,000 to $200,000 yearly for **professional liability (malpractice) insurance**—depending upon risk exposure and discipline.

If you become self-employed, run a seminar, perform treatments, or consult with clients independently from the physician, you will need malpractice insurance. Moreover, if you change your role to act as an independent contractor in the office, you will indeed need to purchase malpractice insurance.

Additional Types of Insurance

All physicians will want to have quality insurance products employed as a good business practice. Regardless of where you are practicing, here are types of insurance coverage that you want to make sure are in place:

- General liability
- Loss prevention—theft coverage for computers and other office equipment

- Business interruption insurance (loss of business income)
- None-owed auto insurance (in case someone is driving your vehicle, or you are driving another's)
- Personal disability insurance (in case of injury and you become unemployed)
- Life insurance

Summary

Typically, office practices function well. However, it is vital that we protect ourselves from unforeseen problems that may arise in our work. It is sensible to use a few safeguards that are easily implemented for the protection of all involved. Remember that everything you do while representing the doctor is a potential risk to the physician. It would be advantageous to speak with the doctor's insurance agent to learn about how malpractice insurance works, and to see exactly how you would be covered in the event of a lawsuit. The most important objective a professional can strive for is to manage risk potential and use problems to create effective control practices and procedures.

Frequently Asked Questions

1. **What does the esthetician do if someone threatens to sue?**

   Report this threat to the doctor immediately, even if the threat seems to be an impulsive response from a procedure. Immediately document the occurrence by stating what was said by all parties involved and list the witnesses. The doctor will then advise you on a course of action. It is most important that you keep meticulous records, document all pertinent information, and keep all files in a safe and an accessible location.

2. **What happens to the doctor if someone sues the esthetician?**

   While practicing under the physician's supervision, you make the doctor liable. We are acting at all times on his or her behalf. It is only if we are performing consultations and treatments independent from the doctor that *we* will be held liable. That means you are receiving financial gain from working under your own business or name.

   In any case, if a client decides to sue the esthetician practicing under the doctor's supervision (in the clinic), the covering insurance company will direct all parties in the claim. Once the lawsuit has begun, it is important to speak only to your employer's legal counsel and the insurance company claims professional regarding the case.

CHAPTER 12

OSHA Made Simple

- Introduction
- Bloodborne Pathogens Standard
- Potential Hazards for an Esthetician Practicing in a Medical Office
- Basic Guidelines for the Esthetician Practicing in a Medical Facility
- OSHA Inspections
- Summary
- Frequently Asked Questions

Introduction

Following government rules and regulations set by the **Occupational Safety and Health Administration** or **OSHA** is imperative regardless of where estheticians practice. These regulations are laws and have been documented in the Occupational Safety and Health Act of 1970, the Chemical Right-to-Know Law of 1983, and the **Bloodborne Pathogens Standard** 29CFR 1910.1030, along with other health and safety regulations as recommended by **The Centers for Disease Control.**

These regulations were developed to protect our health, our co-workers, and the client or patient. OSHA was originally called the **Safety Bill of Rights** and was created as a response to hazards faced by employees in the workplace. The Bloodborne Pathogens Standard was created later in response to the additional hazards of exposure to hepatitis B and hepatitis C virus and human immunodeficiency virus (HIV) faced by health-care workers. Many of the states have chosen to administer the OSHA program as it is; others have adapted the regulations and have created standards that are at least as effective as the federal regulations. The states must enforce and comply with the standards that are at a minimum following the OSHA guidelines.

Bloodborne Pathogens Standard

This standard was created to minimize the transmission of HIV and hepatitis B infections among health-care workers. This covers all employees who can be "reasonably anticipated" to come into contact, because of performing their duties, with blood and **other potentially infectious materials (OPIM).**

While estheticians are at minimum exposure, the term *potential* should resonate as a possibility. Performing extractions, postoperative treatments, facials, microdermabrasion, as we know, all increase the likelihood of exposure. Here are the key elements to the Bloodborne Pathogens Standard.

1. **Universal and standard precautions.** Standard systems have been created to treat all body fluids as if they are infectious, and assume all tissue as being hazardous. Frequent hand washing, wearing gloves, appropriate body protection devices during treatments, and cleanup are essentials to following this rule.

2. **Engineering controls and work practice controls.** Protection devices must be provided by the employer. This includes antiseptic soap, splashguards, masks, eye-flush stations, sharps disposal containers for lancets, gloves, and appropriate labels for biohazardous materials.

3. **Personal protective equipment.** There are precautions in addition to engineering and work practice controls. They consist of lab coats, goggles, masks, gloves, and laundering and cleaning and are also to be supplied by the employer.

4. **Cleanliness of work areas.** The employer is to ensure a work environment that is clean and sanitary. All surfaces must be decontaminated after procedures. In addition, gloves must be worn in all treatments and procedures, and any time during a potential exposure to blood or OPIM (other potentially infected materials). All surfaces must be cleaned with a 10 percent bleach/water solution.

5. **Hepatitis B vaccine.** This must be made available to employees within 10 days of beginning work and is given in three doses over a 6-month period. We are considered a Group One Classification, as we are exposed to body fluids while performing our job in a medical office. Refusing the vaccination is not advisable. If you do decide that you do not want the vaccine, you must sign a waiver.

6. **Follow-up after exposure.** The employer must make a documented confidential medical evaluation detailing:
   • the circumstances surrounding the event
   • the route of exposure
   • the identification of person who was source of exposure
   • immediate washing of the exposed area with soap and water or flush in the case of eye exposure

In addition, OSHA requires:

• The exposed employee be tested for HBV, HCV, and HIV (providing consent is given).
• The source individual's blood is tested for HBV, HCV, and HIV.
• The employee is offered prophylaxis, gamma globulin, or HB vaccine following confidentiality guarantee.
• The employee is counseled regarding precautions to take to avoid transmission.
• OSHA 200 form must be filled out.
• Medical record of employee exposure to be kept for 30 years and confidentiality is guaranteed.

Potential Hazards for an Esthetician Practicing in a Medical Office

The potential hazards for an esthetician working in a medical office are the same as they are for all personnel working in this environment. The team must work together to protect both the public visiting and the staff working in the medical facility. Here are some primary risks to the esthetician in the medical setting.

Needle/Lancet Stick

Needle/lancet sticks may have serious consequences if a client has a communicable disease. It is a possibility that they may not be aware of their condition or share the information with you. Always assume transmission and follow rules for needle stick exposure.

1. **Needle stick exposure, immediately:**
   - **Bleed:** Allow area to bleed
   - **Wash:** Wash and irrigate site vigorously
   - **Cover:** Cover and protect wound

2. **Screen exposure for:**
   - **Severity.**   Was there actual source blood contact with non-intact employee skin or mucous membrane? If yes, check with the physician in the office and follow office protocol.
   - **Source.**   The client reports to your Emergency Medical/Occupational Medicine Facility for appropriate evaluation and screening according to OSHA and your state agency requirements.
   - **Employee.**   You will be directed to the same facility or Emergency Medical/ Occupational Medicine Facility for appropriate evaluation and screening according to the OSHA and state agency requirements.

Airborne Infections

We may become exposed to an airborne illness such as tuberculosis (an infection commonly affecting the lungs, which must be treated with drugs), influenza (flu), or measles without even being aware. Estheticians do not often work in an environment where they encounter patients with a known airborne illness. Personnel caring for patients with these and other airborne illnesses may wear HEPA respirators (lung protection) or other types of protection devices. It is, however, advisable to always wear a mask while performing microdermabrasion, extractions, or chemical peels due to vapor and/or other unknown airborne transmissions. *Always use standard precautions.*

Bloodborne Diseases

Bloodborne pathogen transmissions of diseases such as **hepatitis B** (HBV), **hepatitis C** (HCV), **delta hepatitis**, **HIV/AIDS**, **syphilis,** and **malaria** are potential risks for an esthetician practicing anywhere in the world. These pathogens are undetectable to the naked eye, and some such as hepatitis B can live dry on surfaces for a week. In addition, these diseases can enter your body through an open cut or lesion. Standard precautions are always necessary.

Accidents, Fire, Emergency

Recurrent safety instruction is mandatory in a medical office. Your knowledge of this training will be assessed through routine written and oral examinations, and these documents will be placed in your file. The training will include fire drills, bacteriology/sanitation, eye-wash protocol, evacuations/bomb threats, CPR, patient emergencies, domestic violence safety training, and self-defense instruction. There are unlimited potential situations that may arise while working in the clinic. The key to handling an accident is in using your training, care, and tact. Your office manager or administrator will provide or delegate an appropriate individual to handle filing an accident report, create a clinical emergency protocol, an evacuation policy, and depending upon the type of medical setting, other emergency procedure flowcharts.

Basic Guidelines for the Esthetician Practicing in a Medical Facility

Basic guidelines for an esthetician working in a medical office are the same as they are for all medical staff members. The following is a review of those that will directly affect your daily work space. Avoiding the transmission of disease by using the established standards is the key to maintaining a safe working environment.

Clean your space systematically and routinely.   This is an area where we cannot be too compulsive. Utilize approved cleaning solutions and perform cleansings after each direct contact, treatment, or procedure. Clean all bottles, caps, sinks, and surfaces with a bleach solution of 1 tablespoon to 1 gallon of water. Put all implements in the autoclave after each use.

Hand washing regulations.   Frequent hand washing is the first preventative measure to control the transmission of microorganisms, therefore disease. A standard washing procedure is:

1. A dry paper towel is used to turn on the faucet (sinks are considered contaminated).
2. Wet hands, liquid soap up with fingers pointed down for 2 minutes
3. Use orange stick or brush to clean under nails.
4. Rinse thoroughly without touching faucet.
5. Use paper towels to dry hands. Discard them and then use another to turn off faucet.

You must wear gloves.   Wear gloves for all treatments, procedures, and applications (including makeup). In addition, wear them while cleaning and mixing solutions. Remove gloves immediately after use to avoid contaminating other surfaces via the *inside-out* method. Then perform a thorough hand washing.

Follow standard precautions for disposing of potentially infected material.

1. All **sharps** are put into an approved sharps container.
2. All cotton swabs, used gloves, and other questionable matter are put into an approved red biohazard bag, which is collected and disposed of according to protocol for bio-hazardous material.

Use autoclave for cleaning.   Steam under pressure is the only method for destroying spores and microorganisms.

Read Material Safety Data Sheets.   Create your own MSDS booklet by including all of the material information sheets with which you work. This might include, for example, peels, cleaning solutions, and products. These sheets are provided by the manufacturer detailing ingredients, exposure limits, health effects and warnings of their products. They will contain first-aid information and give you direction on what to do if spills or leaks occur, tell you how to prevent accidents with these materials, and include information on disposing and transporting the material along with regulatory requirements. Have it available and make it useable.

Create a room-cleaning checklist.   This checklist is documentation necessary for use in the clinic (Figure 12–1). It shows the frequency of cleaning—daily, weekly, and 3-month or quarterly—of the esthetic room. This includes all sinks, faucets, floors, treatments product bottles, equipment, vents, walls, ceilings, trash and biohazard red bags, and all other items used in the space.

Understand and use eye-wash protocol.   As always, prevention is the best policy by using appropriate eye guards during the treatment. Accidents do happen, however. The key is getting to an eye-flushing station as quickly as possible. Eye-flush devices can easily be installed onto your existing sink in your work space, and they are inexpensive. Here is an example:

1. Remove the plugs located on top of irrigating device and allow water to flow.
2. Pull stopper upward, which is located on the front of the irrigator that will divert the water through the irrigating holes.
3. Turn water on, test, making sure that it is cool.
4. Water should be adjusted to flow for a minimum of 15 minutes.
5. Client should be adjusted so that the water flow is comfortable, not harsh or too strong, which may cause injury.
6. Refer to appropriate MSDS (Material Safety Data Sheet) on the product for further treatment.
7. Seek medical treatment as indicated.

Your eye-wash station may work slightly differently from this; become familiar with the workings of yours, and test it periodically to remain comfortable with its use.

ROOM-CLEANING FORM

Month of _____

DAILY FREQUENCY:

1. Scrub and clean sinks and faucets_____ (INT)
2. Floors mopped and cleaned_____ (INT)
3. Trash and red HAZMAT cans cleaned, wiped down, and relined _____ (INT)
4. Spillage on walls or doors to be wiped down _____ (INT)
5. Facial bed, microdermabrasion equipment, bowls, countertops to be cleaned after each client/patient _____ (INT)
6. Facial scope _____ (INT)

WEEKLY FREQUENCY:

Clean all air conditioning or heating grills or vents _____ (INT)
1. Clean walls of esthetic room _____ (INT)
2. Clean H_2O steamer and other facial equipment hardware _____ (INT)

QUARTERLY:

1. Clean room ceiling

Week 1 _____
Week 2 _____
Week 3 _____
Week 4 _____
Week 5 _____

Some of these duties may be performed by a professional cleaning service.
OSHA will expect that you have an updated form readily available.

Figure 12–1 Room-Cleaning Form

OSHA Inspections

An inspection by an OSHA representative is conducted without advance notice and cannot be rescheduled. They have the right to enter and inspect any facility at their own choosing. The reasons for their visits are typically in order as follows:

- immediate danger to employees
- fatality or accidents (three or more employees injured)

- complaint filed by someone
- random (can be assigned by computer)

If you are visited by an inspector, you can expect that the individual will present credentials and ask to speak to the administrator or manager of your facility. The inspector will then tell the general scope, purpose, and nature of the inspection as well as discuss the procedures that are to be followed. Your OSHA records, other records, charts, and exam rooms will be viewed, and a general walk around of the facility will be conducted. Employees may be interviewed. At the end of the inspection, violations are discussed with the clinic administrator or office manager.

Always have OSHA regulations posted in appropriate locations in the clinic, do your housekeeping, utilize all personal protective equipment when performing duties and procedures, and follow all rules set forth by standards and regulations, including medical documentation.

If you are visited by an OSHA inspector:

1. Do not panic.
2. Do not volunteer information.
3. Answer questions truthfully.
4. Write down the inspector's name and badge number, the time and date of inspection, and the areas inspected.

Summary

Training and attention to detail serve as excellent prevention of exposure of hazards while practicing in a medical facility. Occasionally accidents will occur, wherein the standards that are set in place provide immediate care for heath-care workers and patients. Practice and encourage universal and standard precautions at work and while out of the office. Transmission of pathogens is often prevented by hand washing.

Frequently Asked Questions

1. **During a routine facial without performing extractions, should the esthetician wear gloves?**

   Universal and standard precautions of the Bloodborne Pathogens Standard makes it a *law* that we wear gloves to perform treatments in the office.

2. **What does the esthetician do if there is an accidental needle-stick poke while performing extractions?**

   In this situation, we follow standard protocol for a needle-stick exposure.

   For needle-stick exposure, immediately
   - **Bleed**
   - **Wash**
   - **Cover**

Screen exposure for:

- **Severity**
- **Source (client)**

The esthetician reports to:

The Emergency Medical/Occupational Medicine Facility for appropriate evaluation and screening according to the OSHA and state agency requirements.

CHAPTER 13

Medical Chart Writing

- Introduction
- Medical Documentation
- Four Basic Types of Chart Writing
- Abbreviations; Symbols; and Identifying Head, Neck, and Chest Regions
- Mistakes and Chart-Writing Etiquette
- Confidentiality
- Summary
- Frequently Asked Questions

Introduction

Estheticians are accustomed to keeping detailed notes on client profile cards, as this information is key to our business, not to mention just plain good customer service. These notes serve as memory for continued product recommendations and treatment plans, and they are a running dialogue between you, the client, and management.

Medical Documentation

Medical chart writing is your formal communication link with the nursing staff and the physician. It also serves as a defense against malpractice lawsuits, as it establishes your professional responsibility and accountability. Keep in mind that a medical chart that you may be adding to may be seen by not only the staff members and physician in your office, but by other physicians, insurance reviewers, lawyers, and judges. It is important that your notes be clear, concise, and well organized.

Depending upon the facility in which you are employed, you may find chart writing practices vary slightly. It is important for you to learn and use approved vocabulary and abbreviations. Using conventional chart-writing methods is necessary for many reasons,

but especially because *it is easier.* It is advisable to request a special chart-writing work-shop with your lead nurse to learn the specifics of your particular office. It is also helpful to take a course in medical documentation. It can be confusing and alarming to co-workers to find that you are not complying with an approved method of charting.

Four Basic Types of Chart Writing

Although there are many methods used for documentation, you will probably encounter one or more of four basic forms: narrative charting, source-oriented charting, problem-oriented charting, and computerized charting.

Narrative Charting

Historically **narrative charting** often included information that was not useful. It may have appeared more like a short story and was difficult to retrieve vital information due to its lengthiness. It did not easily show a relationship between a problem and a resolution. Today narrative charting communicates only essential facts about a client or patient.

Source-Oriented Charting

Source-oriented charting is a form of narrative charting whereby staff members enter their own records. Due to the lack of ease in retrieving information easily, this form of chart writing has typically been replaced by **problem-oriented medical record** keeping.

Problem-Oriented Charting

The **POMR** method is the most common form of record keeping, as it is the most effi-cient. This method utilizes a list of problems, with numbers assigned to each according to priority. Charting with the POMR method is typically made more efficient by using another reduction technique that helps to clarify information in a logical, systematic approach: **SOAP** charting. SOAP is an acronym for the words **S**ubjective, **O**bjective, **A**ssessment, and **P**lan.

The **SOAP, SOAPIE,** and **SOAPIER** methods make medical documentation orderly and retrievable. Information can be accessed easily by looking at the patient's description of their problem or *subjective* viewpoint, then the *objective* observation is documented, then combining the two creates an *assessment,* and then the research takes place for developing a *plan* for treatment. Another look at the model is as follows:

Subjective: the client's perspective
Objective: what is observed
Assessment: evaluation or diagnosis
Plan: what are the future plans, treatments, management

Recently **SOAP** has been expanded to include **I**mplentation and **E**valuation to make the acronym **SOAPIE.** In addition, some have added **R**evision, making it **SOAPIER.** Here is another view of the expanded versions **SOAPIE** or **SOAPIER:**

Subjective: the client's perspective
Objective: what is observed
Assessment: evaluation or diagnosis
Plan: what are the future plans, treatments, management
Implementation
Evaluation
Revision

Example of Actual Chart Notes Using SOAP

Date: 04/07/04
Name: Patient Brown
S: Patient Brown comes in today stating:
  • Her skin feels dry.
  • The dark spots around her eyes are getting darker
O: Exam shows dry skin build-up along nasal labial folds, and dyschromias on the periorbital regions both L and R and on zygomatic region
A: Actinic keratosis and possibly melasma, periorbitally [Remember: as estheticians we do not make a diagnosis]
P: Create home-care regimen. Add glycolic acid for exfoliation, a hydrator for moisture, hydroquinone or kojic blend for lifting pigment, and make an appointment for patient to consult with physician for diagnosis and possible medications.

We typically would not write the letters SOAP (although it is some physicians' preference); the note would look like this in the chart:

04/07/04 Patient Brown states that her skin feels dry on her cheeks and has red spots that peel and never go away. She is also concerned with the "brown spots" around her eyes. A skin analysis shows dyschromias/hyperpigmentation beneath both eyes and periorally. It could be actinic keratosis and **melasma** (pregnancy mask). Will set up an appointment with physician for diagnosis, and prepare a new home-care regimen including glycolic acid for exfoliation, a hydrator for moisture, and a lightening agent to lift pigment.

(Initials)

The HPIP method Another system has been added to this form of charting, which utilizes a similar approach to the SOAP method. It is applied differently, however. The acronym is known as **HPIP,** which is as follows:

H: History
P: Physical Exam
I: Impression
P: Plan

You may see that this is similar to SOAP in that history represents the objective viewpoint, the physical exam represents the subjective viewpoints, the impression shows the assessment or diagnosis, and the plan as the treatment. Therefore, it is not entirely different, and may be easier yet to record.

*Chart Note Using **HPIP** Method*

04/07/04 Patient Brown returns with Grade III acne, has been on AB (antibiotics) both top.[topical] and tab.[tablets] b.i.d.[two times a day][**History Physical Exam Impression,** combined]. We will increase her home-care program by adding BP 10% [benzoyl peroxide] cleanser to the PM regimen, increase the in-office peels to weekly visits. In addition, she will see Dr. Good for an appointment next week to review medical tx [treatment] plan and Rx's [medications] [**Plan**].

(Initials)

Computerized Charting

Computerized charting is gaining in popularity, particularly for nursing staff. It saves time; increases legibility; utilizes clear, concise words; and serves as an excellent networking device. Many hospitals and medical centers use this format for charting. It is expensive and there are patient confidentiality issues, along with computer downtimes that can create problems with its use.

Abbreviations; Symbols; and Identifying Head, Neck, and Chest Regions

For some this may be review. The medical field uses symbols, acronyms, and abbreviations for most written communications. These are conventional, and their use will increase your chances of being understood and respected as a clinician. In addition, it is helpful to reference regions such as nasal region or frontal region to identify a specific area (Figure 13–1).

Here are a few abbreviations and symbols that you will begin to recognize:

Abbreviations

AB	antibiotics	Mg	milligrams
C/o	complains of	Ml	milliliter
C/C	chief complaint	Mm	millimeter
CA	cancer	Min.	minimal
BCC	basal cell carcinoma	Neg.	negative
SCC	squamous cell carcinoma	NKA	no known allergies
5-FU	5-fluorouracil	OTC	over the counter
Derm.	dermatology	p.r.n.	whenever necessary
Dx	diagnosis	Path	pathology
ENT	ear, nose, throat	Pos.	positive
Eval.	evaluation	Postop.	postoperative
F/U	follow up	Preop.	preoperative
Gm	gram	Pt	patient

q.d.	every day		Tx	treatment, therapy
q.h.	every hour		Wt.	weight
q.i.d.	four times a day		Y/O	years old
Rx	prescription		L	left
Sx	symptoms		R	right
t.i.d.	three times a day		A	assessment
tab.	tablet		b.i.d.	twice a day (bis in die)
top.	topically		bilat.	bilateral

Symbols

$\bar{a}$	before		↑	increase or upper
$\bar{c}$	with		↓	decrease or lower
$\bar{s}$	without		Δ	change
>	greater than		Ⓛ	left
<	less than		Ⓡ	right

Mistakes and Chart-Writing Etiquette

Always use a black pen (no pencils, blue-ink pens, felt-tipped pens). Mistakes made in charts are crossed out, not erased or whitened. Instead, draw one line through the mistake; write the corrected version, and then initial. Maintain your objectivity while writing in a patient chart. Write just the facts, not your hunches or feelings, or ideas about a patient. In addition, do not use statements like: "Mrs. Patient is more swollen today than she was at her last appointment." Use the patient's own language such as: "Mrs. Patient stated: 'I feel more swollen today than I have felt for two days.' "

In addition, avoid making value judgments or comments on personality issues while chart writing. If necessary make a note on a separate piece of paper and copy it to the final document when you are certain of what needs to be noted.

As tempting as it might be to go on about a disgruntled patient in their chart, you will be relieved when you do not have to explain yourself at a later date if there is a legal dispute. Keep your words professional, within your scope, and appropriate. If you need to "red flag" this client, put a note on their client profile—not on the patient/physician's medical chart.

Confidentiality

First, it is imperative that we recognize that all dealings with the patient in or out of the office are confidential. Even if you recognize a client or patient in a mall, in the supermarket, or—heaven forbid—at a social function, that person is not going to want you to bring up the fact that you know them from the office. There is nothing more embarrassing than having someone from the office of Dr. Good, the plastic surgeon, ask you how you are getting along with your face-lift, or how your biopsy turned out. Think before you speak. In addition, do not fall into the trap of revealing anything about another patient who has undergone a procedure. People can be coy and cunning about obtaining information. Make your pat answer: "It's confidential."

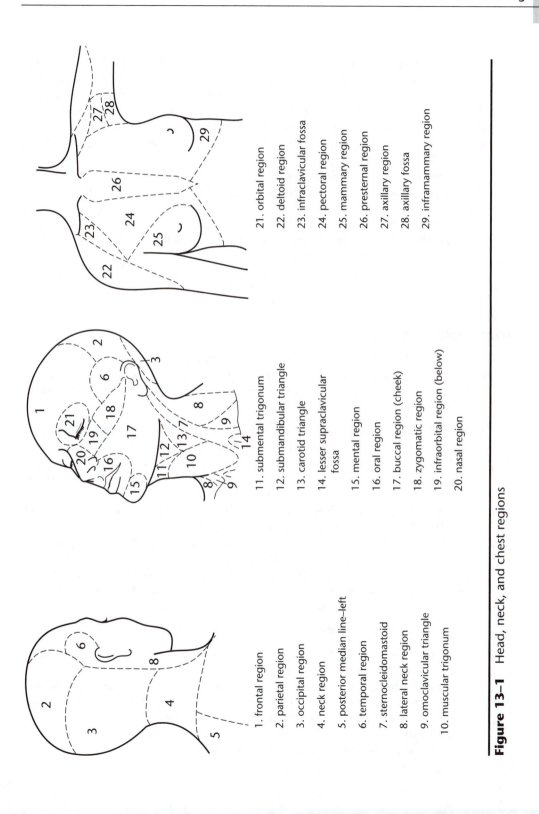

1. frontal region
2. parietal region
3. occipital region
4. neck region
5. posterior median line–left
6. temporal region
7. sternocleidomastoid
8. lateral neck region
9. omoclavicular triangle
10. muscular trigonum

11. submental trigonum
12. submandibular triangle
13. carotid triangle
14. lesser supraclavicular fossa
15. mental region
16. oral region
17. buccal region (cheek)
18. zygomatic region
19. infraorbital region (below)
20. nasal region

21. orbital region
22. deltoid region
23. infraclavicular fossa
24. pectoral region
25. mammary region
26. presternal region
27. axillary region
28. axillary fossa
29. inframammary region

Figure 13–1   Head, neck, and chest regions

In the office you will hear and see confidential information on a daily basis, as you will be privy to charts, consults, and forms that include private documentation about the patient. This information will include the patient's name, physical or psychological condition, emotional status, financial situation, reasons for wanting surgery, and various other very personal points. It is important to remember that you have a legal responsibility to abide by the rules dictated by the confidentiality clause in your agreement to work in a medical office. We have all signed one.

Someone who feels unable to trust that we will keep their information private may not seek the proper care. In addition, they may not give the doctor vital information that may affect the outcome of a procedure. You must also be aware of the behavior of others, as it is easy to forget that a visitor may ask a seemingly innocent question such as: "What did she or he have done?" The same answer applies: "It is confidential information." Protect *everyone*. The wrong answer to that innocent question could also create a loss in revenue when a potential client or patient goes elsewhere. Moreover, an employee or practitioner may even lose a job, a career, or insurance coverage (not to mention be held liable), if she or he fails to keep confidential information private.

Sharing Medical Information

Legally, we estheticians should not be sharing information about a client or patient in any case. Medical personnel are also in breach of confidentiality by sharing information even with a patient's family member unless that patient has agreed to a disclosure. The guidelines are as follows:

- **Share information on a need-to-know basis only to deliver the appropriate care.** Technically, we are not to share information with anyone regarding a client or patient without his or her consent. However, if the information is a necessary part of a procedure or treatment, it is important to share only that which is needed to perform the application.
- **Do not share information with the patient's family unless there is a written consent from the patient.** Unless consent has been given by the patient, other inquiry into the medical status of a patient is not to be given or discussed. This is handled by medical personnel and is confidential. This includes phone calls and face-to-face meetings.
- **Do not discuss information about a patient where others can hear the conversation—such as in a hallway or lobby area.** Visitors can often hear conferences, and this violates patient confidentiality.

Some exceptions to the rule of observing patient confidentiality at all costs would be if:

1. **There is a medical emergency:**   the patient is being transported to a hospital or another location due to an emergency
2. **Domestic abuse:**   It is necessary to allow the doctor to know if someone is being threatened by domestic abuse, so that the individual may get the appropriate help.
3. **If you have a legal responsibility to do so:**   If you are pulled into a legal case you may be asked to reveal confidential information, but it is paramount that you review all of these issues with your administrator and legal defense team.

Confidentiality in Transmitting Medical Records

You will find that medical records are found in a secured location and locked after business hours for a reason. It is the law, and the patient's interest is being protected as well as the treating physicians. With the advent of computers and fax machines, it can be more difficult to retain control of patients' personal information. Some guidelines for protecting confidential information of printed material about patients are as follows:

- Computerized information should be given only on a need-to-know basis.
- Never access information for personal interest.
- Faxing of medical information should be done only in emergencies, not as protocol. Make certain of the fax number to avoid sending the information to the wrong office.
- Do not give information over the phone; it is difficult to verify caller identity.
- Do not release information about the patient to family members, friends, or other health-care workers.
- Do not release information to law offices, insurance companies, or other physicians' offices unless instructed to do so by appropriate personnel in your office.

Typically, these duties will be in the charge of a clerical or medical administrator, but one never knows exactly how a job description may be challenged. Stay abreast of the policies and procedures set up by your administration to avoid the pitfalls of actions, which may have legal consequences. Keep the client, patient, and physician in mind at all times.

Health Insurance Portability and Accountability Act of 1996 (HIPAA)   As of April 14, 2003, federal privacy standards to protect patients' medical records, health information provided to health plans, doctors, hospitals, and other health-care providers has been enacted throughout the United States. The Department of Health and Human Services (HHS) developed this standard to provide patients with access to their medical records and gain more control over how their personal health information is being used.

With the use of computers and fax machines, patient privacy has been in question. At the base of this issue people may be reluctant to share information with their physician or other health-care providers, including pharmacists. A few key standards of patient protection are as follows:

- **Access to Medical Records.**   Patients are able to see and receive copies of their medical records.
- **Notice of Privacy Practices.**   Health-care providers must provide a notice to their patients on how they may use their personal medical information.
- **Limits Use of Personal Medical Information.**   This rule governs health-care providers sharing of information on a *need to know* basis.
- **Prohibits the Use of Patient Information for Marketing.**   Permission must be obtained from the patient to use personal medical information.
- **Stronger State Laws.**   All states must comply with privacy standards.
- **Confidential Communications.**   Patients can request that health-care providers ensure that all communications are kept confidential.
- **Complaints.**   Patients can file formal complaints regarding a breach of confidentiality.

All employees are required to take HIPAA training through their employer, and these rules will be strictly enforced. A complete description of this standard is available at http://www.hhs.gov/ocr/hipaa.

Summary

Note writing on charts can take some skill. Keep it brief and do not allow personal judgments into the text. The key is to give the medical staff enough information about what you have recommended, applied, and observed in the patient's medical chart. Using the standard abbreviations and symbols will become second nature and will shorten the time that you spend trying to explain a methodology.

Frequently Asked Questions

1. **How much information should the esthetician put into a chart?**

   Only what is necessary for the team to see what you have recommended for products, treatments, and the response curve to those items. Use enough information so that the doctor can see at a glance what you have given the patient.

2. **Does the esthetician need to write down everything that the patient says during a phone call?**

   This is a major concern while taking information over the phone. Date, initial, and describe the problem in detail as clearly as you can on a separate piece of paper. Then give the note to the nurse or physician (depending upon the flowchart in your office) for a call back. This note will often be taped to a sheet of paper inside the chart, and will remain as a legal recording of the conversation.

Skin Conditions and Treatments

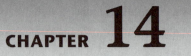

CHAPTER **14**

Skin Conditions

- Introduction
- Physician-Treated Conditions
- Esthetician-Treated Conditions
- Instruments Used to Assess Skin Conditions for Treatment
- Case Studies
- Summary
- Frequently Asked Questions

Introduction

Skin conditions can be socially debilitating to a person who has them, and they can steal the confidence of some of the most stoic. As horrendously as some conditions present, and as frustrating as they are to treat, they are fascinating to study. (See images in color insert.) Some of the many questions that are worthy of contemplation may be:

1. Why do two people with seemingly similar skin types, age, and genetic makeup have entirely different skin? One skin will look smooth, healthy, and beautiful; another in the same family will be plagued with acne, scarring, or pigment changes.
2. Why will some skin gain pigment or lose it, while others will not? How is it that in one square inch on the skin you will find a diverse ecosystem?
3. What treatment should I use on a client sensitive to products that are supposedly made for reactive skin?
4. Which treatments are appropriate for a patient after a procedure?

If you have ever asked yourself these questions and/or wondered about how to care for a pre- or postoperative patient, this section will address some of these issues and offer solutions for some common conditions that you as an esthetician may see in a clinical setting.

Skin conditions such as dehydration, dyschromias, and acne have been successfully prevented and treated by licensed estheticians. As we know, when combined with medical support, conditions that are more severe such as **rosacea** and **actinic** or **solar keratosis** can also be treated by estheticians. New and veteran estheticians alike have trained at conferences and progressed through approved esthetic courses given by dermatologists and plastic surgeons to recognize skin disorders and diseases. Many have as much experience and awareness in recognizing skin disorders and diseases as some general practitioners. Nevertheless, the doctor must make the diagnoses.

Physician-Treated Conditions

Part of being a skin-care professional is recognizing problems and knowing when to refer a client to the doctor. Even an experienced physician may not know the pathology of a given condition until a biopsy is taken. After the physician has made the diagnosis, the appropriate medication or procedure has been given, and the patient is back working with the esthetician, then a treatment plan is created. From there, it is essential to work closely with the doctor to determine the type of treatment and the duration of the program for the patient.

Medical conditions described in this text are those that are treated by the physician; there may be contraindications for esthetic treatments. As clinical estheticians, we may be involved in preparation for a procedure or, later, treating the aftermath of a surgery. The following skin conditions often present in your practice, and you will become adept at recognizing and referring the client for further analysis and diagnosis.

Skin Cancer

Skin cancer is rampant in all forms. The American Academy of Dermatology uses the acronym **ABCD** for self-examination, which represents **A**symmetry, **B**order, **C**olor, and **D**iameter, as a tool for recognizing the difference between **nevi** (moles) and **melanomas.** This helps us in our skin-fitness observations as well. We watch for moles or lesions that are:

- **asymmetrical**—one side different than the other (A)
- showing uneven edges or borders (B)
- appearing in two or more shades (C)
- larger than the others on the client, or 6mm (D)

If your client has a mole that fits one or more of these criteria, there is good reason to send this client to the physician for a diagnosis. It is also important to note that any suspicious mole should be diagnosed by a physician even if it does not meet one of the above criteria. Bleeding, itching, oozing, or a change in texture of a mole, are all reasons to refer the client for diagnosis.

If working for a plastic surgeon or dermatologist, you will undoubtedly see the three major types of skin cancer. They are characterized as follows:

1. **Basal cell carcinoma.**   These are slow growing and are typically caused by sun exposure. In the beginning, they can be small reddish, smooth lesions that mimic **papules.** As they become larger, the centers may invert or have a blister on top. These are found on the face, chest, back, head, and neck. They often are excised or removed with a cryogenic (liquid nitrogen) or a chemical peel.
2. **Squamous cell carcinoma.**   This cancer is more invasive and can metastasize. Caused by sun exposure, it is often found on ears, face, hands, and lips. They are removed by excision, radiation, and scrape and electrodessication (Keir, Wise, & Krebs, 1998).
3. **Melanoma.**   This is the most serious of all three skin cancers. It develops from the melanocytes, and can metastasize quickly and easily throughout the entire body. Its

major cause is UVA/UVB sun exposure. The method for removal is surgery, and it is often followed by chemotherapy. These cancers can be deep and require grafting. If the cancer has spread beyond the site, radiation may be necessary. If melanoma is not caught early, it can be fatal.

Mohs surgery for skin cancer   **Mohs** surgery is often used to remove cancers. Dr. Frederic Mohs developed a specialized technique where the skin cancer is removed and divided into pieces and placed on a microscope slide. Tissue is then marked with colored dye, mapped out, and frozen. Thinner slices are made from the frozen tissue and then examined by the physician. The patient awaits the physician's findings, and if all of the cancer has been removed then the surrounding skin is often closed with sutures. If the cancer is still present, the physician will return to the map and repeat the process again until it is free of cancer cells. Depending upon the stage of the cancer and the extent of the surgery, sutures, skin grafts (thin shave of skin), skin flaps (healthy tissue pulled over site), or **spontaneous granulation** (wound heals by itself) are chosen as methods of wound healing. The physician makes the decision based on the type and size of the wound.

This can be devastating and disfiguring to the patient. Extreme attention to patient education and follow-up are necessary. For severe disfigurements, appearance counseling and group support for facial disfigurement may be helpful. **Let's Face It**, a nonprofit support organization for people with facial differences, is an outstanding resource for those experiencing life-altering facial changes. The Web site address is www.faceit.org.

Protection against skin cancer   All clients, patients, friends, family members, and the general public need to be reminded by estheticians, health-care practitioners, and physicians about the routine use of UVA and UVB protection. This includes personal clothing such as hats, glasses, and UVA- and UVB-reflective fabric garments (www.sunprecautions.com), and sunscreens containing maximum sun protection factors such as zinc oxide and titanium dioxide. In addition, at-risk patients should avoid rays from sun and reflective surfaces such as water, sidewalks, decks, and sand during the hours of 10:00 A.M. to 4:00 P.M. Health-care providers must be trained to recognize cancers and refer clients and patients to a qualified dermatologist or otolayrngologist (head and neck surgeon) for diagnosis; *everyone* should have routine cancer screenings and examinations by qualified physicians.

Staphylococcus/Streptococcus

Staph   **Staphylococcus** *aureus* is a bacterium that can exist on skin or on other surfaces such as in the nose or mouth without symptoms. The problems begin when it invades the tissue through a cut or break in the epidermis. The symptoms can range from pain and swelling around a lesion, small milia-like bumps, or general inflammation in the lymph nodes at any point in the body. Staph infections are typically characterized by inflammation and redness; they can grow in clusters and spread rapidly. A staph infection must be treated with antibiotics; without medication, it will multiply and invade our entire being. New strains, however, are found to be resistant to antibiotics.

Cellulitis is a form of staph, and its origin can be from a **streptococcal** bacterium (see below). Cellulitis is characterized by swelling; skin that feels warm to hot; and sometimes blisters, fever, and headache. A biopsy may be taken, or blood draws can determine the type of infection. Antibiotics are given to treat cellulitis. **Folliculitis** is a form of staph and an infection of the hair follicles. It can create small pustules and sometimes presents as a boil. Larger boils are called **furnicles.** If a client or patient presents with reoccurring boils, they may be diabetic.

It is necessary to recognize these lesions and refer them for proper diagnosis, as you may spread the bacteria unknowingly, and if the patient continues to develop the infection, it may spread to other organs of the body.

Strep   Streptococci are bacteria found within the body and on the skin. Some forms cause disease, and antibiotics are necessary to rid the body of all strep infections. Cellulitis is the most common form of strep infection that we will see in our work. Most other forms are located at sites such as throat and lungs. As mentioned previously, cellulitis can be of staph *or* of strep origin, and presents as an area on the skin that is erythemic (red), inflamed, warm or hot to the host, sensitive, and may appear blistered.

Once the physician determines the bacteria source, the appropriate antibiotic will be prescribed. Eliminate all aggressive home-care products, and in-office treatment plans until the condition has stabilized. In rare cases chills and fever may be associated with cellulitis, and if left too long untreated, some patients must be hospitalized for intravenous antibiotics.

Erysipelas is a form of cellulitis, and can present as rosacea (see page 140) located on the nose and cheeks. It may affect older patients, but it can show up in any age group. The area becomes inflamed or warm and can involve chills and fever. It comes on quickly. It is important to recognize these differences from other diseases such as lupus and rosacea that present with similar characteristics.

Impetigo is another form of strep (it can also be caused by staph), and is characterized by weepy, crusty lesions that grow in clusters. Children often experience impetigo, and they spread it amongst themselves due to a lack of hand washing with soap. Impetigo can evolve into **ecthyma**, which is an advanced, ulcerated form of the bacteria. It is itchy, has pus-filled lesions, and forms dark crusts. This can lead to scars and create severe changes in pigmentation of the affected area.

Seborrheic Keratosis

Seborrheic keratosis is characterized by a flat medium-to-dark-brown raised lesion that has a texture similar to warts. This is often seen on older adults and is not harmful, except the condition can be irritated or bumped by shaving or other habits. The lesions have been known to itch. Liquid nitrogen is most commonly used for the removal of seborrheic keratosis and 5-FU topical chemotherapy works well.

Fungal Infections

Fungal infections are characterized by symptoms, which, like many skin conditions, can mimic others. **Tinea** is the term for fungal infection, of which there are many types found on various parts of the body. Typically, fungal infections may cause itching, swelling, blisters, and scaling. Most physicians will prescribe antiviral medications for fungal infections. **Tinea versicolor** appears as white patches where the production of **melanin** has been compromised. This is often noted on tanned skin, yet it is not directly created by UVA and UVB exposure.

Herpes Simplex Virus

Herpes, an ancient Greek term meaning to creep, is seen in two forms. They are **Herpes Simplex Type I (HSV-1),** the cold sore, fever blister type located periorally (around mouth or around lips); and **Herpes Simplex Type II (HSV-2),** which is considered genital herpes. The only distinction between the two is the lesion site; otherwise they are the same virus and can be transferred through contact.

All facial treatments should be suspended during a HSV-1 type of breakout, and antiviral medication should begin. This is particularly of concern in presurgical procedures, specifically for laser resurfacing, chemical peels, and dermabrasion as the heat generated from these procedures can enliven the virus. For clients who are prone to herpetic breakouts, pretreatment with an antiviral medication for superficial peels and microdermabrasion may be indicated. L-Lysine an amino acid has been helpful as an OTC (over-the-counter) type of drug for the treatment of herpes; beneficial also are nutrition and routine stress relief management. An excellent Web site for your clients and patients to visit is www.herpesite.org.

Rosacea

Rosaceous conditions are on the rise today. A physician must be consulted for medication. Rosacea is characterized often as a hereditary, chronic skin disorder of the sebaceous glands that affects the facial skin and eyes. It is detected by redness accompanying **telangiectases** (spider veins) across the nose and cheeks, which can be slightly raised or distended. It can affect the chin, forehead, and, in extreme cases, the eyes (this is known as ocular rosacea). When treated properly it can become managed and nearly undetectable; if left untreated it may develop beyond repair into disfiguring conditions such as **rhinophima** (bulbous nose). Clients and patients can be directed to www.rosacea.org for more information and support.

Dermatitis

Dermatitis is a term used often as a catchall for various skin ailments ranging from those with known causes to the unknown. As with many types of skin disorders the recipient may experience redness, itching, blistering, scaling, and oozing of fluid from the site. A physician should be brought into the case as it may mimic other disorders and diseases. Sometimes OTC (over-the-counter) medications such as cortisone cream are tried on the lesion first. If the condition persists, the physician may take further action, by doing a workup consisting of a full accounting of home-care product use to determine allergic potentiality. A stronger medication such as an antibiotic may be prescribed to eliminate or manage the condition.

Psoriasis

Psoriasis is a condition where skin cells multiply faster than normal, do not shed, and build up on hands, scalp, and knees. As dying cells move toward the upper layers of the stratum corneum, the increased amount creates red patches, which are also covered with a silverish coating. Treatment for psoriasis is often the use of steroids and cortisone creams. Ultraviolet **light therapy** is also used, along with drugs such as **anthralin** and **methotrexate,** which are anticancer drugs that stop the growth of cells.

Eczema

Eczema is a condition also known as **atopic dermatitis.** It is characterized by a rash that is red, oozes, and crusts. It can be found around moist areas such as under the eye, but also on arms, hands, scalp, and elbows. It often itches and when scratched can create yet another type of infection. Cortisone creams are used to control it, antihistamines are used for itching, and ultraviolet light therapy may also be used along with psoralens (drugs that facilitate light therapy).

Acneic Skin

Levels III and IV, see Kligman's Acne classification. Physicians need to see all clients with advanced cases of acne for medication. Medications such as antibiotics and azelic acid help to stop or slow the growth of p. acnes by reducing inflammation and bacteria. Some advance cases may be given Accutane.

Skin Tags

Skin tags are small flesh-toned skin drops that are loose and often found on the neck, chest, and underarms. They pose no threat other than appearance (although they can become irritated with jewelry) and are often removed with liquid nitrogen or are cut or shaved off.

Xanthomas/Milia (Periocular)

Whitish or yellow-toned fatty deposits around the eye area are called **xanthalasmas.** Neither these nor **milia** (fat or sebum-encapsulated beads just under the skin) located near or around the eye should be removed by the esthetician. Complications can arise—such as bacteria draining into the eye. It is necessary to have a diagnosis and treatment made by the physician as they will typically extract periocular milia, or excise xanthelasmas. Milia located at other sites, however, may be easily removed by a trained esthetician.

Self-Abuse/Excoriation

This condition is characterized by a compulsive, habitual attempt to pick or create trauma to the skin. This disorder creates injuries that usually promote scars. Results from this compulsion can range from appearing like light acne scarring, to severe slashes about the face and other parts of the body. This can be a serious debilitating psychological disorder. It must be followed closely by the physician or a therapist.

Esthetician-Treated Conditions

Beyond the skin types and conditions such as normal, dry, oily, sensitive and combination, you will most likely see advanced conditions, disorders, and diseases. As a clinical esthetician, the types of conditions in which you will be analyzing and making judgments will often become routine. In addition you will work in consort with the physician for the diagnoses and when medications are prescribed.

Dry/Dehydrated Skin

Extremely dry and dehydrated skin presents as if all of the water has been drained out of it. It can look paper thin and lifeless. Sometimes it may be drawn and sallow, yellow, or gray. Often it will have flakiness around the nasolabial (nose to mouth) folds and will show wrinkles more readily. Extreme cases are called **xerosis** (extremely dry skin). This type of dry skin can become barrier impaired, thus leaving it vulnerable to disease and infection.

Photoaged Skin

Photoaged skin appears to have been through major battles in the elements. Parched, lined, pigmented, and at times painful, this type of condition may exhibit actinic keratosis (red lesions, often precancerous and caused by excessive UVA/UVB exposure), on areas such as cheeks, nose, and chin. If properly treated, this skin type responds quickly to medication, exfoliation, nourishment, and treatment.

Actinic Keratosis

Estheticians will find themselves treating this condition, but the client will also need to be referred to a physician for medical care, which often includes biopsies. It is characterized by red or brown, flaky, sometimes raised lesions that will present on areas of the face and body such as cheeks, forehead, nose, chin, hands, or shoulders (areas with maximum exposure to UVA/UVB rays). Actinic keratosis lesions are often precancerous and must not be left untreated.

Oily/Sebaceous Skin

Oily sebaceous skin presents as extremely shiny, large pored, often lumpy or bumpy, and can exhibit donut-shaped lesions—commonly found on areas such as the nose and forehead—called **sebaceous hyperplasia.** These are often harmless, but clients do not like them and often ask to have them removed (a physician-only procedure). This skin condition will oil up within an hour or two of washing, and leave the owner often exasperated trying to fight this excessive oil.

Rosacea

The esthetician will see an increase in rosaceous conditions. A physician must be consulted for medication and thus it is described under Physician-Treated Conditions (see page 137).

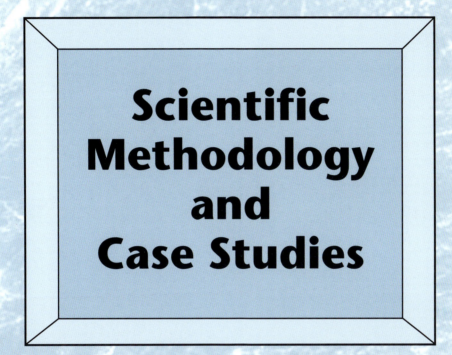

Scientific
Methodology
and
Case Studies

Client A Profile
Grade II Acne

The client in this study is a 22-year-old woman with Eastern European ancestry. She is a Skin Type II, presents with normal to slightly oily orientation. In addition, she has Grade II acne, some roughness, uneven texture and pore size, acne scarring, and slight erythema to some lesions (*observation*). She was generally dissatisfied with the appearance of her skin: she was training to become a nurse and wanted to appear healthy.

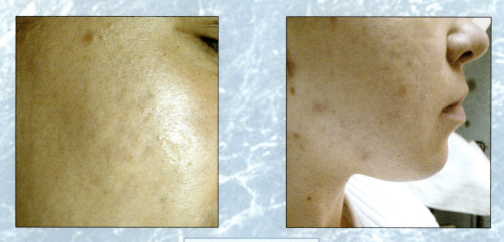

Pre-treatment images

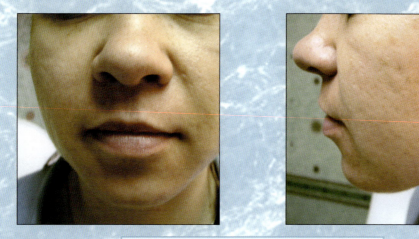

3 weeks home care (see pages 243–244)
2 treatments (see page 244)

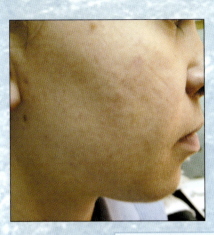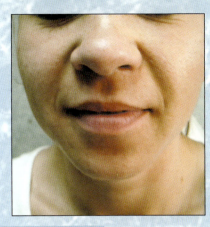

7 weeks home care (see pages 243–244)
6 treatments (see page 244)

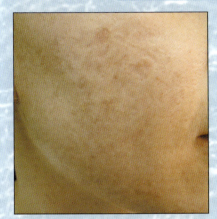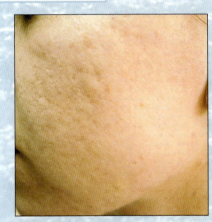

10 weeks home care (see pages 243–244)
9 treatments (see page 244)

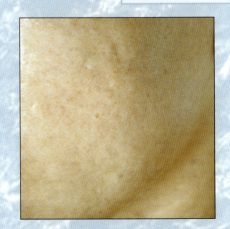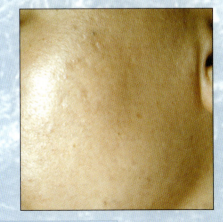

14 weeks home care (see pages 243–244)
13 treatments (see page 244)

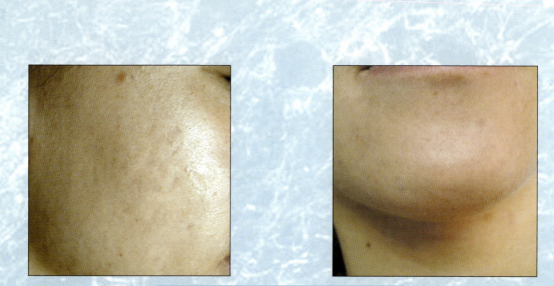

19 weeks home care (see pages 243–244)
18 treatments (see page 244)

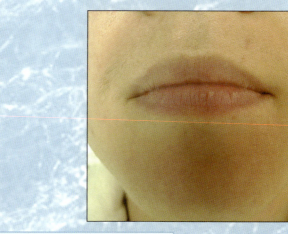

22 weeks home care (see pages 243–244)
21 treatments (see page 244)

Client B Profile
Grade III Acne

Client B is a 24-year-old woman with sensitive, oily, Grade III acne, exhibiting many open and closed comedones, many pustules and papules, several cystic lesions, pigment changes, inflamed skin, and some signs of erythema in general. Fitzpatrick II skin type, some sensitivity, with no known allergies (she suspected an allergy to yeast, but no diagnosis) or other health problems or conditions (*observation*).

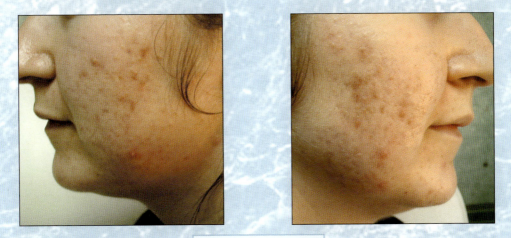

Pre-treatment images

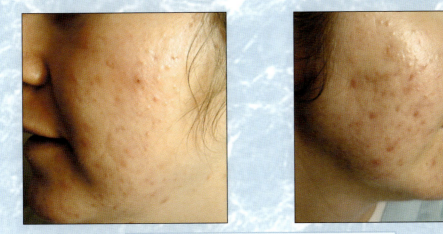

After 3 weeks home care (see pages 245–246)
2 treatments (see page 246)

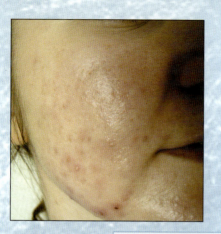
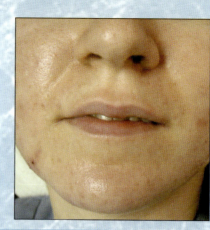

After 7 weeks home care (see pages 245–246)
6 treatments (see page 246)

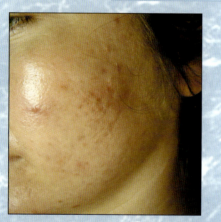
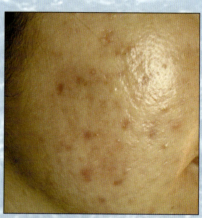

After 14 weeks home care (see pages 245–246)
13 treatments (see page 246)

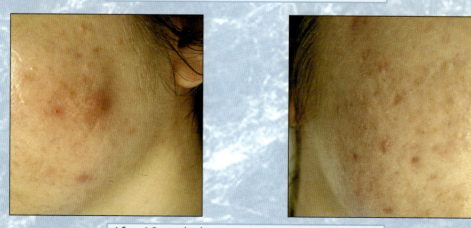

After 18 weeks home care (see pages 245–246)
17 treatments (see page 246)

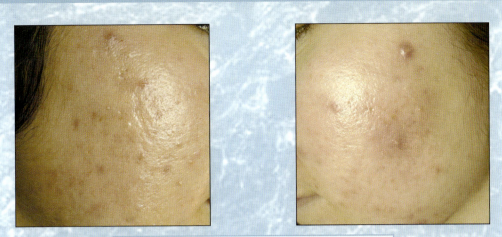
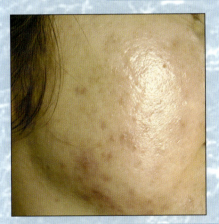
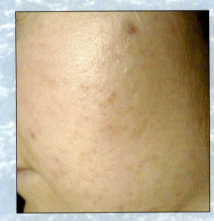
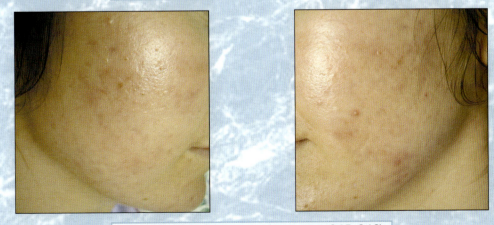

After 20 weeks home care (see pages 245–246)
19 treatments (see page 246)

After 22 weeks home care (see pages 245–246)
21 treatments (see page 246)

After 26 weeks home care (see pages 245–246)
25 treatments (see page 246)

Client C Profile
Grade IV Acne

Client C is a teenage male with Grade IV level acne who had seen a dermatologist, as well as tried oral and topical antibiotics, and OTC drugs and preparations, over several months. According to Client C, none of these remedies had been helpful, and "Nothing is working." He was clearly a candidate for Accutane at first glance, but parents and physician had chosen not to use the therapy at the time. Then he was introduced to the esthetician and admitted to the study. Later, they elected to employ Accutane therapy.

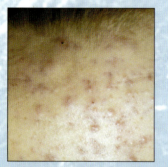 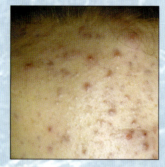 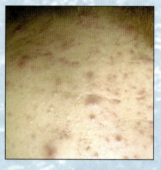

Pre-treatment images

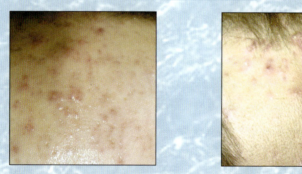

After 5 weeks home care (see pages 249–250)
4 treatments (see page 250)

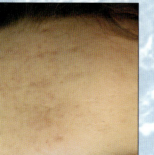 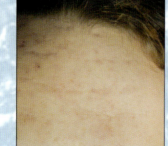 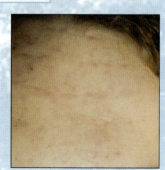

After 8 weeks of Accutane therapy

Client D Profile
Grade III Acne

Client D is a college student with Grade III acne. She came to the clinic via Web site for cosmetic support and for help in clearing up her acne with microdermabrasion. As a college student, the client is under stress, and her response to it did affect her acne. A discussion took place between the client, the parent, and the esthetician, in which the esthetician shared that the microdermabrasion would be one facet of the treatment plan. It would be supplemented by other applications such as peels and home-care products and compliance. In addition, it was determined that the client had no known allergies or general health problems and that she had tried a variety of finer skin-care products, drugs, and OTC preparations to no avail. The treatment plan was laid out and was agreed to by all. The client visits the clinic weekly for multilayer/purpose treatments and skin health-care counseling.

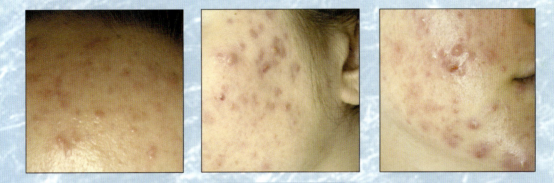

Pre-treatment images

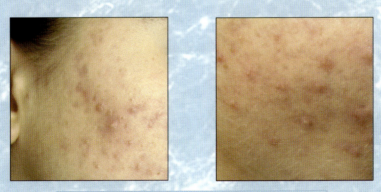

After 4 weeks home care (see pages 251–252)
3 treatments (see page 252)

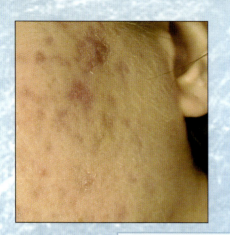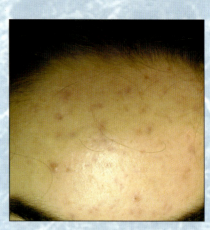

After 4 weeks home care (see pages 251–252)
3 treatments (see page 252)

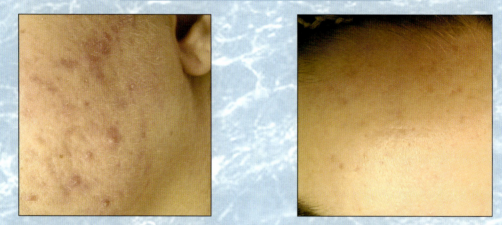

After 10 weeks home care (see pages 251–252)
9 treatments (see page 252)

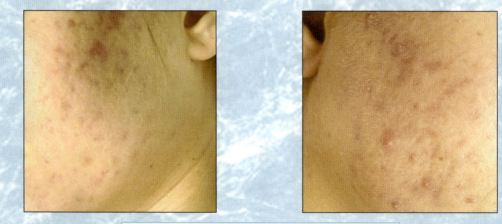

After 12 weeks home care (see pages 251–252)
11 treatments (see page 252)

Client E Profile
Hair Reduction

Client is a female in her early forties, with hirsutism, primarily about the mandible, zygomatic, and mental regions. The hair is dark and coarse on her Fitzpatrick III skin type. She had tried various methods of hair reduction including laser, electrolysis, waxing, tweezing, and shaving, to no avail. She was quite emotional about this hair and its apparent tenacity.

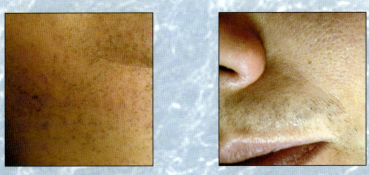

Pre-treatment images

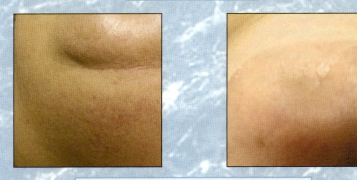

After 1 laser treatment (pages 253–254)

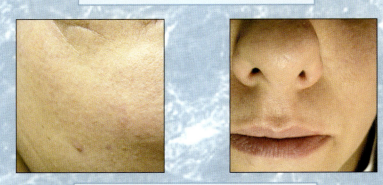

After 3 laser treatments (pages 253–254)

Client F Profile
Hyperpigmentation

Woman in her mid-thirties presents with multiple skin care concerns, including the pigmented area in the buccal region on her left side. Her Fitzpatrick IV skin type and dark hair in that region make it appear deeper than it is; she was using a sunscreen daily. A cautionary measure needed to be observed, as we can create more pigment in the region by overstimulating the melanocytes by aggressively treating it with chemicals that may generate heat, or using the microdermabrader, for example.

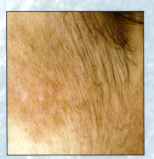

Pre-treatment image

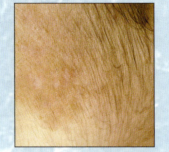

Pre-treatment image

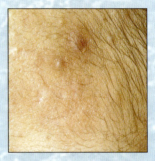

After 3 weeks home care (page 255)
1 treatment (page 255)

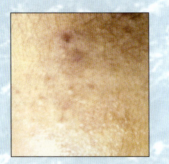

After 5 weeks home care (page 255)
2 treatments (page 255)

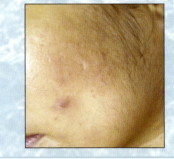

After 7 weeks home care (page 255)
3 treatments (page 255)

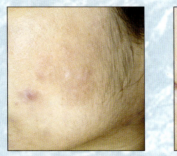

After 9 weeks home care (page 255)
4 treatments (page 255)

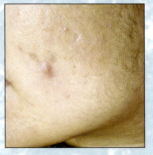

After 10 weeks home care (page 255)
4 treatments (page 255)

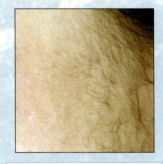

After 12 weeks home care (page 255)
5 treatments (page 255)

Common Skin Disorders

PLATE 1 — **Pustule.** An infected papule.

PLATE 2 — **Nodule.** A solid bump that is normally larger than one centimeter.

PLATE 3 — **Sebaceous cyst.** Enclosure of the epithelium within the dermis that becomes filled with keratin and lipid-rich debris.

PLATE 4 — **Hypertrophic scar.** An elevated scar.

PLATE 5 — **Rosacea.** An inflammation of the skin characterized by chronic diffuse redness, many telangiectasias, and flushing.

PLATE 6 — **Tinea pedis.** Also known as athlete's foot; a fungal infection of the skin.

PLATE 7 — **Allergic contact dermatitis (ACD).** An allergic reaction in the skin due to contact with a particular substance.

PLATE 8 — **Irritant contact dermatitis (ICD).** Dermatitis reaction caused by exposure to an irritating chemical.

PLATE 9 — **Molluscum contagiosum.** A virus belonging to the pox group of viruses; appears in clusters of small flesh-colored papules.

PLATE 10 — **Folliculitis.** Inflammation of the follicle caused by bacteria or an irritation.

PLATE 11 — **Basal cell carcinoma.** Common form of skin cancer that originates in the basal layer of the epidermis.

PLATE 12 — **Squamous cell carcinoma.** Raised, crusty, or wartlike ulcers or bumps on the skin, caused by cumulative sun exposure. It is the second most frequently diagnosed skin cancer.

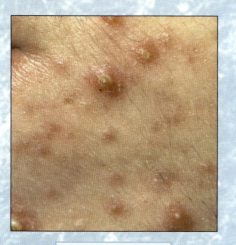

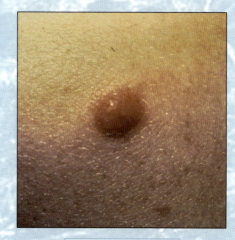

PLATE 1 — Pustule.

PLATE 2 — Nodule.

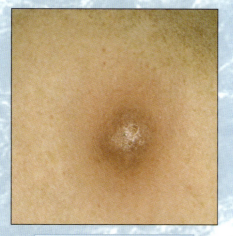

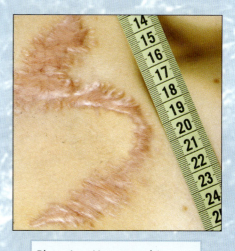

PLATE 3 — Sebaceous cyst.

Plate 4 — Hypertrophic scar.

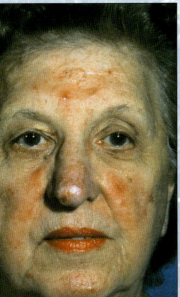

Plate 5 — Rosacea.

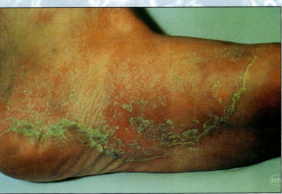

Plate 6 — Tinea pedis.

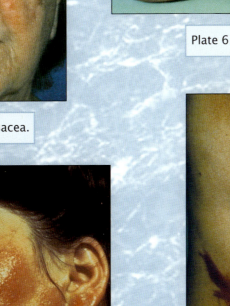

PLATE 7 — Allergic contact dermatitis (ACD).

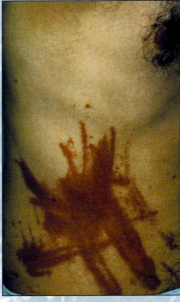

PLATE 8 — Irritant contact dermatitis (ICD).

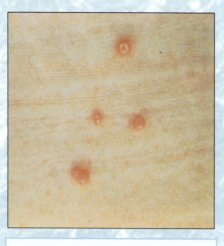

PLATE 9 — Molluscum contagiosum.

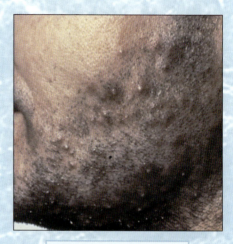

PLATE 10 — Folliculitis.

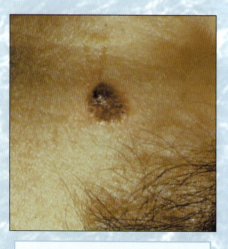

PLATE 11 — Basal cell carcinoma.

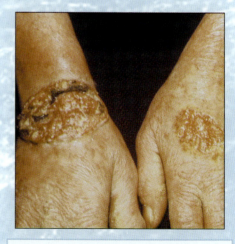

PLATE 12 — Squamous cell carcinoma.

Today estheticians have experience with soothing and calming treatments and skin-care products for home-care use along with camouflage therapy. In addition, many medical offices have laser therapy available to lessen or eliminate telangiectases and general redness.

Acneic Skin

Acne is attributed to three main factors: microorganisms, hormones, and inflammation. All types have one thing in common, an enlarged hair follicle plugged with oil and bacteria. The noninflammatory types of acne are open **comedones.** The inflammatory types are closed comedones, papules, pustules, cysts and nodules. They develop as our bodies' own natural response to a regular fixture on our skin—a bacterium known as *Propionibacterium acne* (P. acnes), which can thrive in sebum-enriched environments. Fortunately, today we have medications, treatments, and products to address the effects in all stages.

Hormonally Challenged Skin

This is without a doubt one of the most difficult conditions to manage because of the lack of stability in hormonal activity. This condition affects various populations and mostly presents in teenagers (both girls and boys), pregnant women, and perimenopausal women.

Once sebaceous glands are stimulated by androgens (male hormones present greater in males, but in females also), they will produce more **sebum.** We see more propionbacterium acnes (P. acnes) with this condition. This hormonal surge creates an inflammation in the hair follicle. Thus, everything aligned along the base of the follicle including increased sebum, dirt, and grime becomes trapped by the enlarged follicle. Bacteria can survive in an anaerobic environment (with no oxygen to dry it up), hence a pustule ensues. In addition, teenagers' cells are shedding faster than those in the latter years, so they tend to bond together, clogging the follicle.

New medications, treatments, and products have dramatically changed the formation of hormonally challenged skin, and when full compliance is observed, these outbreaks can be greatly minimized. In advanced cases of acne (levels 3 and 4) and in extreme cases of rosacea, medication called **Accutane** also known as **Isotretinoin** (vitamin A) is prescribed. This medication is used when all other methods—antibiotics and topicals—have failed. Isotretinoin decreases sebum released by sebaceous glands and increases cell renewal. The physician will monitor the patient closely with monthly visits and blood draws, as there are side effects associated with taking this medication.

Pigmented Lesions

Pigmented lesions are technically called **dyschromias.** They can present **hyperpigmentation** (more pigment)**,** or **hypopigmentation** (lost pigment and appears white). Pigment and its changes are created by **melanocytes,** which are small active melanin-producing cells located in the basal layer of the epidermis and in the upper layer of the dermis. Their intelligence can sense danger caused by UVA, UVB, and UVC (the ultraviolet rays that emit radiation), which cause damage at all levels of the skin. When under attack the melanocytes will create more melanin, which will rush up like small umbrellas to protect the upper layers of the epidermis. Another pigment related condition is melasma. Often referred to as Pregnancy Mask, melasma is found around the periorbital bone and on the perioral region. Its cause is related to hormones and can be a challenge to treat because these melanocytes are deeper and often located in the upper dermis.

A freckle, a brown spot, or a tan are all examples of hyperpigmentation. A loss of pigment can be incurred by trauma to the skin through these rays as well. Tinea veriscolor (loss of pigment due to tanning or other trauma to the cells) is often present on skin when a person has sustained significant sun exposure. However, some children may acquire this condition at an early age. This is even more reason to strengthen our resolve to utilize sunscreens at all ages. **Vitiligo** is an extreme condition of a loss of pigment and exhibits as pure white spots on the skin.

Self-Abuse/Excoriation

The esthetician's role in treating this condition—characterized by a compulsive, habitual attempt to pick or create trauma to the skin—is to refer the client to a physician. Often such clients will not seek medical help on their own, so if they come to see you, there is hope in their getting the help that they need. Unfortunately, you may see a fair amount of people seeking help for this in a medical office.

Do not provide hands-on treatments for these clients, as they are noncompliant. They may unconsciously use your treatment or products as a trigger to harm themselves. This can be a serious debilitating psychological disorder, and again, must be followed closely by the physician, or a therapist. (See page 141).

Instruments Used to Assess Skin Conditions for Treatment

Assessment is paramount to the success of a given treatment or procedure. Again, while we are not making the diagnosis, we do analyze the skin and make *assessments*. Have the physician see your client if they exhibit any of the disorders that are potentially disease-bound and require medication.

While an esthetician may make headway in treating acne grades I, II, and III in some cases, it is responsible to have medical intervention in grades III and IV. Patients with rosacea should be seen at the first opportunity, as medication is part of the management for this condition. Do not think or allow the client to believe that your products and treatments alone will resolve these problems. You may be able to help them *manage* their condition, but a physician must be in partnership to minimize the potential of the advancement of the condition.

Another reason for having a diagnosis made by the physician is that often if a patient exhibits one type of condition, he or she may also have a **subclinical** condition. This is a condition which is undetectable to the naked eye and may exist underneath the skin. The physician will have the training, experience, and knowledge to suspect an additional underlying condition and will treat accordingly or prophylactically (using precautionary measures).

There are five primary instruments used to analyze skin conditions, which will guide you toward a treatment plan. They are:

- Fitzpatrick Skin Typing
- Glogau Photodamage Classification
- Rubin Photodamage Classification
- Kligman's Rosacea Classification
- Kligman's Acne Classification

Fitzpatrick Scale

As we learned in basic training, one of the first tools to utilize in assessment is the **Fitzpatrick Skin Type** scale. It will serve as a guide in determining the strength of the treatment and the type. Fitzpatrick Skin Types are as follows:

- **Skin Type I.**   Always burns, never tans; this skin type will often have blue or light green eyes, may have **ephelides** (light freckles), or **lentigines** (light to darker pigmented lesions) a blue/pink undertone to the skin, and is usually a blond or a redhead. These individuals do not usually have problems with pigment and tolerate peels well. They may, however, develop erythema after treatment and may hold more redness or color after laser resurfacing
- **Skin Type II.**   Always burns, turns slightly tan; this skin type has limited protection from burning rays, and the skin may appear slightly warmer than that of type I. This skin type may have ephelides, or lentigines but will usually not develop pigment problems with peels, and they are good candidates for aggressive peels and laser resurfacing. They will have light-to-medium colored hair, and light-to-medium blue or green eyes.
- **Skin Type III.**   Usually does not burn, but tans easily; this skin type may exhibit a tendency toward hyperpigmentation following peels and procedures, but it will tolerate treatments well. It may be important to pretreat this skin type for hyperpigmentation with a lightening aid prior to doing a more aggressive type of treatment. The individuals will have darker eyes and usually darker hair.
- **Skin Type IV.**   Rarely burns, tans effortlessly; this skin type is definitely prone to pigment changes and is often not a candidate for laser resurfacing. These types will have dark eyes and dark hair. It is necessary to lower the amount of glycolic acid in a home-care or treatment product and definitely to do pretreating prior to peeling. Special considerations to the type of treatments must be observed to avoid post-treatment inflammatory hyperpigmentation (pigment changes created by trauma, injury, and chemicals such as peels or product).
- **Skin Type V.**   Dark pigmented skin, rarely burns, deeply pigmented; this skin type is definitely at risk for hyperpigmentation and hypopigmentation and is not a candidate for laser resurfacing or deeper peels. This skin type will have black eyes and hair and will scar easily, and possibly has a serious propensity for **keloids** (raised worm-like scars).

- **Skin Type VI.**   Darkest of skin types, can hypopigment, hyperpigment, and keloid. You must watch peeling procedures carefully and use lighter percentage performance agents in home care and in treatment. Tolerates classic European facials well, as well as light exfoliation. Do not overstimulate melanocytes by overbrushing, vacuuming, or otherwise abrading the skin (such as with microdermabrasion); this could result in hyperpigmentation.

Glogau Classification for Photodamage

The **Glogau Photodamage Classification** system presents four levels of photodamage. They range from minimal to extreme and are as follows:

Type I	No wrinkles—you see no wrinkles, at rest or while moving	Early photoaging • Mild pigment changes • No keratosis • Minimal to no wrinkles • 20s–30s or younger • Minimal acne scarring • No to minimal makeup
Type II	Wrinkles only in motion—you see them only when the person is talking, laughing, frowning, etc.	Early-to-moderate photoaging • Lentigines, other pigment changes showing • Wrinkles forming • Light keratosis • Nasolabial lines beginning to form • 30s–40s • Minimal makeup
Type III	Wrinkles at rest—you see the wrinkles when the person is not moving	Advanced photoaging • Hyperpigmentation, telangiectases • Keratosis • Wrinkles even when not moving • 40s–50s • Makeup always worn • Acne scarring shows through makeup
Type IV	Wrinkles as predominant characteristic—you see only wrinkles	Severe photoaging • Sallow-ashy skin color • Prior skin cancers • Wrinkles all over • Makeup not worn—sets in cracks • Severe acne scarring

Rubin's Classification of Photodamage

Dermatologist Mark G. Rubin has created a method for determining the level of photo-damage (Rubin, 1995). The categories are as follows:

Level 1

Alterations are in the epidermis only. These changes are primarily superficial pigment changes, roughness, lentigines, a dull or ashy appearance, and increased thickness. This client will benefit from a superficial peeling such as glycolic acid and a steady home-care program combining including AHA and/or BHAs, nourishers, antioxidants, and sun-screens.

Level 2

Alterations are in the epidermis and papillary dermis. These conditions may include all of those seen in level 1, as well as actinic keratosis, stronger pigmentation values, flat sebor-rheic keratosis, and an increase in wrinkles. This client will benefit from medium-depth peels such as TCA (trichloracetic acid) and a more aggressive home-care program includ-ing retinoids and hydroquinone.

Level 3

Changes are not only in the epidermis and papillary dermis but also in the reticular der-mis. This will be the most severe level of photodamage, and skin will be leathery, yellow in color, and exhibit open comedones. This client likely would benefit from laser resurfac-ing and possibly other cosmetic procedures along with a progressive home-care program depending upon age and sensitivity to performance and active agents.

Kligman Rosacea Classification

Dermatologists Albert M. Kligman and Gerd Plewig developed a method for classifying rosacea. It is as follows:

1. **Stage I** consists of erythema (redness) about the nasolabial folds, cheeks, and glabel-lum (forehead). Skin seems to itch, burn, and react to all forms of cosmetics.
2. **Stage II** presents as inflammation, pustules, and papules, and pores seem larger; con-dition may spread over other parts of the face including hairline and chin.
3. **Stage III** is the most serious form of rosacea and presents with large nodules; skin has an orange-peel appearance and becomes coarse.

Kligman's Acne Classification

1. **Grade I** is open and closed comedones with transitory blemishes.
2. **Grade II** is a few larger open and closed comedones accompanying a few pustules and papules.
3. **Grade III** is acne exhibiting many open and closed comedones, many pustules and papules, can show several cystic lesions, pigment changes, is inflamed, shows some signs of erythema (redness) and is painful.

4. **Grade IV** exhibits all of the above including advanced stages of cystic acne, scarring, inflammation, and erythema (redness). This level puts the patient at risk for further disease and both physical and mental health problems.

Case Studies

The following case studies will provide you with instrument classification use, general home-care plan information, and in-office treatment applications. They are organized according to SOAP specifications and could be transferred to the client/patient's chart as such.

CASE I

Client A is a Fitzpatrick II skin type, exhibits III Glogau, or Level 2 Rubin classification, and is 45. She could use an aggressive treatment plan bimonthly, which includes chemical peels, microdermabrasion, and pharmaceuticals, as she is not at risk for hyperpigmentation. Including a retinoic acid product three or four times a week, along with routine exfoliation would be beneficial to her keratosis. Daily hydrating elements such as serums and moisturizers for nourishment containing antioxidants and sunscreens, UVA and UVB protective clothing, hats, and sunglasses would be indicated as preventative measures. In addition, she could use comprehensive makeup support, such as a non-commedogenic foundation and mineral powder to even out skin tone. This is an ideal candidate for a reparative treatment plan with a forward focus on age management.

CASE II

Client B is a Fitzpatrick IV skin type with a classification I orientation. This 25-year-old male client enjoys relatively clear skin, has medium brown skin, and has no wrinkles or keratosis, and thus minimal photodamage. This client could benefit from a routine treatment plan of a deep pore-cleansing facial including steam, galvanic/deincrustation, vacuum, light massage, extractions, mask, high frequency, and hydration. He could also benefit from a home-care program including a lower-level benzoyl peroxide cleanser to alternate with his regular one, to keep pores clean and free of debris. He could also use daily a light moisture/hydrator containing a sunscreen with antioxidants (without minerals such as zinc oxide and titanium dioxide, as they will appear white on his bronze skin).

A light, lower-concentrated glycolic peel could be traded for the deincrustation step, and a microdermabrasion could replace the vacuum. One word of caution, however: we do not want to stimulate melanocytes in this skin type creating postinflammatory pigmentation. Special attention must be given to strength and depth of these more aggressive treatments on higher pigmented clients.

Summary

Always factor in the classification and skin type as a context when creating a program. The classifications are excellent measurements to use for your treatment and home-care recommendations; they are easily understood when communicating with medical personnel and colleagues. Physician direction, patience, diligence, and compliance are necessary to affect these skin conditions, as they will be more challenging than what you may see in another environment.

Frequently Asked Questions

1. **How does the esthetician determine which instrument to use and when?**

We will always start with the Fitzpatrick Skin Type instrument first. This is protocol in your initial skin analysis. Once the Fitzpatrick type has been determined, depending upon the issue that the client has presented to the esthetician, you will next use one of the photodamage classifications, and then treat accordingly.

2. **Why will a Fitzpatrick Skin Type III or above pigment more easily with some products and treatments?**

The more pigment a skin has, the more likely it will be to pigment further. Higher Fitzpatrick Skin Types have larger melanocytes than the lower-level types, thus making it more prone to trauma, injury, and stimulation. Higher Fitzpatrick skin types will pigment much more easily with aggressive home-care programs containing high levels of AHAs or BHAs, and will be more prone to postinflammatory hyperpigmentation resulting from aggressive treatments such as microdermabrasion or chemical peels. It is advantageous to pretreat higher Fitzpatrick skin types with lightening preparations prior to in-office treatments.

CHAPTER 15

Tried-and-True Treatments

- Introduction
- Informed Consent
- Skin Type–Specific Home-Care Protocols and In-Office Treatments
- Actinic Keratosis
- Rosacea
- Summary
- Frequently Asked Questions

Introduction

This chapter will focus primarily on treatments such as peels and microdermabrasion and on pharmaceuticals for more advanced skin conditions. It by no means suggests that you leave behind the routine facials and therapeutic treatments that you learned in your basic training. As with all good clinical work, assessment, planning, and following protocol are the key elements to a successful outcome. The following three points illuminate the importance of evaluation and creating an appropriate treatment plan.

1. **Watch the combination of elements in treatments.** It is important to note that if we use aggressive acid peels and microdermabrasion, we do not also apply brushes, massages, heated steam, or herbal exfoliates to the skin after these treatments. Once you become adroit at handling various skin types, conditions, and treatment applications, you will learn which elements of a routine facial will be complementary and which to avoid. It is of the utmost importance that we do not exceed our training, experience level, or knowledge and licensure in the clinical setting.

2. **Do not overtreat.** You can be creative in your treatment plans, but make certain that you do not overtreat, thereby creating a wound (and ultimately a scar) to a slightly abraised epidermis. This can happen. For example, if you want to use a standard facial approach to your treatment, selecting an enzyme for exfoliation that would be compatible with the masks and steam that you may use would be your obvious choice. You would not want to use steam after a chemical peel. Moreover, if you are using glycolic acid to exfoliate, there is no need to also use other deincrustation methods

such as the **galvanic treatment.** In addition, you do not want to apply a chemical or microdermabrasion to a freshly laser-resurfaced area. We will visit this in more depth in Chapter 17, under postoperative treatments.

3. **Make certain that your treatment plan is compatible with the prescribed medication.**   Obtain from the doctor the contraindications of a given medicine that the patient is using. For example, a patient taking Accutane for acne would not be a candidate for a glycolic peel or microdermabrasion until they have been off the medication for at least a year or have been cleared by the physician for this procedure.

We need to get into the habit of checking to make sure that a treatment plan is compatible with what is already being prescribed. This may involve calling the patient's dermatologist, plastic/cosmetic surgeon, or clinical esthetician.

One of the many exciting features of treating clients in a clinical setting is that you are able to design *complete* programs for them. Such a program ranges from home-care products to office treatments, to medical support, and then back to the maintenance phase needed, to achieve long-lasting results. When you begin to see the positive changes—which often occur quickly—it is thrilling for both the client and the esthetician, and physicians are delighted when they are able to trust that their patients are nurtured and progressing.

Informed Consent

Upon determining the type of treatment—and its risks, efficacy, and frequency—make certain that the patient fully understands the plan and is willing to comply with both in-office and home-care components. Before any treatments are applied, all risks should be visited and major questions brought out for discussion with the patient, and an **Informed Consent Sheet** (a form signed by the client or patient indicating that they understand the risks and are willing to have the treatment) must be signed by the patient. The form does not need to be lengthy, too wordy, or full of legalese. It needs to describe briefly:

- what treatment you are applying
- purpose of the application
- potential risks
- release of liability if it does not work or there is an unforeseen problem associated with the treatment

Shown here is an example of a basic consent form (Figure 15–1), which you may adapt and make legal/compliant according to your state regulations. (Figure 15–2 may also be adapted.)

This section covers clients and patients using products in a manner consistent with the plan created by the esthetician and physician.

It is the opinion of many clinical estheticians that starting the client on a home-care regimen is a natural first step. We learn about the habits of a client through this process, as described in Chapter 1. We need to know if rules will be followed and we want the skin to be in optimum condition. We never want to send a client off having had an aggressive chemical peel without having been properly prepped for such a treatment.

TREATMENT CONSENT FORM

I _____ am authorizing _____ to perform _____ a superficial facial treatment for the purposes of _____. I understand that there are minimal risks and they have been explained to me in detail. I accept this treatment of my own free will, and understand that no guarantees are given to me.

I may experience _____ and it may require more than one treatment to achieve these results _____. (initial)

I may experience redness or dryness from this treatment _____. (initial)

I also understand that I should not use glycolic, retinoic acid, retinol, or high concentrations of vitamin C for 3 to 4 days after my treatment _____. (initial)

If an unforeseen condition arises from my having had this treatment, I will immediately contact the office _____. (initial)

TREATMENT SPECIALIST	SIGNATURE	DATE
_____	_____	_____
_____	_____	_____
_____	_____	_____
_____	_____	_____

*This form is for educational purposes only, it claims no legal assumptions.

Figure 15–1   Informed Consent—Option A

Skin Type–Specific Home-Care Protocols and In-Office Treatments

The following home-care protocols and in-office treatment plans are presented as a guide as you meet a client's needs based upon skin type and condition. Use this guide only for reference. It does not take the place of advanced training by a credentialed qualified training instructor or the physician with whom you are connected.

Dry/Dehydrated, Hyperpigmented, Photoaged Skin

Dry, dehydrated, photoaged skin, which also exhibits dyschromias, is often a primary focus for estheticians working in a medical setting. This skin type regularly present for advanced clinical care, and it can be treated successfully with in-office treatments and

INFORMED CONSENT FOR PEELS

Initial   I, _____ authorize _____ of
Your Medical Office/Facility Name, to perform the following peel:

❑ Glycolic   ❑ Lactic (AHA)   ❑ Salicylic   ❑ TCA   ❑ Jessner's

_____ 1. This process involves application to the affected skin area with a cotton swab or
small brush. Depending on the solution, it may be left on for up to ____ minutes. This
is determined by product strength, skin type and condition, sensitivity, age, or prior
use of any exfoliating agent.

_____ 2. While other peels are neutralized and removed during treatment, I understand that
TCA and Jessner's peels are applied in ____ layers and not removed.

_____ 3. In order to receive maximum results, more than one application may be required,
thus, it may be recommended that I participate in a series of treatments. My program
is customized based on the advice of the physician and/or esthetician.

_____ 4. Rate of improvement depends on my age, skin type and condition, degree of sun/
environmental damage, pigmentation levels, or acne condition. I will follow pre-
and/or postpeel instructions and maintain appointment schedules exactly as
prescribed, including home care.

_____ 5. I acknowledge that no guarantee has been made about the results of the procedure.
Although it is impossible to list every potential risk and complication, I have been
informed of some possible benefits, risks, and complications which may include, but
are not limited to, the following:
  • Softer, smoother skin
  • Reduction in the appearance of lines and wrinkles
  • Reduction in acne lesions
  • Swelling and redness
  • Scabbing or peeling of treated skin and surrounding areas
  • Prolonged skin sensitivity to wind and sun
  • Areas of persistent increased or decreased pigmentation

_____ 6. Any potential risks and complications could result in the need to discontinue the
treatment. In this case, an alternative recommendation(s) will be suggested. It is very
rare that a permanent disability occurs. If the need arises, I authorize my skin care
professional to perform such required treatment or procedure. I also agree to immediately inform the skin professional if I have concerns, or am overly uncomfortable
during treatment, or after I return home.

_____ 7. I agree to inform my skin professional when I introduce new medication(s) and/or
product(s) during the course of the treatment. I attest that I have had an opportunity
to ask questions and have questions answered to my satisfaction.

_____ 8. I certify that I am over the age of eighteen (18), that I am not pregnant or nursing, on
Accutane, or taking any other medication that may be contraindicated to having this
procedure. I have read and will follow to the best of my ability any and all instructions.
I understand the potential risks and complications, and choose to proceed after careful consideration of the possibility of both known and unknown risks, complications,
limitations, and alternatives.

Patient's signature_____ Date _____

Esthetician's/Physician's signature_____ Date _____

Figure 15–2   Informed Consent—Option B

consistent home care. These clients are usually interested in products and treatments and will often go to great lengths to achieve a healthier, younger appearance.

Home care   A home-care program for a Rubin's Classification Level II and III dry, dehydrated, photodamaged, pigmented skin type Fitzpatrick I–III at a minimum should consist of the following:

A.M.

1. A cleanser containing an 8% to 10% alpha-hydroxy acid product with a pH of 3.5 or above (not too irritating). It should serve to hydrate in a lotion, milk, or cream form. A toner is often requested by this client and can be utilized to remove excessive dirt, makeup and cleanser. Exfoliation is only one fraction of what the photodamaged skin needs. Cleansers containing amino acids (super-hydrating proteins), copper (good for wound healing) (Procyte 2001), allantoin (for soothing), are all excellent choices for step 1.
2. A moisturizer containing:
   - **Exfoliant**—glycolic, malic (apple), lactic (milk), salicylic (wintergreen leaf) acids, or papaya enzyme
   - **Hydrator**—amino acids, hyaluronic acid, marine algae
   - **Lightener**—kojic, hydroquinone, bearberry, arbutin
   - **Antioxidants**—vitamins C, E, and A or **alpha lipoic acid**
3. A sunscreen with zinc oxide and or titanium dioxide

P.M.

1. The cleansing routine could be the same as the morning.
2. Retinoic acid, hydroquinone, or glycolic acid combination, for cell normalization, pigment lightening, and exfoliation respectively. This could be used every other night until well tolerated. On opposite nights use a hydrating cream containing ingredients such as chamomile or azulene, copper, and/or allantoin, for calming. This evening program would serve as preparation for in-office peels and some procedures such as laser resurfacing.

Fitzpatrick IV and V skin types do not usually exhibit this level of photodamage because of the pigment protecting the skin. Creating a modified version of this program with lower levels of AHAs and sunscreens that do not contain the whitening effects of the minerals would be excellent. In addition, do not overstimulate the melanocytes by using aggressive home-care products with a low pH.

In-office peels   Treatments for this type of skin condition yield great results. In most cases evidence of improvement are immediate if the skin has been ignored, is parched, and in need of exfoliation and hydration. Tried-and-true treatments will begin to improve the barrier function of the skin while slowly burning off the damaged skin (Table 15–1). They may be used in combination, or individually, depending on your experience and client need. After-care is as important as the peel. Depending upon the treatment that you apply, look at standard protocol for specific post-peel/treatment instructions.

Type of Peels	Benefit of Peels
Glycolic Peel	The glycolic peel can be used for a light exfoliating treatment on this skin type. It lifts dead cellular debris, which can enhance hydration and penetration of moisturization. It can also be the first step in a multilevel treatment, and using a lower-level preparation can give you many cues as to how the skin will respond to a more aggressive approach later. Perform this peel weekly or every other week for 6 to 8 weeks depending upon damage and tolerance. Then meet with the doctor for follow-up to determine the next plan.
Microdermabrasion	The microdermabrasion will eliminate surface buildup, stimulate circulation, and create an open field for the next layer of a peel, and for a hydrator to penetrate more readily, and to temporarily tighten the skin through a slight inflammation. Perform this treatment bimonthly for 8 to 10 weeks, then follow up with the doctor.
Enzymatic Peel	Enzymes found in papaya (papain), pineapple (bromelain), or pumpkin will slowly dissolve dead skin cell buildup (proteins/keratinization). This treatment can be very conservative and can be performed along with a routine standard facial indefinitely. However, it may not be enough to affect photodamaged skin beyond improvements seen after 2 to 3 months.
Trichloracetic Acid (TCA Peel)	A TCA peel can be beneficial particularly for photodamaged skin, which also has a loss of elasticity, is hyperpigmented, and needs lightening. This requires some preparation and is not indicated for Fitzpatrick V or VI skin types due to its potential to keloid, pigment, and scar. *This peel is physician-applied or directed.* The TCA peel is highly effective for photodamaged skin. Lower levels 10%–15% can be performed three to four times a year, whereas higher levels 20%–30% may be performed once a year.

(See Chapter 18 for peel protocols)

Table 15–1   Peels for Dry/Dehydrated, Photoaged Skin

Oily Skin

Treatments for oily skin that is also acneic (see pages 156–158) and hormonally challenged (see pages 158–160) are a large part of your business. Oily skin knows no age or gender boundary. In addition to treating the most difficult cases, you will find that if you can improve measurably the skin fitness of someone fighting acne, you will win not only loyal clients, but their friends and relatives will flock to you.

If the skin is clear and oily, we can affect the skin by applying standard protocols of a routine facial, which may combine an AHA/Beta or microdermabrasion application. On this skin, we are using primarily light water-based gels, acidic-astringent–type formulas, masks, and exfoliants aimed at cutting oil and equalizing the sebaceous activity or production. The skin may also require the use of performance agents such as benzoyl peroxide or salicylic, glycolic, and azelaic acids for deep pore cleansing and acneic lesion control.

Home care for oily skin

A.M.

1. Cleanse with a water-based citrus, AHA and or BHA gel or light lotion cleanser and follow with companion toner.
2. Spray with Isolutrol marine-based algae product used for controlling oil.
3. Apply performance agents AHA/BHA hydroxys, benzoyl peroxide or a sulfur-based product for exfoliation and oil control, and hyaluronic acid for nourishing.
4. Use a light oil-free sunscreen containing antioxidants and zinc oxide with **SPF** of at least 30.

P.M.

1. Repeat A.M.
2. Repeat A.M.
3. Repeat A.M.

Oily skin in-office peels   These treatments are to be used as a guide and are training and experience dependent (Table 15–2). In addition, it is necessary to use assessments based upon the instrument classifications to determine which peel/treatment to apply to a specific condition based upon Fitzpatrick Skin Type, photodamage levels and types, and Kligman's Acne Classification.

Oily Acneic Skin

If the acneic condition is a Grade I or II, and in the Fitzpatrick I or II range, we will be more aggressive with acids with the client than if they are in the III, IV, V, or VI color range. We do not want to bring up more pigment, creating postinflammatory pigmentation in darker skin. Otherwise, oily skin with acne can tolerate weekly treatment plans, and if the client is experiencing Grade III and IV types of acne, they should be referred to the physician for medical support as well. Common forms of medications may be oral, topical, or a combination of both. These medications may include clindamycin phosphate erythromycin, tetracycline, tretinoin, adapolene, sulfur, and resorcinol. This skin type will benefit from all of the treatments mentioned, but it is always advisable to start with the lightest treatment to obtain a benchmark. That way you will slowly learn how much the client can tolerate, and you will learn much about their skin.

Home care

A.M.

1. Cleanse with a water-based citrus, AHA, BHA, benzoyl peroxide, lactic acid, bentonite, azelaic acid, or combination cleanser.
2. Spray with Isolutrol marine-based algae product used for controlling oil.
3. Apply performance agents AHA/Beta hydroxys, benzoyl peroxide, or a sulfur-based product for exfoliation and oil control and anti-inflammation. Hyaluronic acid is good for nourishing, and azulene or bisabolol (chamomile) for soothing.

Glycolic Acid	A glycolic peel can be used alone or in concert with other elements for oily skin. When used alone it is best as a low pH solution to dry with a high concentration of glycolic acid. It is best used on skin which is aged 25 to 55 years.
Salicylic Acid	Salicylic acid peels can be used to fight oil and bacteria. Always patch test and watch for allergies to aspirin.
Microdermabrasion	Microdermabrasion can be used successfully on oily skin for exfoliation, and to even skin tone. Not for use directly on cysts or pustules.
Jessner's Peel	Both Jessner's and modified Jessner's can be used successfully on oily skin, and they serve to lighten pigmented areas (always patch test this peel).
Enzymes	Papaya (papain), pineapple (bromelain), and pumpkin provide excellent exfoliation of dead skin cells that may be contributing to an acneic condition. They are an excellent choice for sensitive oily or acneic skin and provide hydration as well.
AHA/TCA Microdermabrasion Combination	AHA or light TCA peels along with microdermabrasion can be applied in layers by performing the microdermabrasion first, and then the glycolic or TCA. A full assessment should be made, and a consult with the physician prior to performing this advanced peel. The combination peels require advanced training and pretreatment with skin lighteners and retinoic acid as well.

(See Chapter 18 for peel protocols)

Table 15–2 Oily Skin Peels

4. Use a light oil-free sunscreen containing antioxidants, zinc oxide with SPF of at least 30.

P.M.

1. Repeat A.M.
2. Repeat A.M.
3. Repeat A.M.

This client may also be using antibiotics both orally and topically. If a topical antibiotic is prescribed by the physician, apply it after cleansing. In addition, warn the client about increased photosensitivity and potential yeast infections. Recommend eating yogurt or taking acidophilus tablets.

In-office peels   These peels are to be used as a guide and are training and experience dependent (Table 15–3). In addition, it is necessary to use assessments based upon the instrument classifications to determine which peel/treatment to apply to a specific condition based upon Fitzpatrick Skin Type, photodamage levels and types, and Kligman's Acne Classification.

Glycolic Acid	A glycolic peel can be used alone or in concert with other elements for oily acneic skin. When used alone it is best as a low pH solution to dry with a high concentration of glycolic acid. It is best used on skin which is aged 25 to 55 years.
Salicylic Acid	Salicylic acid peels can be used to fight oil and are good bacteria fighters. Always patch test and watch for allergies to aspirin.
Microdermabrasion	Microdermabrasion can be used successfully on oily acneic skin for exfoliation, and to even skin tone. Not for use directly on cysts or pustules.
Jessner's Peel	Both Jessner's and modified Jessner's can be used successfully on oily acneic skin, and serves to lighten pigmented areas (always patch test this peel).
Enzymes	Papaya (papain), pineapple (bromelain), and pumpkin provide excellent exfoliation of dead skin cells that may be contributing to an acneic condition. They are an excellent choice for sensitive acneic skin and provide hydration as well.
AHA/TCA Microdermabrasion Combination	AHA or light TCA peels along with microdermabrasion can be applied in layers by performing the microdermabrasion first, and then the glycolic, salicylic, azelaic or low level TCA. A full assessment should be made, and a consult with the physician prior to performing this advanced peel. The combination peels require advanced training and pretreatment with skin lighteners and retinoic acid as well.

(See Chapter 18 for peel protocols)

Table 15–3   Oily Acneic Peels

Hormonally Challenged Skin

Hormonally challenged skin is not unlike acneic skin, but it is difficult to control the hormones which are driving the acne by swelling the hair follicle and trapping bacteria and debris along the shaft. Products and treatments for this skin type are similar to those for treating acneic skin, but they can be coordinated to align with menses, be it mid cycle, or 8 to 10 days prior to starting menstruation. Use the protocol for acneic skin and adjust accordingly.

No skin is more dynamic than that of the acne prone which is hormonally charged. It can change midstream. You will need to have multiphasic products, both aggressive and nurturing; combination treatments, with many elements working synergistically; and medical intervention perched to help this often-exasperated client.

For the older dehydrated, hormonally compromised skin, treatments and products that work for dry dehydrated skin are excellent choices. In addition, you may consider using products for sensitive skin containing ingredients such as azulene and allantoin since they are known for comforting reactive skin. Here are a few tips for hormonally challenged skin at different stages.

Teenagers and Accutane   Teenagers are especially vulnerable to acne and the psychosocial issues surrounding having unclear skin. Depending upon the stage of the acne, physicians and parents will put teenagers on Accutane therapy (vitamin A) to shrink sebaceous glands, slow down acneic activity and for scar management and to lesson the lesion frequency. These clients will require a different type of program, as they will be unable to use AHAs BHAs, retinol, or retinoic acid. They will be under direct supervision of a physician and will typically be prescribed a nonactive cleanser and an emollient moisturizer. You will not want to perform acid peels or microdermabrasion on teenagers undergoing Accutane treatment.

Pregnancy   Pregnancy and lactation are contraindications for AHAs, BHA, and enzymes. Light forms of microdermabrasion are acceptable for treatment in Fitzpatrick Type I–III; however, in Fitzpatrick Type IV, V, and VI the use of moor mud, clays, and sulfur masks are safer due to the potential of postinflammatory pigmentation.

Have a full line of products without performance agents or active agents, such as clay, sulfur-based, and citrus products along with treatments such as light microdermabrasion and gentle papaya enzymatic masks with extractions available for your clients who become pregnant. Remove them from acids and aggressive products at once. It is not so much that these ingredients are dangerous; it is simply that it is unethical to test them on pregnant women. If you design treatments that include massage and hand and foot treatments for mothers-to-be, you will booked for weeks ahead. Watch aromatherapy, however, as some women have morning sickness that will last all day.

Perimenopausal   The perimenopausal period is considered the 10 to 15 years before the actual passage into menopause. Susan Love, M.D., describes in her book titled, *Dr. Susan Love's Hormone Book, Making Informed Choices About Menopause* (Love, 1998), that even though transitory, symptoms arising from the perimenopausal period can actually be worse then those in menopause. The changes that one begins to experience during this phase of life include symptoms that are related to the skin.

This period usually begins in the mid-to-late thirties. In some clients, the skin dries up; in others, the first signs of acne appear. You will need to meet the changing need in the client as she travels through this important time. Many good products are on the market for this age group and they fall under the umbrella of antiaging. Keep in mind the basics:

• cleanse
• exfoliate
• hydrate and nourish
• protect

This goes for in-office treatments as well. You may find this client beginning to ask about surgical procedures such as blepharoplasty (eyelift) and texture-smoothing procedures such as laser or photo rejuvenation. Develop a comprehensive program that includes home care, in-office peels, and alternative health therapies including massage/body work, yoga, diet, exercise, and working with colleagues on a referral basis. This client is your mainstay, along with those in menopause and beyond. You will have this client for many years if you set the groundwork in place now.

Menopausal Menopause brings about changes in the life of women that are positive, empowering, and liberating. One of those changes is the cessation of menstruation or . . . *no more periods.* This is exciting for most, particularly if a woman has a positive outlook on her life. Christiane Northrup, M.D., states in her book *Women's Bodies, Women's Wisdom,* that if you have not dealt with certain issues in your earlier years, they will present themselves for resolution during menopause. It is inspiring to pass through this phase of life, and to become aware of oneself both in growth, and in acceptance of our limitations.

Do keep in mind that women who are perimenopausal or menopausal may be experiencing hot flashes, in which case you do not want to use your warm or hot mittens, or wrap them up in your finest down comforter. They will throw them off (not to mention become cranky with you). Stay in the room at all times, to avoid undue strain or stress on this client, who may require cool cloths, ice water, or the need to get up off a table at a moment's notice. Migraine headaches or allergies can be brought on by scents (always ask about aromatherapy); however, light, soothing scents such as rose, rosemary, lavender, or **sage** are all good for relaxation during a treatment. Massage, lymphatic drainage, and shiatsu are excellent when used in combination for this client.

Postmenopausal Women who are postmenopausal may still get an occasional hot flash; always check first on the temperature to meet the need of the client. If heat is to be used during the treatment, such as steam or mittens, they will usually tell you if they cannot tolerate it as it may bring about a hot flash. This client is usually quite comfortable with most techniques, although do not overstimulate or exfoliate the skin; it may be thinning and will bruise easily. If microdermabrasion is used, make sure that it is with the lowest setting and pressure. If you use acid peels, apply lighter versions with higher pH levels, and make sure to superhydrate the skin with a mask and nourishing hydrators after treatment.

Actinic Keratosis

Actinic keratosis (AK) is an advanced condition and will require medical intervention. It usually presents in Fitzpatrick I and II and occasionally III types. While some AK may not be precancerous, if left untreated it may turn into skin cancer. The physician will be brought into the loop as early as possible. If you have a client that you suspect has actinic activity, which many with photodamage will, set up your treatment plan with the doctor.

The doctor may prescribe a topical gel or a cream called 5-fluorouracil or 5-FU. This treatment is applied topically according to the depth and amount of the actinic keratosis. Some patients are instructed to use this in a full-out aggressive program of daily use for

6 to 8 weeks, whereas others are instructed to use it in a **pulse method** (intermittently applied) weekly or biweekly.

With the pulsed or intermittent program, it can be used in conjunction with other topicals such as glycolic, lactic, salicylic, and retinoic acids. Some esthetic treatments supporting patients undergoing this treatment are proving to be beneficial. AHA and BHA peels, microdermabrasion, and hydrating nourishing masks are offering additional penetration, exfoliation, and comfort.

Daily Use of Medication Prescribed by the Physician

If your patient is using 5-fluorouracil medication *daily* as prescribed by the physician, you will not be treating the patient for the duration of the treatment phase. The patient will be given a topical steroid by the doctor for soothing and comfort. It is the nature of this treatment to burn off the skin, and it looks charred. This will last for several weeks, and the patient is instructed to see the physician during this time to make certain that the treated areas are free of infection. Sometimes a patient will develop a staph infection and will need to be given an antibiotic.

Weekly 5-FU Program with the Addition of Home-Care Products

Pulsed or intermittent treatments will yield slower results, but if the physician determines that a less aggressive approach to apply the 5-FU is indicated, these two methods can reduce morbidity to the patient while increasing comfort and encourage the necessary behavioral changes in lifestyle. The patient becomes much more aware of appropriate skin-care practices while following this regimen—providing that it is simple.

Home care

A.M.

1. Cleanser/toning—AHA, or combination AHA and beta hydroxy acid, or an enzyme such as papaya or pineapple, with hydrating and moisturizing ingredients such as glycerin or an oil (remember this skin is dry and often dehydrated) such as **evening primrose oil** (fatty acids . . . good for hot flashes too!)
2. Hydrating moisture cream or lotion containing AHAs, BHAs, or a combination, along with amino acids, antioxidants, allantoin, and/or bisabolol (chamomile derivative) for soothing
3. Apply a sunscreen with a minimum of a 30SPF, containing zinc oxide and titanium dioxide.

P.M.

1. Cleanser/toner same as A.M.
2. Moisturizer same as A.M.

Once a week apply 5-FU in place of night moisturizer.

Biweekly 5-FU Program

Home care

A.M.

1. Cleanser/toner program same as for weekly
2. Moisturizer same as for weekly
3. Sunscreen daily, rain or shine, same as for weekly

P.M.

1. Cleanser/toner program same as for A.M.
2. Moisturizer same as for A.M.

Twice a week apply 5-FU in place of night moisturizer.

Esthetician-Guided and -Treated Program for Actinic Keratosis

As we might imagine, an esthetician-guided program is highly recommended and diligently followed by the patient with AK. The opportunity for the patient to learn about their skin is provided and carried out by the esthetician by a combination of home-care protocols and in-office visits. The esthetician will have time to educate this patient and to give helpful hints about whether they are following their home-care program.

Currently there are two pulsed-treatment methods being followed where the patient comes in for treatments weekly or biweekly. These treatments consists of a thorough cleansing, a lower concentrated (70%) buffered glycolic peel, and an application of 5-FU. The patient is encouraged to come in at the end of the day so that they may just leave the treatment in place throughout the night. The home care is routine, similar to the home treatment unassisted by the esthetician.

Weekly Esthetician-Assisted Program

Home care

A.M.

1. Cleanser/toner—same as above
2. Moisturizer
3. Sunscreen

P.M.

1. Cleanser/toner
2. Moisturizer

In-office visit with esthetician

1. Cleanse.
2. Apply peel prepping solution.

3. Apply light glycolic peel (70% high pH, buffered) 4 minutes to start.
4. Remove peel.
5. Apply 5-FU.

Leave on.

Patient goes back to regular program the next day.

Biweekly Esthetician-Assisted Program

Home care

A.M.

1. Cleanser/toner
2. Moisturizer
3. Sunscreen

P.M.

1. Cleanser/toner
2. Moisturizer

In-office visit with esthetician

1. Cleanse.
2. Apply peel prepping solution.
3. Apply light glycolic peel (70% high pH, buffered) 4 minutes to start.
4. Remove peel.
5. Apply 5-FU.

Leave on.

These treatments are experimental and must be supported by the physician. The results are slower as indicated, and the peels may not be appropriate for more advanced cases of actinic keratosis. These treatments are excellent prepatory phases for more advanced treatment of actinic keratosis, such as daily 5-FU or laser resurfacing.

Rosacea

Medical treatment for rosacea (see image in color insert) is necessary to avoid permanent damage and will be determined by the physician depending on the stage that the patient is experiencing. Once the diagnosis is made by the physician, the appropriate treatment plan may be initiated and followed by both the patient and the esthetician. Typically, the physician will prescribe a topical antibiotic treatment, which is commonly called metronidazole. Metrogel, Metrocream, Metrolotion, and Noritate are all brand names of this medication. If the patient is experiencing a flare, an oral antibiotic such as tetracycline, Minocin/minocycline, or erythromycin may also be prescribed. In extreme cases of stage III type rosacea, **isotretinoin** or Accutane (an oral vitamin A medication) may be prescribed.

These medications work by slowing down the sebaceous activity and shrinking the glands. Once the condition is under control it is much easier to maintain, and under medical supervision you may introduce a comprehensive skin-care program to this patient. Stress, diet, and exercise all contribute to the flushing condition of rosacea, and can be modified to relieve some of the symptoms.

Stress

Stress will increase flushing by increasing the body's "fight-or-flight" recognition by stimulating our sympathetic nervous system. The vascular system will begin to ignite by sensing automatically the rise in adrenaline. As the heart rate goes up, the arteries, veins, and capillaries increase in blood flow. In the case of the patient with rosacea, this will present as fully dilated facial vessels, and sometimes an accompanying burning sensation. Looking for ways to combat stress in the patient with rosacea is paramount to their comfort.

Diet

Diet also plays a role with the rosacea patient. Sugar (including alcohol), caffeine, spicy foods, super-high carbohydrates, and heavy meals can all contribute to the flushing by stimulating blood flow as well. It is important to reduce or eliminate these foods in favor of slower-acting foods such as complex carbohydrates and proteins, and to drink more water to flush the system.

Exercise

Choosing forms of exercise that may be cooler in nature such as water sports, yoga, or Pilates, performed in a cooler room might be a good alternative to overstimulating the vascular system. Outdoor activity will stimulate the vascular system just as much as indoor exercise will. Make certain that if the patient chooses to spend time skiing, snowboarding, or any other outdoor sport that he or she cover all exposed areas with a sunscreen containing zinc oxide and/or titanium dioxide and wear hats, gloves, and appropriate eyewear. When returning to a warm room, one should acclimate slowly, not all at once.

Treatments

Home care for stage I or II rosacea with a **dry skin type**

A.M.

1. Cleanser/toner—This lotion or cream cleanser should be calming and soothing and include ingredients such as sodium hyaluronate (water binding, nonirritating), arnica (for reducing inflammation), green tea (soothing/antioxidant), and papaya (exfoliating).
2. Medication—antibiotic/antifungal lotion or cream

3. Hydrating/moisturizing lotion or cream containing amino acids (proteins). The Mark Lees Sensitive Science line is excellent, particularly the Soothing Cleanser and Toner, and Calm and Restore. Other important ingredients are antioxidants, such as alpha lipoic acid and vitamin E, and, if flare is under control, a lower concentrated AHA with a high pH for exfoliation.
4. Sunscreen containing zinc oxide, titanium dioxide
5. Mineral makeup as a base

P.M.

1. Cleanser/toner—same as A.M.
2. Medication—same as A.M.
3. Moisturizer—same as A.M.

Home care for stage I rosacea or II with an oily skin type

A.M.

1. Cleanser/toner—gel or light lotion based with a light sulfur base (anti-inflammatory, antibiotic), or lower level AHA with a high pH (not as irritating) at 3.5–3.8
2. Medication—gel, lotion, or cream
3. Hydrating gel with soothing ingredients such as allantoin, hyaluronic acid, and lower-level AHA with high pH, and Calm and Restore by Mark Lees
4. Sunscreen lotion with antioxidants such as pycnogenol (pine), (bioflaviods), and zinc oxide
5. Mineral powder makeup

P.M.

1. Cleanser/toner—same as A.M.
2. Medication—same as A.M.
3. Hydrator—same as A.M.

Home care for extreme cases of stage III rosacea This is under direct supervision of physician only.

A.M.

1. Cleanser. Some physicians will recommend Cetaphyl; Toleriane products by La Roche Posay are excellent for skin undergoing Accutane treatment.
2. Medication—oral; this is often Accutane, an oral medication that dries the sebaceous system and is a contraindication for most treatments and products.
3. Protector—Vaseline is used on lips (they become very dry), and often a moisturizer such as Lubriderm, or Calm and Restore by Mark Lees, or Toleriane Facial Fluid, by La Roche Posay.

P.M.

1. Cleanser—repeat A.M.
2. Medication—repeat A.M.
3. Hydrator—repeat A.M.

Again, this patient is under the direct supervision of the physician, usually a dermatologist. Regular blood draws are made to ensure that this medication is not adversely affecting the organs of this patient. It is a controversial medication, but it has made a positive change in the lives of many who have undergone treatment.

In-office treatment for rosacea in stage I   The key to treating this skin type is to not overtreat. You will need to compartmentalize this treatment by sectioning the facial areas and using two or three treatments on the appropriate areas, all in one setting. Frequency should not be greater than every 4 to 6 weeks, depending upon the amount of flushing the patient is experiencing, and the amount of control they have with medication and home-care compliance. When treating this patient . . . do *not* use the following:

- **Massage:** it will always create more erythema
- **Steam:** it will always create more erythema and often will increase flare, if you must spray, use a cool spritz
- **Brush or microdermabrasion on the butterfly area (nose, cheeks):** it is too aggressive for this skin type and will increase likelihood of more erythema
- **High levels of AHAs and BHAs with a low pH:** as rosacea becomes under control, lighter levels of these ingredients can benefit, but they must be used with caution and at a higher pH level

Rosacea can be treated by an esthetician when appropriate applications and materials are used. If the patient is not flaring, has minimal erythema, and is enjoying a reasonably clear phase, here is an example of a soothing, exfoliating, hydrating treatment:

1. Cleanse with a non AHA/BHA appropriate to the skin type of client
2. Apply a hydrating mask to nose and cheek area (always test patch first; if it burns, remove it). It may contain azulene (enriched chamomile), aloe, bisabolol, and licorice extract for soothing, as well as honey for hydration.
3. The outer areas of the face may well tolerate an exfoliating treatment while the mask that you have applied is setting. You may use a low-level, high-pH, buffered glycolic peel such as MD Forte, 70%, on the outer perimeters, forehead, and neck for 3 minutes to start. Alternatively, you could use a noncrystal **microdermabrader** on the outer regions such as the frontal, temporal, mandible, and mental regions for exfoliation. Just make certain that you do not use either of these methods on the rosacea-affected areas.
4. When you have completed using the exfoliating treatments on the outer areas, apply the hydrating soothing mask over the entire areas that have been given treatment by the peel or the microdermabrader.

5. While this mask is setting up on the full face and neck, microdermabrade the hands and arms, and follow with a hydrating mask on those as well.

6. Remove mask from face and neck first. With a larger cotton tip applicator, briskly follow with a light brush of liquid nitrogen to cool and soothe, follow with a copper hydrating gel (Procyte 2001) for healing. Apply a moisturizing sunscreen with an SPF of at least 30, containing antioxidants, zinc oxide, and titanium dioxide.

7. Then remove mask from arms, and follow with hydrating copper gel, amino acid lotion, and/or moisturizing sunscreen containing antioxidants and an SPF of at least 30.

8. Apply mineral makeup with zinc and titanium dioxide for more protection.

Summary

When in doubt about a treatment or an assessment, always consult the physician. Risk management practices are necessary for the health of your practice. Make certain to obtain an informed consent document as protocol. Look for contraindications prior to recommending a home-care program or an in-office treatment plan. Hormonally challenged skin is not unlike other types of skin, and can be treated with the same treatments, once classification instruments have been applied.

Frequently Asked Questions

1. **How does the esthetician determine how aggressive to be on a given classification or skin condition?**

   The basic rule of thumb is a test patch. Start lighter than you would if this client had been with you a while, and expect subclinical conditions. There are often surprises and sometimes clients can be allergic to a preparation. Think: slow and methodical. Document everything.

2. **It seems that hormonally driven skin conditions are the most difficult to treat; what can the esthetician do to help the client with this problem?**

   It is true, hormonally driven acne and rosacea flares can be difficult to treat. Maintain a positive attitude for the client, and remind them that they have been clear before. Tell them that you understand how disheartening this is for them, and that you are there to support them.

   Go back through the home-care program and see if you need to change some preparations. Check on compliance. Tweak in-office treatments to accommodate change in condition. Consult with the physician, and set up appropriate follow-up appointments.

CHAPTER 16

Treatments, Home Care and Self-Care for Health-Compromised Clients

- Introduction
- Lupus
- Cancer
- Bleeding Disorders
- Parkinson's Disease
- Multiple Sclerosis
- Diabetes
- Communicable Diseases
- Summary
- Frequently Asked Questions

Introduction

Clinical estheticians will often be visited by people with health-compromising disorders and diseases. For each of these special clients, it is of great relief to find a caring, well-trained, and experienced skin-care professional who understands how to treat those with health issues. This may mean directing a self-care program at home, in addition to what their physician is providing. Often we find that people with health problems have no skin-care support and can be greatly comforted by just a few steps, which may include home-care products and in-office treatments.

The following conditions are commonly seen in the practice of the clinical esthetician. As always, prior to treatments, obtain permission from the attending physician and/or the physician with whom you are associated.

Lupus

Lupus or **Systemic Lupus Erythematosus (SLE)** is an autoimmune disease, which means that the body's immune system attacks its own healthy cells (Rothfield, 2000, p. 11). It is a chronic rheumatic disease, in which the connective tissue throughout the body becomes inflamed. The cause is unknown. The symptoms of lupus are swollen, painful joints, skin rashes, sensitivity to sun, high fever, hair loss, purple hands and feet, and fatigue. These symptoms can change drastically from day to day. The rashes are typically on the upper parts of the body, but they will generally present in the butterfly area on the nasal and **zygomatic** regions. This is often confused with rosacea, may itch, and have small lesions or a rosaceous type of flare or inflammation to the skin.

Medical Treatment for Lupus

Depending upon the severity of the disease, people with lupus will be treated with aspirin or ibuprofen for mild cases, and for more severe cases Vioxx® or Celebrex® may be prescribed. The goal in treatment will be to decrease inflammation. In more advanced cases, where internal organs have been affected, a steroid may be introduced to slow down the body's immune system and thus the attacks on the healthier cells.

Increase in photosensitivity   Clients with lupus will at times be extremely sensitive to light and sun. A sunscreen containing broad-spectrum protection against UVA and UVB rays, along with minerals zinc oxide and titanium, would be essential for daily use. In addition, broad-brimmed hats, sunglasses, and long-sleeved clothing are necessary to protect from the heightened sensitivity that patients may experience.

Raynaud's Phenomenon   Raynaud's Phenomenon can also appear on the extremities of a person with lupus. The condition is characterized by extreme vascularity (redness), primarily on the hands, and may include small ulcers on the tip of the fingers (Provost, 1995, p. 15). It is often caused by exposure to cold or emotional stimuli. The hands may feel painful, numb, or prickly, or they may burn. Raynaud's Phenomenon is also seen in people with scleroderma (an immune system disorder) arthritis, and pulmonary hypertension (high blood pressure within the lungs). The treatment focuses on protecting the body from extremes in temperature—particularly cold—and the use of vasodilators.

Skin Care and Treatments for Clients with Lupus

As an esthetician working in a medical office, you almost certainly will encounter a client presenting with lupus. Women between the ages of 15 to 45 are the most common ones to be struck with lupus. African-American women are three times as likely to develop the disease, and the rate is similarly high among Hispanics, Asians, and Native Americans (White, 2001, p. 983).

You need to determine the severity of the disease by having the physician evaluate the client before you begin a treatment plan. If the condition is not severe, you may proceed with a treatment plan that may mirror the care given a patient with sensitive or rosaceous skin. This would include both home care and an in-office treatment as follows.

Home care   Home-care protocol would consist of products containing hydrating, soothing, and calming ingredients containing high levels of UVA and UVB protection, along with mineral zinc oxide and titanium dioxide. Depending upon skin type and condition, some ingredients that you may find in products beneficial in a home-care regimen for a client with lupus are given below.

A.M.

Cleanser: green tea extract, allantoin, papaya, red clover, licorice
Antioxidant: alpha lipoic acid, vitamin E, low levels of **vitamin C, selenium,** or **beta carotene**
Hydrator/Moisturizer: sage, **phospholipids,** evening primrose oil and **lecithin, linoleic acid, dimethicone** for barrier protection
Environmental/Sunscreen Protection: zinc oxide, titanium dioxide

P.M.

Cleanser: same as A.M.
Gentle Exfoliant: retinol, papaya, pineapple, lactic acid
Hydrator: amino acids, linseed oil, hyaluronic acid, **copper peptide**

In-office treatments

1. Cleanse with tepid water and gentle cleansing agent.
2. Apply a gentle enzymatic or vegetal peel/mask to face, neck, and chest (if desired).
3. Mist periodically with slightly warm water, while allowing mask to set up.
4. If hands are not affected, cleanse and apply light microdermabrasion, then apply hydrating mask to hands and arms. If hands are affected, eliminate microdermabrasion and give a gentle hand massage while facial peel/mask is on.
5. Remove enzyme peel/mask and apply hydrating mask with a light massage.
6. Remove mask from hands and apply amino acid lotion or hydrating cream with sun protection.
7. Remove facial-hydrating mask.
8. Apply serum containing antioxidants, hyaluronic acid, and/or copper gel.
9. Apply hydrating moisturizer.
10. Apply environmental protection with zinc oxide and titanium dioxide.
11. Apply mineral powder as appropriate or indicated by client.

A shoulder massage is also of benefit, as people with lupus may be under a great deal of stress due to the limitations created by this disease. Work closely and communicate with your client and they will let you know how they are feeling when they come for treatment. Tune in. It may be that you need to vary your treatments for them often.

Cancer

Most of us have been affected directly by cancer, or we know of someone who has been. Cancer means "wild growth of cells" (McCutcheon, 2002, p. 3). These prolific cells begin to eat up all of the normal cells and take their place in the body. They do not replace the normal processes of the healthy cell; they just multiply and feed off the host.

Any area in the body can develop this disease, which if left untreated can eventually spread, or **metastasize** and can ultimately take the life of the person afflicted. Cancers have different structures and some are slower growing than others. Nevertheless, all need some form of treatment. If there is a positive aspect to having a fast-growing cancer, it is that it can be detected more readily, as it grows faster than normal cells. The faster the detection, the faster the treatment can begin to save a life.

The average survival rate for all cancers has increased to 60 percent; major improvements have been made in detection of breast, prostate, and colon cancer. Furthermore, treatments are evolving and becoming more effective and less painful; it is estimated that within 10 years survivors of *all* cancers will ultimately reach 85 percent to 90 percent (Jordan, 2002).

Dealing with the Emotional Aspects of a Client with Cancer

As with other health issues, a clinical esthetician will need to become adept at treating and understanding both the physical and emotional aspects of those clients with cancer. A client may become emotional about hair loss on the head, eyebrows, and lashes; become fearful about upcoming treatments; or focus on their own mortality. It is important that you remain compassionate, objective, dependable, and calm while working with such a client. You may need to change your treatment plan and home-care recommendations often.

Facial and body treatments can be of great relief to a person going through cancer therapy. One must be flexible, however, because depending on the severity, stage, or nature of the disease, the appointments must be given only when the patient is feeling well enough, and the red and white blood cell counts are where they are recommended to be by their physician. If the patient needs to cancel or miss an appointment, just let it go. It will be necessary to become acquainted with the physician and consult routinely. This is the only way that we will learn how best to take care of these special clients. Each person will require a slightly different program.

Skin Care for Clients with Cancer

Home care   Home care for cancer patients is essential because their skin becomes very dry with treatments such as chemotherapy, radiation, and surgeries. The skin may also darken, scale, flake, lose pigment, develop erythema and sores, swell, or become jaundiced (yellow). It is vitally important that we do not give them anything with active agents such as retinoic acid or higher levels of bleaching aids, which may affect the blood. Do not use AHAs, BHAs, or other exfoliants in home care. Keep the program simple and meet the needs of your client by not overtreating them.

A.M.

1. Cleanse with a gentle rinse-off cleanser that is also moisturizing.
2. Apply a moisturizer with antioxidants, azulene (chamomile), and amino acids for hydration.

3. Use environmental protection such as sunscreen with zinc oxide and titanium dioxide.
4. Mineral powder and makeup as appropriate and desired by client.

P.M.

1. Repeat A.M.
2. Repeat A.M.

If health and interest-level is apparent, you could suggest a moisturizing mask containing sodium hyaluronate (water binding/hydrating) or calendula extract (for healing, soothing and calming).

In-office treatments   In-office therapeutic treatments may consist of a soothing, hydrating facial, with procedures that are not too long or involved. Sometimes this client may become nauseated, so check in and make sure he or she is comfortable. Have a glass of water standing by, and an empty container to use if the client becomes ill. If a client does become ill, stand by, get cool cloths for the forehead, and make certain that the individual does not fall. When appropriate have the client lie back down for a few minutes before trying to get up. Reassure that everything is just fine; there may be embarrassment about messing up your floor or treatment bed.

You can design many treatments for your clients with health issues. Just keep in mind that stinging or burning from a peel or microdermabrasion is too harsh for them in their present state, and prolonged steaming can be nauseating for some. *Do not leave the room* during the treatment. Offer treatments that are soothing and relaxing, such as:

1. Cleanse with a gentle cleanser containing lavender.
2. Apply a light exfoliating mask that is hydrating and complements the lavender scent of the cleanser.
3. Perform a gentle massage (facial).
4. Apply a soothing hydrating mask.
5. Cleanse and perform a hand massage.
6. Apply a mask to the hands.
7. Remove the facial mask.
8. Apply hydrating serum with hyaluronic acid, lipids, and antioxidants.
9. Apply moisturizer.
10. Remove mask from hands.
11. Apply environmental protection SPF30 with zinc oxide and titanium dioxide to face and hands.

Terminal Cancer Patient

This patient will teach you much about peace, love, and patience. The reality of working with someone terminally ill is truly life altering. Often the patient will have come to terms with their mortality and will be helping family and others to cope with the eventuality of their leaving. It is fine to ask questions. Offer to go to their home if they are unable to see you in the clinic. A soothing hand and foot massage would be wonderful for this patient. Bring along a CD or tape with music that is relaxing and pleases them.

Often family members are exhausted and emotional, so you may be able to help them as well with stress by offering a complimentary visit for a treatment. By now a **hospice** may be involved and attending nurses may give you guidance on what to use or not to use in the way of massage product. Some patients may also enjoy a light shoulder or scalp massage. Each individual is unique. One person may want her nails polished; another a hand and arm massage. Just your presence may be of great comfort. These patients will often slip in and out of sleep. Some may speak of dreams they are having and may have difficulty discerning between the dreams and reality. This is normal. They may be in pain, in which case the attending nurse, physician, or hospice worker will help to relieve it through medications such as morphine. Use your intuition and allow the nurse, physician, family member, or the hospice volunteer, to guide your movements by gently showing them what you are doing. If the patient is uncomfortable with any of your movements, stop at once, be silent. Quietly leave and turn the patient back over to their caregiver.

If such patients have been your clients, it will mean much to them and to the family that you are able to help them at this time. It is fine to cry, and to say that you love them. Make visits short, and let the family know when you are available, and that they can depend on you. For more information about cancer, visit www.cancer.com.

Bleeding Disorders

This section was written with the help of Barbara Evans Forss, a woman with Factor VII-deficient **hemophilia,** who volunteers as an educator and advocate for anyone living with a rare, inherited bleeding disorder.

Bleeding disorders are primarily hereditary defects in the clotting system. Plasma proteins (also called clotting factors), are greatly reduced or nonexistent in hemophiliacs, the majority of whom are males with Factor VIII- or IX-deficient hemophilia. Other, rarer factor deficiencies may affect both males and females in equal numbers. Another more common bleeding disorder, affecting males and females and known as **von Willebrand's disease (vWD),** may actually be present in as much as 2 percent of the population, according to studies sanctioned by the National Hemophilia Foundation.

All bleeding disorders have one thing in common: the blood does not clot efficiently. A bump, bruise, or cut might have major consequences to this person, so it is important to be aware of this client's special circumstances.

Since most people who have been diagnosed with a bleeding disorder also use a variety of medicines and methods to self-treat, it is very important to listen to the client. Most hemophiliacs regularly infuse clotting factor, and many people with vWD use a variety of coagulation medicines. They are accustomed to managing their bleeding episodes, are quite knowledgeable about their condition, and may have much to teach you about its symptoms and complications.

What is of great concern, however, is the client who may be unaware of an underlying bleeding disorder. Hemophilia was once considered only a male disorder and was usually diagnosed at birth, when a newly circumcised male would hemorrhage. Most women to-day are routinely dismissed and misdiagnosed for a bleeding problem, even unusually heavy or long menses, or other bleeding symptoms, as it is often said that "women are supposed to bleed."

Use a Conservative Approach to Home Care and Treatment

It is extremely important to use a conservative approach in all product use, treatments, and home-care recommendations with these clients. A thorough history of bleeding episodes should be taken, so that any symptoms of excessive bleeding should lead you to suspect an undiagnosed bleeding disorder. These include:

* excessive bleeding after brushing teeth, flossing, or dental work
* unusually heavy periods and/or long duration
* nosebleeds
* bruising
* joint pain

Guidelines to Assisting People with Bleeding Disorders

As estheticians we are traveling into uncharted territory when treating those with bleeding problems. Here are a few guidelines:

* Patch test everything you use or sell to the client.
* Do not perform extractions, unless the client has been prophylactically treated with their clotting medication, or you have it available in the clinic.
* Do not use microdermabrasion, vacuum, stiff brush, or other device that may bruise or overstimulate the blood circulation.
* Refrain from using products containing salicylic acid as they may penetrate and create blood thinning. This client does not take aspirin or any of its by-products, as they may penetrate and create blood thinning.
* For in-office peels, use enzymatic products and those that are not too aggressive, such as papaya. Perform the treatment manually rather than by using machines. Treatment would include a light facial massage, masks, light enzyme peels, fine cool mist, and light hand and arm massage. Eliminate the prolonged steam as it may create too much vascular activity, and *do not leave the room.* You want to stay nearby at all times.
* Home-care products may contain lower levels of AHAs, antioxidants, hydrators, and sunscreens with zinc oxide and titanium dioxide for protection.
* Vitamin E is not recommended for internal use; it too will thin the blood.
* Make certain the individual's white blood cell count is high, otherwise they are more vulnerable to infection (they will know what their count is).
* Use samples with disposable containers for treatments.

If your client does begin to bleed because of a treatment, get them to medical attention immediately. Do keep in mind there is a fragileness to the capillaries, which increases with age.

It is a good idea to have the phone number of the client's hematologist readily available when performing a treatment. More information on bleeding disorders can be found by visiting the National Hemophilia Foundation's Web site: www.hemophilia.org, or calling toll-free 1-800-42-HANDI.

Parkinson's Disease

Parkinson's disease is a progressive disorder that affects muscle control and balance. Patients with Parkinson's disease have lower levels of dopamine, a complex chain reaction from in-house chemicals, which give messages within the central nervous system, telling muscles to move, stop, or make other physical decisions. Dopamine also affects blood pressure and controls output from the pituitary gland (Grogan, 2001, p. 304). Eventually, the disease makes it difficult for the patient to control all movement, which becomes involuntary. The patient will jerk, exhibit tremors, or shake, and will have difficulty with memory functions such as focus and recall.

Skin Care for Clients with Parkinson's Disease

In the early stages, clients may benefit from home care and in-office treatments, which are basic and soothing. Eventually, an individual with Parkinson's will need direct care and continual home support, and the client may not be able to come in for treatments. Work closely with the caregiver, and supply product to meet the changing needs. Depression is often another symptom of Parkinson's and will need to be addressed by the support team. In addition, if in doubt about a specific treatment or product, check with the physician in charge.

Home care

A.M.

1. Use appropriate cleanser to skin type; it should be soothing and calming and can be removed with a soft warm cloth or easily rinsed.
2. Hydrator: some clients may have dry skin, in which case a moisturizer with an emollient base with amino acids and antioxidants would be beneficial along with a 30SPF. If client has oily skin, use a gel preparation.
3. If a hydrator does not contain sunscreen, use one with zinc oxide and/or titanium dioxide with a 30SPF.

P.M.

1. Repeat daytime regime.
2. Use hydrator appropriate for skin type.

In-office treatment   An in-office treatment for a client with Parkinson's will depend entirely upon the stage of the disease. If the client is comfortable reclining, you may be able to perform a facial using an abbreviated application of a massage and mask. Hand and foot massages are excellent choices for this client, and will lower stress levels. Steam may prove to be too active and not necessarily soothing to this client. One treatment idea is as follows:

1. Cleanse with product appropriate to skin type.
2. Apply a clay mask for deep cleansing; you may dampen the mask occasionally to keep it from completely drying out.
3. While the clay mask is setting, do a soothing hand massage, then apply moisturizer with sunscreen.
4. Next, use a hydrating, soothing mask with an aromatherapy element—such as lavender for calming, sandalwood for soothing, or geranium for relaxation.
5. Apply a light effleurage type of massage 2–3 minutes, then remove mask.
6. Apply hydrator, moisturizer, and sunscreen to face, neck, and chest if gender appropriate.

Due to involuntary movement by this client, refrain from performing extractions, which could endanger both you and them. *Do not leave the client unattended.* For further information on Parkinson's Disease visit www.parkinsonsdisease.com.

Multiple Sclerosis

Multiple Sclerosis—or MS as it is called—is an autoimmune disease where the myelin sheaths (insulators) of the nerves are attacked by the body's own cells and are replaced by scar tissue, which interrupts the passage of nerve impulses (Keir, Wise, & Krebs, 1998, pp. 241–242). Typically, the central nervous system, the brain, and the spinal cord are affected. This creates loss of balance, tremors, bowel and bladder problems, foot dragging, and extreme weakness. This disease is often misdiagnosed because it mimics so many other afflictions. A client with this diagnosis may feel a loss of control and may benefit from stress-relieving treatments.

Skin Care for Clients with Multiple Sclerosis

While heavy massage would not be indicated, a simple facial or hand and foot massage may be beneficial in soothing the client and provide a necessary element of touch, which may feel calming.

Home care   Home care for a client with MS needs to be simple in nature and easy to apply. As stress begins to take its toll, and frustration with the condition sets in, the client needs to find outlets to release a buildup of emotion. This client can regress, and then go into a type of remission. Stress relief is key to helping those with MS.

A.M.

1. Apply a citrus cleanser appropriate to skin type; this citrus scent can also be a mood elevator.
2. Use a hydrator, again appropriate to skin type; gel for oilier skin and a cream or lotion formula for normal or drier skin, respectively.

3. The use of a sunscreen is necessary for the health and protection of the barrier mantle of the skin (30SPF).

P.M.

1. Repeat A.M.
2. Repeat A.M.

In-office treatment   Depending on the stage or condition of the disease, the client may be having difficulty getting into the chair. Ask if it is acceptable to have the client moved onto the facial bed. (Always have assistance doing this.) Begin by giving a light, soothing shoulder massage, thus relaxing the neck and shoulders. Then:

1. Cleanse.
2. Gently apply a deep pore-cleansing mask or scrub with spherical granules (depending upon skin type).
3. Use a light steam for 3–5 minutes (no longer).
4. Remove deep pore-cleansing mask.
5. Apply hydrating, soothing mask with chamomile or basil for uplifting and soothing muscles.
6. While the mask is setting up, give the client a hand and arm massage with a massage lotion complementary to the mask.
7. Remove mask, and apply hydrator, moisturizer, and sunscreen to face and hands.

Always make certain that you stay in the treatment room, and close to the client. *Do not leave them unattended.* For more information visit, www.nationalmssociety.org.

Diabetes

Diabetes or *diabetes mellitus* is a metabolic disorder of the pancreas (White 2001, p. 960). The food we ingest begins a complex chemical journey as it is processed into the system. Of the food we eat, 100 percent of the carbohydrates, 58 percent of protein, and 10 percent of fat is broken down into glucose/sugar (White 2001, p. 906). The hormone insulin, which lowers blood sugar by allowing the cells of the body to absorb glucose from the blood (Grogan 2001), is delivered from the pancreas. In diabetics, this does not happen. Depending on the severity and type of diabetes the nutritional and medication needs vary.

Types

There are two types of diabetes:

Type I   Type I diabetes is insulin-dependent and requires routine medication to avoid excessive blood sugar levels or hyperglycemia. If the patient does not receive routine amounts of insulin, this type of diabetes is fatal.

Type II   People with Type II diabetes have some insulin deficiencies, but modifications in diet and exercise will improve the body's own natural insulin balance. This type of diabetes is the most common form; it is often created by obesity.

Clinical considerations   In the clinic, we will see both types. Treatments and products for Type II diabetes will typically follow those that would be normally offered given the skin condition, age, **Fitzpatrick Skin Type,** and history of the client.

For diabetes Type I however, we must take special precautions. We need to avoid treatments and products that can potentially create barrier impairment. Due to metabolic processes and the constant battle to stabilize the sugar levels, diabetics do not typically heal well, and, through the impaired healing process, they are more susceptible to infection. Bacteria, viruses, and fungi proliferate in glucose/sugar; therefore keeping the epidermis intact is essential. Finding a simple hydrating home-care program is beneficial, as the skin is often parched, flaky, and rough. Ingredients such as amino acids, hyaluronic acid, silicones, and zinc oxide, and titanium dioxide for UVA/UVB protection, would be helpful to supplement moisture loss and protect against environmental factors. Avoid sugars such as polysaccharides and glycolic acids.

Skin Care for Diabetics

Home care

A.M.

Cleansing: sodium laureth-5 caroxylate (super-mild surfactant), or sodium lauryl sulfate; allantoin or azulene (chamomile) for a soothing cleanser
Hydrating: sodium hyaluronate, hyaluronic acid, alanine or arginine (amino acids that are emollient and humectants), dimethicone
Environmental protection: zinc oxide, titanium oxide, amodimethicone (amino acids bonded with dimethicone silicone to protect barrier)

P.M.

Cleansing: repeat A.M.
Hydrating: repeat A.M.

Exfoliation products are not used, due to potential irritations and barrier impairment. This would include AHAs BHAs, and enzymes (low-level enzymes could be patch tested, but you should check with the client's physician).

In-office treatments   In-office treatments for diabetics should be focused on improving circulation. Swedish massage and reflexology along with bodywork such as Reiki and Trager, craniosacral, lymphatic drainage, and shiatsu are good choices. One approach to treatment would be:

1. Cleanse: soothing/calming cleanser (not exfoliating)
2. Apply hydrating mask containing lipids (for barrier improvement), azulene, elastin, collagen (soluble)

3. Do lymphatic drainage.
4. Apply antioxidant treatment containing vitamin E, alpha lipoic acid (prevents sugar's toxic effects by not allowing sugar to attach to protein/collagen (Perricone, 2000, p. 124).
5. While the mask is setting up on face, throat, and chest, massage hands and arms with essential oils such as lavender for calming or orange blossom for stimulating (have client select based on personal choice).
6. If time allows, a foot massage or reflexology treatment could follow for improved circulation.

To find more about diabetes go to Web site www.diabetes.org.

Communicable Diseases

The next two conditions are listed as self-care only. Individuals with hepatitis and HIV/AIDS are not offered in-office treatments. Special considerations and training are required to offer care to those clients with these progressive conditions, which are considered communicable diseases.

Hepatitis

Hepatitis is a virus, which causes an inflammation of the liver. There are five types of hepatitis: Type A, Type B, Type C, Type D, and Type E. Type A and E are transmitted when an infected person goes to the rest room, does not wash, and then prepares food. Type B is associated with body fluids; and both B and C are transmitted through broken skin or needle-stick punctures. Type D is a more severe version of B.

As health-care workers we often hear about types B and C. They are easily transmitted through exchange of body fluids such as during sexual intercourse, sharing needles, and in some cases touching a surface which may be infected. Hepatitis is serious, and it is of great concern to us as skin-care professionals. Vaccines for hepatitis B can be obtained and are mandatory for clinicians; they should be protocol for estheticians working in any setting.

Hepatitis B and C are often treated with **interferon,** a type of chemotherapy. Clients with hepatitis will exhibit a yellow tone to their skin, will feel nauseous, have headaches, and will generally fatigue easily. Help them with a home-care program after contacting their physician to determine their needs. It may be that they have allergies or cannot tolerate certain agents such as herbal preparations or exfoliants.

Home-care programs for clients with hepatitis

A.M.

1. A cleanser with kaolin clay or grains would be beneficial.
2. Use hydrator with soothing properties, such as allantoin or chamomile.
3. Encourage daily use of a sunscreen protector with zinc oxide or titanium dioxide for UVA/UVB refraction.

P.M.

1. Repeat A.M.
2. Repeat AM.

A body hydrator would be helpful for this client as well. You may offer a soft net scrub along with a citrus bath gel for an uplifting bath experience. An apple cut in half (remove seeds and stem) can be very refreshing on skin while bathing, followed post-bath by a body hydrator without AHAs or BHAs. These can be too caustic for the sensitive skin condition of a person with hepatitis. For more information visit, www.cdc.gov.

HIV/Acquired Immune Deficiency Syndrome

HIV is human immunodeficiency virus, which is the virus that causes acquired immune deficiency syndrome or AIDS. We have all heard of this horrific disease by now, and much is being done to eradicate its potential to take the life of its host. When a person gets HIV the virus kills the T4/CD4 cells, which are cells that help us to fight infections. An unaffected person will have around 600 T4/CD4 cells, and an HIV-infected individual may have a much lower amount and eventually none. At this point, the disease has become AIDS. Without medication, such individuals will develop many illnesses, including cancer, pneumonia, and serious skin infections such as Kaposi's sarcoma, which is a rare form of skin cancer. Most of these potentialities have been thwarted due to the advent of drug intervention, which fosters an ability to maintain the body's immune system.

Home care for clients with HIV/AIDS   To assist clients with HIV in a home-care program is a true blessing. Although they are not able to come in for treatments, we can do much to help them to feel and look their best. As mentioned previously, maintaining strength and a healthy immune system is the goal. They will have dietary, medical, and emotional needs that will be met by their health-care professional. The esthetician's role is to provide them with an appropriate skin-care program that they can administer themselves.

A.M.

1. Use cleanser with an uplifting scent such as citrus or herbal essences.
2. Apply nourishers with hyaluronic acid and antioxidants such as vitamins C or E, or grape seed extract to fight off **free radicals.** Squalane or cermides offer lipids to improve the skin's barrier functioning.
3. Apply sunscreen with zinc oxide and titanium dioxide to protect as a physical barrier against UVA/UVB penetration on sensitive, vulnerable skin. These need to be used rain or shine, and daily.

P.M.

1. Repeat A.M.
2. Repeat A.M.
3. Two to three times a week, use a mask for a light exfoliation. This could contain oatmeal, cornmeal, or clay. In addition, body lotions with a soothing chamomile scent and arnica could help with inflammation on joints and feet.

Always check with the physician prior to offering a program to an individual with special needs. There may be underlying conditions that need to be addressed. Some herbs may interfere with medications, so use of them must be approved prior to starting the regimen. Many people with HIV know what they are supposed to use, but always support their continued interest in research and the potential for interactions with preparations. For more information visit, www.cdc.gov.

Summary

Caring for clients with special health problems will often be among the most endearing experiences that you will have. These individuals have acknowledged a sense of mortality, have learned patience, and are unusually optimistic. They will bring much to you in the way of personal and professional growth, and they typically are generous with their time and knowledge. You may learn a great deal while treating them.

Frequently Asked Questions

1. **How does the esthetician move a larger patient in a wheelchair onto the treatment bed?**

   Always enlist the help of others while moving a patient from a wheelchair to the treatment bed, even if you feel that you can do it alone. This gives the client more security and comfort, and is the safest approach to use.

2. **What does the esthetician do if a client with special considerations presents with lesions that does not look familiar?**

   Surprisingly, this happens often. Do not frighten the client by running out of the esthetic room, but rather ask the client:

   • how long they have had them.
   • if they have expanded or grown.
   • whether they are causing pain or itching.

   Defer to the physician after gaining this information.

CHAPTER 17

Pre- and Postoperative Care

- Introduction
- Preoperative Care
- Postoperative Care
- Pre- and Postoperative Treatment Plans
- Laser Resurfacing
- Rhytidectomy (Face-Lift) and Forehead Lift
- Blepharoplasty (Eyelift)
- Liposculpture/Liposuction
- Summary
- Frequently Asked Questions

Introduction

In pre- and postoperative care, we are working more closely with the physician and the patient than at any other juncture. Attention to detail and adherence to procedure protocols, including patient education, will often determine the outcome of a procedure, as well as patient satisfaction.

For clinical estheticians, assisting in pre- and postoperative care provides a connection to another human in a way that encompasses a full range of emotion, for both the patient and the esthetician. We take a client from a skin-care consultation, through to a cosmetic surgery consult, on to a treatment plan and applying the treatment, then on to the preoperative consultation, surgery, postoperative follow-up appointments and postoperative treatments, to camouflage makeup, to routine skin care. The loop takes many turns and creates opportunities for growth. Every patient will be a challenge, and some challenges are easier met than others. We never want to become complacent while dealing with patients, as we must anticipate and fully appreciate each of their own experiences.

Preoperative Care

Prior to surgery, people tend to be nervous about the forthcoming procedure, and many have a difficult time concentrating on very detailed information. Make certain that you have written protocols to send along with them for home use, and that they are certain about how to prepare for the procedure. It is important to take cues from the patient, and do not overload them with too much information in one setting. Reassure the patient that it is normal to be anxious, nervous, and worried. In addition, recommend that they convey all concerns to the doctor.

While preparing the patient for a surgery, it is required by the physician that you determine whether the patient is taking supplements, medications, or eating foods that may interfere with the surgery. An increase in bleeding time or a decrease in coagulation may occur if certain herbs, supplements, drugs, or foods are not eliminated from the patient's diet 3 weeks prior to surgery.

The following list (Table 17–1) provided by R. Emil Hecht, M.D., of The Center for Facial Plastic and Laser Surgery, Bellingham, Washington, has been compiled through medical research, clinical experience, and anecdotal evidence.

Postoperative Care

After surgery patients can be in varying degrees of pain. Medical personnel will always see the patient postoperatively, tend to the immediate needs of the patient, and administer appropriate postoperative treatment. Depending upon the type of surgery, the protocols of a given physician, and the experience of the esthetician, the esthetician is brought back into the scenario to perform therapies. These may include massage techniques to reduce swelling, to calm, and to soothe; treatments for hydration, protection, and camouflage; and typically a new-product orientation for home-care compliance.

Pre- and Postoperative Treatment Plans

Well-designed pre- and postoperative home care and in-office treatment plans are at the core of preparing a patient for surgery. The products and treatments used in either pre- or postoperative stages are aimed at conditioning the skin to heal. In the preoperative phase, conditioning includes increasing the skin's metabolism and reducing the cellular debris on the surface. Postoperatively the goal is to decrease inflammation, moisturize/nurture, and soothe. In both phases, we hydrate and protect the skin from UVA and UVB rays emitted by the sun. Here are treatment plans for the most common procedures.

Note: **Universal Precautions** *(as defined by OSHA) apply in all clinical environments. You must wear gloves while performing treatments. Both clients and patients appreciate this measure.*

Laser Resurfacing

Strict rules apply to the patient undergoing a laser resurfacing procedure. They must fully understand that the outcome of their surgery is highly dependent on their willingness to follow all protocols set forth by the medical team. All phases of the preoperative and postoperative stages are labor-intensive and hands-on for the patient.

Discontinue Before Surgery
IMPORTANT NOTICE

FOODS:
garlic, onion, ginger, cayenne pepper, papaya, pineapple (contains bromelin), turmeric (contains curcumin), Chinese black mushrooms

SUPPLEMENTS:
vitamin B6 (40mg), bromelain, vitamin C (3000mg), curcumin, vitamin E (400I.U), essential fatty acids (fish oil, flax oil, borage oil, black currant oil, etc.) magnesium (500mg), selenium (200mcg).

HERBS:
feverfew, ginkgo, panax ginseng, proanthocyanidins, (picnogenol from grapeseed or pinebark extract, bilberry, etc.).

ASPIRIN or ASPIRIN-LIKE PRODUCTS:

Advil	Coricidin "D" Decongestant	Nuprin
Aleve	Coricidin Demilets or Medilets	Pabirin Buffered Tablets
Alka-Seltzer Plus Cold	Coricidin Tablets	Pacaps
Medicine	Counter Pain	Pamprin
Anacin	Darvon with A.S.A.	Panalgesic
Anaprox	Darvon N with A.S.A.	Percodan
A.P.C. Tablets with Batabital	Dristan	Percodan Demi Tablets
A.S.A. Compound	Defort-Deful	Persistin
Arthritis Pain Formula	Dolor	Phensol
Arthritis Strength Bufferin	Ecotrin	Quiet World
Ascriptin	Empirin	Analgesic/Sleeping Aid
Ascodeen-30	Empirin with Codeine	Robaxisal Tablet
Aspirin Tablets	Emprazil	SK-65 Compound Capsules
Aspirin Suppositories	Equagesic	Sine-Off
Aspergum	Excedrin	Sodium Salicilate
Bayer Aspirin	Feldene	St. Joseph's Aspirin for
Bayer Children's Chewable	Fiorinal	Children
Aspirin	Fiorinal with Codeine	St. Joseph's Cold Tablets
Bayer Children's Cold Tablets	Goody's Headache Powder	Supac
Bayer Timed Release Aspirin	Indocin	Synalgos
Buff-A Comp Tablets	Liquiprin Tablets	Synalgos-DC Capsules
Bufferin	Midol	Tolectin
Buffadyne	Momentum Muscular	Triaminicin
Cama Inlay Tablets	Backache Formula	Trigesic
Cheracol Tablets	Monacet	Vanquish
Clinoril	Motrin	Viro Med
Congesperin	Naprosyn	Zoprin
Copron Capsules	Norgesic Forte	Zomax

Should you inadvertently take any of these products, please notify our office promptly as we may have to postpone your surgery.

Table 17–1   Pre- and Postoperative Vitamin Herb Cessation List

Before Surgery—at 8 Weeks

Home care   A prelaser kit is used as described:

- **AHAs** and or **BHAs** (alpha and beta hydroxy acids) for exfoliation
- **Hydroquinone** (medical grade melanocyte-suppressant skin lightener). *Note: There are other nonmedical grade lighteners such as licorice extract, kojic acid, bearberry, and mulberry, for those patients allergic to hydroquinone, but keep in mind these agents must also be tested for patient sensitivity.*
- **Hydrating moisturizer with amino acids** (enhances water retention), vitamins C or E, alpha lipoic acid or green tea extract (antioxidants help to neutralize free radicals), hyaluronic acid (natural moisturizer with water-binding capabilities)
- **Tretinoin/retinoic acid** (Retin-A, Renova, Activa) a vitamin A derivative stimulates growth of fibroblasts, which are tiny spindle-shaped cells present in connective tissue from which collagen and elastic fibers are formed. It is also used for exfoliation on the upper layer of the stratum corneum (N. Michalun, M. Michlaun, 2001, p. 232).
- **Environmental protector/sunscreen** containing at least an SPF of 30, and physical barriers such as zinc oxide, titanium dioxide, **parsol 1789 (avobenzone),** and broad-spectrum chemical sunscreens, such as **octyl methoxycinnimate,** and **benzophenone-3 (oxybenzone)**

A.M.

1. Cleanser
2. Lightener (hydroquinone)
3. Moisturizer/hydrator with AHA and or BHA
4. Sunscreen with 30SPF

P.M.

1. Cleanser
2. Lightener
3. Retinoic acid
4. Moisturizer/hydrator

In-office treatments   At 8 weeks before surgery, you may begin a treatment plan that will change and adapt to the needs of the patient's process. This plan will be followed until 4 weeks after surgery. The patient's skin type, classification (level or degree of photo-aging), and physician protocol will determine the plan that you will follow. Use one of the following:

- **Superficial chemical peel such as AHA, BHA or Jessner's** (a combination of AHA, BHA lactic acid, and resorcinol, depending upon preparation) are best applied by starting with the lowest concentration, gradually increased as the patient tolerates. These peels will help to stimulate the home-care program by exfoliating the upper layers of the epidermis and serve as an additional skin-lightening measure. Make certain the patient stops using retinoic acid the day before, and 3 days after, a peel.

- **Microdermabrasion** (mechanical exfoliation/polishing of the skin with the use of crystals or other abrasion hand piece) can be used as an alternate to chemical peels. This is an excellent modality in superficial exfoliation for very strong, oily, thick, skin that has had extreme sun exposure. Make certain that the patient stops using retinoic acid 2–3 days prior to and after a microdermabrasion treatment.
- **Enzyme peels:** enzymes such as **papain** (papaya), or **bromelin** (pineapple) will dissolve keratin (remove the buildup of protein/dead skin cells), thereby softening and aiding in the hydration of the skin. Papaya is the gentler of the two and is often used on very sensitive skin.

Closer to Surgery

At 6 weeks preop

- Continue home care with prelaser kit.
- Continue in-office treatment with chemical peel or microdermabrasion.

At 4 weeks preop

- Continue home care with prelaser kit.
- Continue in-office treatment with chemical peel or microdermabrasion.

At 2 weeks preop

- Continue home care with prelaser kit.
- Continue in-office treatment with chemical or microdermabrasion.

At 1 week preop

Home Care: Change in Protocol

We now drop the bleach and tretinoin or retinol from the program using:

- cleansing regime.
- moisturizer with AHA ingredient such as glycolic, lactic, or combination.
- sunscreen.

3 days preop

Home Care

Antiviral medication: patient begins to take medication to suppress herpetic breakout (cold sores); routine as prescribed by physician. In addition, a homeopathic form of **arnica** can be taken to reduce swelling—providing the physician has prescribed this herb, and the patient does not have a heart condition or other special health problems related to the circulatory system.

In-Office Treatment

Apply a soothing, hydrating facial treatment, using cool steam, high frequency, light-to-little massage, and sunscreen. At this point, the patient's skin has become conditioned, and we do not want the patient's skin to be overtreated the day of surgery.

After Laser Surgery

Days 1–5 postop   **Silon dressing** is a special type of dressing which is applied to freshly ameliorated/lasered skin. Petroleum ointment is then used on unaffected areas such as lips and around the eye area. Instruct patient to call the office if this dressing falls off. They may need to have it replaced. Continue taking anti-viral medication as directed.

Days 5–10 postop   Once the physician removes the dressing, the patient begins to apply solution soaks every 2–3 hours as indicated by physician. (Solution is usually 1 teaspoon vinegar to 1 cup of water.) This is followed by an application of petroleum ointment. *This must not dry out!* Keep well lubricated.

Some physicians are using a copper peptide ointment and cleanser for the first 10 days, omitting the use of the dressing and petroleum ointment. Each physician will dictate the use and application based on research and preference.

Home care days 10–15 postop

Postlaser Kit

Once the patient's skin has **re-epithelialized** (has regained intact epidermis), and the patient has been given instruction by the physician, you may begin:

- gentle cleanser
- hydrocortisone for itching
- squalane-for moisturizing (light emollient, plant lipid)
- copper peptide cream, lotion, or gel (enhances wound healing)
- sunscreen

Days 15–30 postop

- Continue home-care products using hydrating moisturizers, copper peptide cream, and sunscreen with SPF of at least 30.
- Camouflage therapy: use mineral powder makeup for this step. It contains titanium dioxide and natural pigments, which are much less irritating to the new skin than over-the-counter brands of makeup. Patients may exhibit pustules and milia, which may be gently extracted.

One month postlaser   Most patients will be tolerant of a light exfoliating AHA (less than 5% glycolic, with a high pH 3.5) product if directed by a physician at this point.

Often the skin is still peeling, and this product will help to further the healing. However, all in-office treatments should be directed toward hydrating and soothing for up to 3 to 6 months. Avoid using warm steam on a postlaser patient. Continue to remind patients in every visit to use sunscreen and to avoid the sun.

Note: Do not use microdermabrasion, glycolic, salicylic, or lactic acids on a postlaser patient, until indicated by physician.

Rhytidectomy (Face-Lift) and Forehead Lift

The face-lift or forehead lift requires preparing the patient for surgery. If patients receive continued support throughout both phases, they tend to be less anxious and will feel as though their experience is less isolating.

Before Surgery

As with the laser-resurfacing procedure, the patient tolerates the postoperative phase much better if the skin is brought to its optimum condition, with well-orchestrated home-care and in-office treatment programs. It is beneficial if you can start these protocols 8–10 weeks prior to the surgery date, but if you do not have that much time, they can be modified. In addition, if the patient is having a combination of procedures—such as a face-lift and laser resurfacing—the esthetician would combine both treatment plans.

Home care at 8 weeks preop   Depending upon skin type and classification, have client use at a minimum products containing the following:

- **Cleansers:** AHAs, BHAs, or enzymes for exfoliation; chamomile or allantoin for soothing
- **Exfoliators:** AHAs, BHAs, vitamin A derivatives such as retinol or retinoic acid, enzymes such as papaya/papain and pineapple/bromelain
- **Hydrators/moisturizers:** alpha lipoic acid/amino acids (hydrator); hyaluronic acid (hydrator); bioflavonoids, green tea (antioxidant/free radical fighter); vitamins C and E (antioxidants)
- **Eye cream:** alpha lipoic acid (hydrator); vitamins A, E, C (antioxidants); arnica (reduces swelling); sodium hyaluronate (moisturizing agent)
- **Sunscreen:** titanium dioxide (physical barrier against UVA/UVB rays); zinc oxide (physical barrier against UVA/UVB rays); parsol 1789/avobenzone (a chemical ingredient with broad-spectrum protection against UVA rays); octyl methoxycinnamate (a chemical ingredient used in a wide variety of sunscreens)

A.M.

1. Cleanser
2. Exfoliant
3. Hydrater/moisturizer (sometimes exfoliants and moisturizers are combined)
4. Sunscreen

P.M.

1. Cleanser
2. Exfoliator
3. Hydrator/moisturizer

In-office treatments   Treatments for forehead and face-lift may include a combination of classic facials and peels, which can be applied every other week. **Manual lymphatic drainage** (a soothing, stimulating treatment to reduce swelling and anxiety, described on page 194) can be added to the following treatments, or begun as a stand-alone treatment at a minimum of biweekly, 2 weeks in advance of the procedure date.

At 8 weeks before

Apply treatment appropriate to skin type. At a minimum, include the following:

1. Cleansing: remove makeup with a gentle cleanser.
2. Exfoliation: apply chemical peel, microdermabrasion, or enzyme peel.
3. Extractions: gently perform extractions to pustules, whiteheads, blackheads, and milia.
4. Hydration: use a combination of amino acids (enhances water retention in the skin), lipids/ceramides (form a protective barrier in epidermis to reduce moisture loss), copper peptide gel (for wound healing).
5. Protection: apply a sunscreen with antioxidants after every treatment.

Closer to Surgery

At 6–3 weeks preop

- Continue home-care regimen.
- Continue in-office treatments once a week.

At 2 weeks preop

- Continue home-care regimen.
- Continue in-office treatment, add **manual lymphatic drainage** (rhythmatic treatment to help reduce swelling through improving circulation, therefore lymphatic fluid flow).

1 week preop

- Continue home-care regimen.
- Apply two manual lymphatic drainages spaced 2–3 days apart.

Note: For patients with rosacea follow protocol, except use medication Metrogel, Metro-lotion, and Metro cream (Metronidazole topical antibiotic used to fight symptoms of rosacea such as redness and swelling), first after cleanser. Then use a moisturizer containing chamomile/azulene, alpha lipoic acid (antioxidant and anti-inflammatory), and sunscreen. In addition, use enzyme peel for exfoliation instead of more aggressive peels for in-office treatment.

After Surgery

Week 1 postop

Home Care Immediately after Surgery

Patient rests. Tylenol is taken for pain. Patient keeps jaw movement at a minimum, by having liquid meals. Cleansing is performed by using a warm, soft cloth on all nonbandaged areas. A light hydrating moisturizer can be used.

In-Office Treatment

- Postoperative appointment 2–3 days after surgery
- Patient comes in for postoperative appointment with the physician. If drains have been used, they are removed (sometimes used to avoid potential hematomas). Bandages are often replaced with a **facial bra** to enhance healing of newly placed skin, muscles, and nerves.

Days 8–15 postop

Home Care Once Bandages Are Removed

- Keep gentle cleansing regimen (avoid using product on all suture and staple sites).
- Clean suture sites with a hydrogen peroxide and water solution (mix equal parts) and apply antibiotic ointment.
- Moisturize and hydrate (avoid suture and staple sites).
- Use sunscreen with minimum of 30SPF (avoid suture and staple sites).

In-Office Treatment

- Patient sees nurse and physician for suture and staple removal.
- Patient sees esthetician for manual lymphatic drainage and camouflage therapy as directed by physician.

2 weeks postop

Home Care

- Continue with home care.
- Apply camouflage makeup.
- Patient applies scar-management product with ingredient such as allium cepa (onion extract) to act as anti-inflammatory and antikeloid (hypertropic raised scar that looks like a worm) measure. Silicone scar tapes and liquid preparations are used readily for scar management.

In-Office Treatments

- Continue manual lymphatic drainage, two per week, 3 days apart.
- Apply soothing facial mask such as **azulene** (German chamomile). Patients often need some exfoliation at this point; you may use an enzyme (papaya) mask. Avoid chemical

peels, microdermabrasion, heat/steam or any treatment that may be too aggressive at this point.

- Physician will usually see the patient for another postoperative visit during this time.

3 weeks postop . . . and beyond

Home Care

- Most patients can return to their presurgery home-care regimen at this point. They can use AHAs, BHAs, hydrating moisturizers and sunscreens.

In-Office Treatments

- Many patients will feel some numbness located near or at incision sites. Manual lymphatic drainage is applied as part of a routine facial treatment.

Blepharoplasty (Eyelift)

This treatment plan may be modified if performed in conjunction with another procedure. For example, laser resurfacing is often applied periorbitally (around eye area) on lower lids to tighten the skin around the eye after the fat deposits have been removed. Follow laser-resurfacing protocol if indicated.

Before Surgery

Home care at 6 weeks preop

- On face, routine skin care as followed for **rhytidectomy** and forehead lift
- Eye cream containing arnica or cucumber extract (reduces swelling), hyaluronic acid, and amino acids (hydration), bioflavonoids (antioxidants), and sunscreen

Note: If patient is having laser resurfacing add hydroquinone (lightener) A.M. and P.M.; retinoic acid (collagen stimulation and cell normalizer) P.M. only.

In-office treatments at 4 weeks preop   Add to routine facial one of the following:

- Microdermabrasion: use periorbitally for exfoliation and stimulation, followed by hydrating eye mask containing evening primrose oil (hydrating and improves barrier climate), chamomile, allantoin (soothing), and/or **ladies' thistle** (wound healing). Follow with appropriate hydration and sunscreen.
- Use a light glycolic peel for exfoliation, lightening, and hydrating. Depending upon skin type and classification, follow with appropriate hydrator and sunscreen.

At 3 weeks preop

Home Care

- Continue with home care (prelaser kit if indicated).

In-Office Treatment

- Continue with exfoliation treatment and eye mask.

At 2 weeks preop

Home Care

- Continue with home care as indicated.

In-Office Treatment

- Continue eye treatment.

1 week preop

Home Care

- Continue as indicated. If having laser resurfacing, stop using hydroquinone and retinoic acid

In-Office Treatment

- Use hydrating eye mask treatment only the last week.

After Surgery

Days 1–7 postop

Home Care

- Apply eye drops as indicated by physician.
- Topical antibiotic at suture site (if directed by physician).
- Tylenol for pain as directed by physician.

In-Office Treatment

- Nurse or physician removes sutures at 5–7 days.
- If laser procedure was performed on lower lids, physician removes bandage/sheeting at day 5 (if it has not fallen off). Apply postlaser soaks (1 teaspoon vinegar to 1 cup H_2O), then keep well lubricated with petroleum. If using copper ointment, apply every 3 to 4 hours after soaks.

Days 7–12 postop

Home Care

- If laser surgery was performed, patient follows protocol using postlaser kit items: hydrocortisone, squalane, or copper peptide cream, and sunscreen.
- If not, use hydrating eye cream and sunscreen.

- If indicated by physician, light camouflage may be applied (if appropriate products are used such as mineral-based powders).

In-Office Treatments

- Follow-up visit with physician
- Camouflage makeup for bruising as directed by physician

2–3 weeks postop

Home Care

- Return to hydrating eye cream as followed in presurgery protocol.
- If laser resurfacing, continue following postlaser protocol.
- Continue camouflage makeup.

In-Office Treatment

- Do manual lymphatic drainage (if no laser).
- Apply a hydrating/soothing eye mask as complement to routine facial treatment.

Note: Do not use microdermabrasion, glycolic, salicylic, or lactic acids on freshly amelio-rated (laser) skin. These treatments can resume only after several months, as indicated by physician.

Liposculpture/Liposuction

Liposculpture or liposuction can be enhanced by applying several massage techniques that aid in the stimulation of fluid preoperatively and reduce swelling postoperatively. The treatments are as follows.

Endermology

Endermology is a body treatment given before and after liposuction to help stimulate the reduction of adipose tissue (fat) in areas, such as the buttocks, thighs, and calves. The endermology machine provides a slight vacuum to the affected areas, thereby increasing blood and lymph to those areas and thus reducing the incidence of bruising and swelling associated with liposuction. Varicose veins, heart and circulatory problems, and diabetes can all be contraindications for this treatment. Use only as directed by physician. It can be performed every 10 days for 6 weeks before surgery on hips, buttocks, thighs, and calves.

Massage—Ayurvedic, Manual Lymphatic Drainage, Swedish Massage

The positive effects of massage on the pre- or postoperative patient are being realized in health-care settings throughout the world. Massage preoperatively can reduce anxiety; postoperatively, it naturally serves to increase the circulatory system and thus help the patient release fluids and swelling created by the surgery. Creating a sense of well-being in the patient, it is both calming and stimulating simultaneously. In addition to being a stress reliever, massage is a form of both internal and external communication and a means of eliminating toxins that have built up in the body. As with all treatments, it is important to work closely with the physician, for input as to when these applications may begin or end, prior to or after a surgery.

Manual lymphatic drainage   Lymphatic drainage is a treatment that is used pre- and postoperatively to stimulate the movement of fluid in the connective tissues, therefore reducing inflammation and increasing relaxation. This treatment was originally created by Dr. Emil and Estrid Vodder in 1932 as they practiced physical therapy in France. They discovered that by applying a treatment that included light, rhythmatic manipulation to their patients suffering from chronic sinus and bronchial problems, the patients would heal much faster.

This treatment also emulates a wave-like sensation, which soothes muscle tension and the nervous system, and creates a deep relaxation not present in other types of massage or other treatments. It is excellent for pre- and postoperative procedures. Facial lymphatic drainage requires advanced training and takes regular practice to master.

Ayurvedic massage   Ancient Ayurveda massage techniques offer a personal approach to treatment which focuses on root causes rather than on the treatment of symptoms. It is helpful in restoring balance to the body through the use of specific oils to body type.

The Ayurvedic practitioner is trained in complementary medicine and looks at the whole health care plan for the patient pre- and postoperatively, including diet, exercise, meditation, herbology, and rejuvenation. Melanie Sachs, author of *Ayurvedic Beauty Care, Ageless Techniques to Invoke Natural Beauty* says, "Touch awakens the tissues so that the body and mind connect and become more fully aware of the need for healing in a particular area."

This is especially important in the postoperative stage, and countless patients will tell you how much better they feel as a result of massage whether they consciously understand what has taken place or not. They will feel better.

Summary

As with all procedures, strict adherence to pre- and postoperative protocols defines the eventual outcome. As patient educator, the clinical esthetician has a great opportunity to increase and enhance the effectiveness of surgical procedures; you can give the patient the much needed support before, during, and after a procedure. The cycle then continues as the patient then become the client again, and resumes routine visits for education, products, treatments, and subsequent procedures.

Treatments at a Glance

Procedure	Preop Treatment	Postop Treatment
Face-lift/rhytidectomy	MLD Routine facial Microdermabrasion Chemical peels	MLD Soothing facial Camouflage
Eyelift/blepharoplasty	MLD Routine facial Microdermabrasion Peels: pretreat if laser	MLD Calming facial Camouflage Posttreat if laser
Forehead lift	MLD Routine facial	MLD Soothing facial Camouflage
Laser resurfacing	Chemical peels Microdermabrasion Prelaser kit	Postlaser kit Soothing/hydrating facial
Liposuction	MLD Endermology	MLD Endermology
Breast augmentation	MLD	Breast manipulation Scar management
Breast reduction	MLD Ayurvedic massage	MLD Scar management
Abdomectomy (Tummy tuck)	MLD Ayurvedic massage Herbal wraps	MLD Swedish massage Scar management

Note: Treatments listed on this chart are given as simply a guideline, and postoperative treatments are to be administered only after sufficient healing has taken place as recommended by the physician.

Frequently Asked Questions

1. **If the esthetician sees a problem with the manner in which a patient is preparing for a surgical procedure, what is the appropriate protocol?**

   The esthetician as patient educator should reiterate the original preparation plan to the patient and ask for full cooperation. Explain that the results are dependent on following the treatment plan, and that the doctor is expecting the follow-through. Some surgeries may have to be canceled if the patient is noncompliant.

2. **Is it necessary to do all of these steps pre- and postoperatively?**

   Every office will have its own procedure/protocol for pre- and postop surgical care based on the interest, recommendation, or requests of the physician. It will be important to follow the steps detailed by your medical personnel. It is in your interest, however, to continue your own education, present new information to the staff as appropriate, and keep up with the science behind introducing new protocols.

CHAPTER 18

Standard Protocols for Peels

- Introduction
- Glycolic Peel
- Jessner's Peel
- Salicylic Acid Peel or Beta-Hydroxy Peel (BHA)
- Microdermabrasion
- Enzymes
- Trichloracetic Acid or TCA Peel
- Summary
- Frequently Asked Questions

Introduction

It is important for you to determine the best possible treatment for your client based on his or her needs and your experience level. At any time that you feel the needs or desires of a client or a patient are beyond your scope or comfort level, it is best to admit that, bring in the physician, do a less complicated treatment, or refer the client to another practitioner. It is best to create boundaries that you are not willing to cross, rather than be sorry about an outcome that could have been prevented.

Be sure to check with state licensing guidelines to determine which strength or levels of chemical peels you are to administer as an esthetician. As you know, in working in a physician's office you may have access to much higher levels of acids—and you may be adroit at utilizing them—but you are not licensed to apply them.

Each manufacturer has its own idiosyncrasies with respect to compounding. Therefore it is important to know what the pH of a given peeling product is, and how that presents in the peel. For example, a nonbuffered 15% glycolic peel with a pH level of 1.0 is going to be much more aggressive than a buffered compound with a 3.8 pH containing the same percentage of glycolic.

Buffered or neutralized products will stabilize the value of the glycolic. When introducing a nonbuffered product it is much more difficult to measure the depth of peel you are going to achieve. Should you use a nonbuffered solution? It fully depends upon your experience level and the skin type that you are peeling.

A lower pH level will always yield a more caustic reaction in the realm of chemical peeling. For a thicker, oily, problem-prone skin type, this may be your best choice; conversely, a thinner, dryer skin type will tolerate a buffered, higher pH preparation.

Glycolic Peel

The client should use at least 8% glycolic home-care products for a minimum of 2 to 3 weeks prior to treatment. In all cases, the longer, the better. In addition, if he or she were a Fitzpatrick III through V, it would be a good idea to add hydroquinone, kojic, or another skin-lightening product as a prophylactic measure to quiet melanocytes. This applies to all chemical peels.

Performing a Glycolic Peel

You will need:

- your peel product in a glass container
- brush (most estheticians like and use a stiff fan brush)
- water
- glass bowl
- cleanser
- timer
- stripping solution (acetone or acetone combination)
- gauze 4 × 4s
- gloves
- consent form

Objective   Your objective with a glycolic peel is to perform a superficial exfoliation of the stratum corneum. The peel has reached its optimum use when the skin has turned slightly pink or pink. If you notice that some areas are turning pink much faster than overall general skin, you will neutralize those areas with water. If you notice the skin is turning white, *remove peel immediately* as the skin is frosting and unless you are experienced with these peels, you are approaching a much deeper peel. (Some skin types are more prone to frost than others, i.e., Asian or light olive, also are prone to hyperpigmentation.)

Contraindications:

- anyone on Accutane should wait for at least a year posttreatment and get physician recommendation. There can be some subclinical conditions (not seen or detected by the naked eye) such as a potential to keloid or scar.
- herpetic breakout (cold sores)
- open wounds, acne lesions, or bleeding from a lesion
- pregnancy and/or lactation are also contraindications.
- cancer

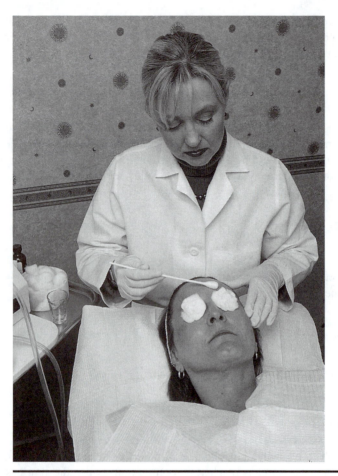

Figure 18–1   Esthetician applying a glycolic peel

- autoimmune diseases
- diabetes
- bleeding disorders

Procedure
1. Cleanse face, throat, chest, or all areas to be treated.
2. Apply stripping solution to eliminate oil, which will keep peel from penetrating (if skin is extremely dry or sensitive, skip this step).
3. Set timer for 3 minutes for first peel.
4. Starting at forehead, paint glycolic upward toward hairline, and follow around in a counterclockwise fashion as you stand behind the client. Save periorbital and throat areas for last.

5. Watch for "hot spots." If some areas exhibit persistent erythema (redness), dilute with water. You are looking for an even peel.
6. Remove with warm water and 4 × 4 (gauze works best).

Postpeel

Treat as follows:

1. A light cryogenic treatment calms the skin after a peel: use liquid nitrogen on a large cotton swab (shake excess thoroughly) and briskly brush over treated area. Clients love this part of the treatment (you must exercise extreme caution while using liquid nitrogen, and you must be fully trained by dispenser of cryogenic product and medical personnel).
2. Then apply a light hydrating serum containing hyaluronic acid, antioxidants, chamomile, or an additional soothing serum.
3. Then apply a moisturizer without performance agents (i.e., glycolic, salicylic).
4. Then provide a sunscreen. Sunscreens containing micronized zinc oxide or titanium dioxide are best for creating a physical barrier against UV rays.
5. Mineral powders and makeup can be applied providing that the makeup is of good quality.
6. Remind client not to use performance agents (glycolic, retinol, retinoic acid, or higher levels of l-ascorbic acid vitamin C) for up to 3 days after a peel.

Jessner's Peel

A **Jessner's peel** is often a combination of two or more chemicals such as glycolic and salicylic, or glycolic, lactic, salicylic, or resorcinol in combination with any of the peeling agents mentioned. This peel is excellent for hyperpigmentation, acneic/problematic skin, or aging skin, and on most skin types up to a Fitzpatrick V. Always test patch this peel 48 hours prior to administering the full peel. If your Jessner's preparation contains salicylic, always check to make sure that the client is not allergic to aspirin. (Salicylic acid is derived from the same wintergreen plant as aspirin.) Also, do not apply to a client with a bleeding disorder.

To prepare the skin, the client should use at least 8% glycolic home-care products for a minimum of 2 to 3 weeks prior to treatment. In all cases, the longer, the better. In addition, if he or she were a Fitzpatrick III through V, it would be a good idea to add hydroquinone, kojic, or another bleaching product as a prophylactic measure to quiet melanocytes. This applies to all chemical peels.

Performing a Jessner's Peel

You will need:

- your peel product in a glass container
- brush (most estheticians like and use a stiff fan brush)
- water

- glass bowl
- cleanser
- timer
- stripping solution (acetone)
- gauze 4 × 4
- gloves
- consent form

Objective   The objective of the Jessner's peel is to exfoliate the upper layers of the stratum corneum, dry up acne lesions, and fade hyperpigmentation in superficial cases. If your Jessner's peel contains glycolic acid, you may create hyperpigmentation if the product is left on too long (postinflammatory hyperpigmentation), if the client is prone to hyperpigmentation (Fitzpatrick III–V), or if skin was not appropriately prepped with hydroquinone (bleach).

Contraindications

- anyone on Accutane
- pregnancy, lactation
- herpetic breakout

- cancer
- autoimmune diseases
- diabetes

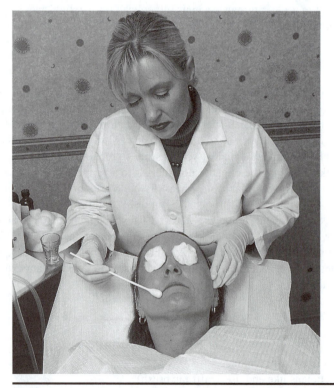

Figure 18–2   Esthetician applying a Jessner's peel

- extremely sensitive skin, rosacea
- thin-skinned Fitzpatrick I
- allergy to aspirin or salicylites

- open wounds or lesions
- bleeding disorders

Procedure

1. Cleanse face, neck and chest or areas to be treated.
2. Apply a stripping solution to eliminate oil (which will keep product from penetrating).
3. Set timer for 2 minutes for one layer.
4. Starting at forehead, paint Jessner's peel upward toward hairline and follow in a counterclockwise pattern as you stand behind the client.
5. Depending upon skin type and condition, you may want to apply a second or third layer. Allow 2 minutes in between layers. Jessner's peels may vary, so your level of experience will dictate the type of peel product you are using, as well as the amount of product that you apply. It is recommended that you use only product that is within your state's licensing code.
6. Once peel has been applied in one or two layers watch for "hot spots" (red areas) or "frosting" (completely white). If you are inexperienced and you see either one of these conditions, remove the peel with water or the approved neutralizer.

Postpeel

1. A light cryogenic treatment calms the skin after a peel by using liquid nitrogen on a large cotton swab (shake excess thoroughly) and briskly brush over treated area.
2. Apply a light hydrating serum containing hyaluronic acid, antioxidants, chamomile, or an additional soothing serum.
3. Apply a moisturizer without performance agents (glycolic, salicylic, retinol).
4. Then add a sunscreen. Sunscreens containing micronized zinc oxide and or titanium dioxide are best for creating a physical barrier against UV rays.
5. Mineral powders work well postpeel and with zinc oxide and or titanium dioxide. If Fitzpatrick III or above, the powders will not work on darker pigmented skin as the minerals will look ashy. Just use appropriate sun protection.

Salicylic Acid Peel or Beta-Hydroxy Peel (BHA)

The objective of a **beta-hydroxy peel** is to exfoliate the upper layers of the stratum corneum, dry up acne lesions, and fade hyperpigmentation in superficial cases. If your client is allergic to aspirin, this peel is contraindicated for them. Also, do not apply to a client with a bleeding disorder. This peel is excellent as a bacteria fighter, and is helpful in Grades I, II and III types of acne. Fitzpatrick III and above may find it too active, as sensitive skins will. Test patch always.

Performing a Beta-Hydroxy (BHA) Peel

To perform a beta-hydroxy acid peel you will need:

- your peel product in a glass container
- brush (most like and use a stiff fan brush)
- water
- glass bowl
- cleanser
- timer
- stripping solution (acetone)
- gauze 4 × 4
- gloves
- consent form

Objective   Your objective with a beta-hydroxy acid peel is to perform a superficial exfoliation of the stratum corneum. The peel has reached its optimum use when the skin has turned slightly pink. If you notice that some areas are turning pink much faster than overall general skin, you will neutralize those areas with water. If you notice the skin is turning white, *remove peel immediately* as skin is frosting; unless experienced with these peels, you are approaching a much deeper peel. (Some skin types are more prone to frost than others, i.e., Asian or light olive, also are prone to hyperpigmentation.) Always test patch 48 hours prior to peel.

Contraindications

- Anyone on Accutane should wait for at least a year posttreatment.
- herpetic breakout (cold sores)
- open wounds, acne lesions, or bleeding from a lesion
- pregnancy
- allergy to aspirin
- cancer
- autoimmune diseases
- bleeding disorders

Procedure

1. Cleanse face, throat, chest, or all areas to be treated.
2. Apply stripping solution to eliminate oil, which will keep peel from penetrating.
3. Set timer for 3 minutes for first peel.
4. Starting at forehead, paint beta-hydroxy upward toward hairline, and follow around in a counterclockwise fashion as you stand behind the client. Save periorbital and throat areas for last.
5. Watch for "hot spots." If some areas exhibit persistent erythema, dilute with water. You are looking for an even peel.
6. Remove with warm water and 4 × 4.

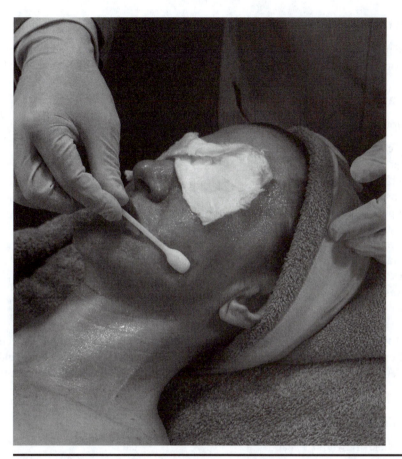

Figure 18–3   Esthetician applying a BHA peel

Postpeel

Treatment is as follows:
1. A light cryogenic treatment calms the skin after a peel by using liquid nitrogen on a large cotton swab (shake excess thoroughly) and briskly brush over treated area.
2. Then apply a light hydrating serum containing hyaluronic acid, antioxidants, chamomile, or an additional soothing serum.
3. Then apply a moisturizer without performance agents (i.e., glycolic, salicylic).
4. Then provide a sunscreen. Sunscreens containing micronized zinc oxide or titanium dioxide are best for creating a physical barrier against UV rays.
5. Mineral powders and makeup can be applied, providing that the makeup is of good quality.

Microdermabrasion

Microdermabrasion is one of the best peels we can offer our clients today. It is safe for most skin types and conditions, it is easy to administer, and the results are predictable.

Performing a Microdermabrasion

To perform a microdermabrasion peel you will need:

- a machine
- water
- bowl
- cleanser
- stripping solution (not used for extremely dry skins)
- eye goggles (yours and client's)
- face mask (yours)
- crystals—salts or other to meet the specifics of your machine
- gauze 4 × 4
- gloves
- consent form

Objective   The goal is controlled shedding of the stratum corneum using approved particles. (Some machines use no crystals and dermabrade by using a stainless steel hand piece with diamond chips embedded into the head of the piece, which slightly abrades the surface of the epidermis.)

Contraindications

- Accutane use within 1 year
- herpetic breakouts
- rosacea; sensitive, thin skin
- open lesions of any type; type III or IV acne
- telangiectases (small red veins)
- cancer
- diabetes
- autoimmune diseases
- bleeding disorders

Procedure

1. Cleanse face, throat, chest, and any or all areas to be treated.
2. Apply stripping solution to normal to oily skin types to eliminate all excess oil from surface for better peel.
3. Don goggles (both you and client) if using crystal/particles.
4. Put on mask (yours).
5. Start at left eyebrow, pulling hand piece back to hairline on forehead, making full contact of skin to aperture (typically at a 45-degree angle)
6. Proceed counterclockwise until you work around the face. Turn down power on periorbital and neck regions.

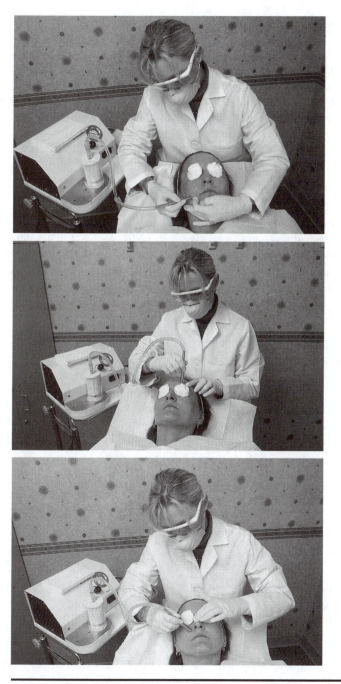

Figure 18–4 Esthetician performing microderabrasion

7. Cleanse, being certain to remove all of the crystal, if you have this type of machine.

8. Begin to hydrate with an antioxidant serum containing hyaluronic acid, then use a hydrating moisturizer on dry skin, oil-free hydrator on oily skin, and a sunscreen appropriate to skin type.

9. Mineral powder is fine to use posttreatment. However, instruct your client to avoid performance agents for up to 3 days. That includes retinol, retinoic acid, glycolic, and beta-hydroxy/salicylic acid.

10. If you have an extreme case of hyperpigmentation, you may use hydroquinone immediately after the peel, and then hydrate and apply sunscreen.

Enzymes

There are many types of enzymes to use today. They are an alternative or, in some cases, a necessary change from doing acid peels. An enzymatic peel exfoliates the stratum corneum by dissolving built-up proteins and cellular debris. Common types of enzymes used are pineapple, papaya, or pumpkin. Some enzymatic peels can be very strong, even though many practitioners consider them lighter fare. Papaya enzymes are excellent on sensitive skins, and they can be combined with other components during a standard facial and can be used on most patients with rosacea.

Performing an Enzymatic Peel

You will need

- your peel product
- brush (most like and use a stiff fan brush)
- water
- glass bowl
- cleanser
- timer
- gauze 4 × 4
- gloves
- steam
- consent form

Objective   Your objective with an enzyme peel is to perform a superficial exfoliation of the stratum corneum, soften the surface tissue, and increase hydration.

Contraindications

- Accutane use
- herpetic breakout
- open lesions
- cancer patients
- diabetes
- autoimmune diseases

Procedure

1. Cleanse face, throat, chest, or all areas to be treated.
2. Starting at forehead, paint beta-hydroxy upward toward hairline, and follow around in a counterclockwise fashion as you stand behind the client. Save periorbital and throat areas for last.
3. Set timer for 10 minutes for first peel.
4. Steam if skin is not too rosaceous or sensitive.
5. Remove with warm water and 4 × 4.

Postpeel

The treatment is as follows:

1. A light cryogenic treatment calms the skin after a peel: use liquid nitrogen on a large cotton swab (shake excess thoroughly) and briskly brush over treated area.
2. Then apply a light hydrating serum containing hyaluronic acid, antioxidants, chamomile, or an additional soothing serum.
3. Then apply a moisturizer without performance agents (i.e., glycolic, salicylic).
4. Then provide a sunscreen. Sunscreens containing micronized zinc oxide or titanium dioxide are best for creating a physical barrier against UV rays.
5. Mineral powders and makeup can be applied, providing that the makeup is of good quality.

Trichloracetic Acid or TCA Peel

Trichloracetic acid is a powerful chemical agent. It can create scarring if not handled properly. When done well, you will have a hard time finding a better result short of laser. Check with state regulations to determine whether you should be performing this peel and at what strength. Most states will allow a 10% TCA peel to be performed by estheticians while working in a physician's office, but this is clearly enough to create a problem if put into the wrong hands.

Performing a TCA Peel

You will need:

- your peel product in a glass container
- water
- glass bowl
- cleanser
- timer
- stripping solution (acetone)
- gauze 4 × 4
- gauze pad for applying TCA
- gloves

- cold packs to apply after the peel
- Consent Form
- antiviral medication (pretreatment if herpetic prone)

Objective   The objective of applying a TCA peel is to revitalize and rejuvenate the epidermis by peeling off the uppermost layers of the stratum corneum. With pretreatment of a minimum of 3 weeks, utilizing a combination of bleach, AHAs, retinol, or retinoic acid, you will lessen the potential for hyperpigmentation, and the skin will be conditioned to heal at a faster rate. In addition, your client will want to take an antiviral medication 3 days prior and 3 days after the peel. Much higher concentrations of this peel are often used by physicians, and it can be applied in conjunction with the laser.

This peel is performed by administering several layers in very thin applications to the areas being treated. Typically, the skin will turn white or frost, giving an indication of the depth of the peel. It is important to wait approximately 2 minutes between each layer to fully allow acid to complete the task and for the comfort of the patient. Optimum peeling occurs when the acid has turned the skin white in a uniform manner.

Special care should be offered several weeks ahead of the treatment. The client or patient should be scheduled for two appointments prior to the treatment and two after treatment, or as indicated.

During the first two appointments you will assist the client by providing proper home-care products and protocols to secure compliance. The first appointment is for a consultation and product recommendation, the second to clarify any questions and to make sure they are using the pretreatment regimen (AHAs, bleach, retinol or retinoic acid, and sunscreen). You may be able to ward off any problems if you actually see the patient and how they respond to direction (this is a good rule of thumb preoperatively as well).

The second two appointments will be to follow up on the peel, and to make certain that they are following the postpeel protocol. Look at this peel as if it is a surgical procedure. It is not to be taken lightly.

Contraindications

- Accutane use
- herpetic breakout
- open lesions
- pregnancy/lactation
- cancer
- autoimmune diseases
- diabetes

Procedure

1. Cleanse.
2. Apply eye covers.
3. Apply stripping solution.
4. Starting at forehead, apply peel evenly and carefully until all areas are covered.
5. Wait 2 minutes.
6. Reapply peel.
7. Wait 2 minutes.

8. Reapply peel.
9. Wait 2 minutes
10. Some areas will be turning white. Apply peel only to areas that are not turning white and wait to see if they come up.
11. Then wait again.
12. Apply cold compresses to the affected area.
13. Then apply Vaseline or an occlusive ointment.
14. Client uses a predetermined gentle cleansing solution and ointment until full peeling has taken place, which may be up to 5–6 days.

Unless you have experience, you should stop here. Obviously if you are working beside a qualified nurse or physician then you can continue, but it is important to stay within the esthetician license.

The client should use a cleanser and other skin-care products without active ingredients or performance ingredients (AHAs, retinol, larger levels of vitamin C) for at least 3 weeks. You will be able to tell patients at their second posttreatment appointment when they may resume their routine.

Summary

The key to peeling and applying treatments is in the preparation. These protocols are to be used for reference purposes only. Having advanced training is necessary, and complete adherence to the policies and direction of the attending physician and state regulations is absolute.

Making good judgments using classifications and skin typing for peel and treatment selection, preparing the skin, obtaining consent, and methodical application and follow-up care are all considered rudiments in having a positive outcome. Utilizing these methods will build your repertoire in helping diverse skin challenges.

Frequently Asked Questions

1. **How does the esthetician know whether the peel they are applying is buffered?**

   Manufacturers' data information sheets will delineate whether the peel is buffered. You can also call a manufacturer and ask for specifics on peels. The firm should have, and be willing to send you, the Material Safety Data Sheets (MSDS) on their products. If you are not sure about a preparation, wait until you have enough information to make an informed decision to use it.

2. **How long after surgery can the esthetician use manual lymphatic drainage on a rhytidectomy (face-lift) patient?**

   Usually after the sutures and staples come out—at about day 8. The physician will make the initial determination. Once you are familiar with healing phases and procedures, you will recognize the appropriate time frame on postoperative treatments.

CHAPTER 19

Small Procedures and Special Clinics

- Introduction
- Injectibles
- Lip Augmentation
- Lasers and Laser Safety
- Photorejuvenation/Light Therapy
- Telangiectases/Laser Spider Vein Treatments
- Laser Hair Reduction
- Summary
- Frequently Asked Questions

Introduction

Estheticians, medical assistants, nurses, and patient-care coordinators are adroit at scheduling appointments, receiving funds for procedures, and—depending upon the licensing laws of your particular state—in performing treatments or procedures.

Small medical procedures such as vascular laser therapy, injectibles, and lip augmentations will be administered by medical personnel. In states where light therapy or laser hair reduction may be performed by a clinical esthetician, the physician must be present. This is necessary, as liability is always an issue when working in the clinic.

Special Clinics/Small Medical Procedures

One-day clinical events can be fun, lucrative, and easy to plan. Regardless of whether the esthetician, the physician, or the nursing staff is actually applying the treatment, the challenge is in the details of creating a well-executed special clinic or event. Use of staff resources will help tremendously in setting up ancillary profit events and you will not need to bring in extra help for these clinics if you train, develop proficiencies, and are aware of the skill and proper licensing that your current staff member may possess. All positions, duties and supplies must be decided well before the patients arrive. Clients and patients can feel the tension between staff members when details are not well planned or executed.

Retain Informed Consent as Protocol for all Small Medical Procedures

Risk management dictates all participants (including staff members) will sign a consent form, for all small procedures, and will follow instructions as per provided by the physician. If your patient is returning for subsequent treatments such as in the case of Botox or laser hair reduction, you need not use a different form for each procedure. Create a form that has several blank signature and date lines, to keep a running list (Figure 19–1).

Injectibles

Injectibles are primarily administered by the physician; however, a physician's assistant or RN may also train to apply the product. Materials such as **Botox** are used for the purposes of paralyzing an overzealous corrugator muscle; and collagen, fat transfers, and synthetic materials are fillers used to enhance a deflated area such as in the case of deep **rhytides**, or wrinkles, augmenting thin, small lips, or acne pocks and scars, respectively.

Rather than debate the effectiveness, controversy or other issues surrounding the various types of injectibles available today, the following discussion of them will be perfunctory and assumes that the physician or practitioner with whom you are associated has done his or her research, has made the best decision for the client, and has extensively trained in a hands-on fashion with the material being used.

Keep in mind that products come and go in all areas of the industry. Essential to maintaining a healthy practice is allowing the clinical trials to take place prior to use. Jumping on the newest or latest untried material can prove to be catastrophic to a well-respected office, and it can cause a lack of trust of you and your services.

Botox

The bacterium *Clostridium botulinum* produces seven different toxins. As we know, *Botulinum Toxin Type A,* or *Botox*, is a serum that blocks neuromuscular (nerve cell in muscle) activity. It is a nontoxic serum that, when injected into a facial muscle such as the **corrugator** (forehead between the eyes) will weaken the overdrawn muscular activity, decreasing the ability to frown and thus eliminating a fatigued, angry, appearance. It has been used successfully for wrinkles in this country for 10 years. For 30 years physicians have been using Botulinum Toxin Type A in treating **strabismus** (eyes that are misaligned) and **blepharospasm** (uncontrollable blinking). It has recently been introduced as a remedy for migraine headaches and for **hyperhidrosis,** or excessive sweating, by blocking the nerves to sweat glands.

Botulinum Toxin Type B, or **Myobloc** has been approved to treat **cervical dystonia** (neck muscles contracting abnormally causing pain). Once injected into the muscle, Myobloc creates relief to the sufferer almost instantaneously. Some of its benefits have proven to be as effective as Botox; however, it has not been cleared by the FDA to treat wrinkles at the time of this writing. Two key facts about Botox are provided below.

CONSENT FORM FOR BOTOX

Patient Name: _____

To the patient: You have the right to be informed about your condition and treatment so that you may make the decision whether or not to undergo the procedure after knowing the risks and hazards involved. This disclosure is not meant to scare or alarm you; it is simply an effort to better inform you so that you may give or withhold your consent for the treatment program.

I have requested that _____ attempt to improve my facial expression lines with Botox. This is a trademark for botulinum toxin. These injections have been used for more than a decade in children and adults to improve the problem of muscle spasm of the facial muscles. This toxin has also been useful to correct double vision due to muscle imbalance. Injection of minute amounts weaken the muscle and prevent frowning, crow's feet, and expression lines. Although the results are usually dramatic, I have been informed that the practice of medicine is not an exact science and that no guarantees can be or have been made concerning expected results in my case.
Initial if true _____

The solution is injected with a small needle into the muscle. You see the benefits develop over the next five to seven days. Less frowning will be possible.
Initial if true _____

Side effects and complications have been minimal. Occasionally, slight swelling, and/or bruising may last for several days after the injections. Rarely, an adjacent muscle may be weakened for several weeks after an injection. I have been advised of the risks involved in such treatment, the expected benefits of such treatment, and alternative treatment, including no treatment at all.
Initial if true _____

I understand that several sessions may be needed to complete the process to obtain desired results.
Initial if true _____

I agree that this constitutes full disclosure, and that it supersedes any previous verbal or written disclosures. I certify that I have read, and fully understand, the above paragraphs, and that I have sufficient opportunity for discussion and to ask questions.
Initial if true _____

Figure 19–1   Botox Consent Form

CONSENT FORM FOR BOTOX

FIRST PROCEDURE:

_____
Patient Signature   Date   Staff Signature

SECOND PROCEDURE:

_____
Patient Signature   Date   Staff Signature

THIRD PROCEDURE:

_____
Patient Signature   Date   Staff Signature

FOURTH PROCEDURE:

_____
Patient Signature   Date   Staff Signature

FIFTH PROCEDURE:

_____
Patient Signature   Date   Staff Signature

Figure 19–1   Botox Consent Form *(continued)*

Keep it in the fridge   One of the first few things that we learn about Botox is that it is perishable. It needs to be used within the allotted time, and it needs to be refrigerated. It is best to inform clients and patients that you have set aside a specific date for injections; that way you are not subject to drop-ins expecting their dose on demand. Once you are able to train your patients for these clinics, the day will run smoothly. Depending on your practice size and availability to perform Botox injections, you may want to have regularly scheduled appointments weekly, bimonthly, or monthly.

Make sure to book solid appointments   Once you determine how many people will be coming to the clinic, you can order the serum accordingly. It is best to have the serum arrive the day prior to the clinic date.

Be certain to notify all participants in advanced of their scheduled appointment time, as a no-show on this date can be a loss in revenue that cannot be made up. It is good to have a waiting list just in case someone does have to cancel with you; that way you will not waste the serum.

Indications   The primary cosmetic use of Botox Botulinum Type A, in a cosmetic application, is to paralyze the muscles that create wrinkles in the forehead (frontal region both vertical and horizontally), periorbitally, upper lip and marionette, and platysma (neck).

Contraindications

- herpetic breakout
- autoimmune diseases (lupus, arthritis, non-Hodgkin's lymphoma, where the body identifies its own cells as foreign bodies and attacks them)
- cancer
- any communicable disease
- diabetes
- bleeding disorders
- keloid or connective tissue problems
- Accutane use within 2–3 years

Collagen

Collagen products range from the effective to the ineffective. You will receive varied opinions about product, and most physicians have their favorites; those physicians are of course bound by laws that prohibit them from using products that have not been approved by the FDA or sufficiently clinically researched.

Injectible collagen comes in the form of animal: bovine (cow), porcine (pig), human (the client's own), or harvested from cadavers. It works by injecting the material to raise depressed skin to meet the surrounding skin. Depressed or wrinkled skin creates a shadow, and the darkness makes lines appear deeper. When a line is brought closer to the surface, either from underneath or from outside, the skin will look lighter, therefore smoother. As in all camouflage work, light comes forward, dark recedes.

Watch for unrealistic expectations. Most patients or clients find these injections bearable, but they often complain that the implanted collagen does not last long enough. It is also worth noting that once a client becomes used to a fuller lip or smoother depression it is difficult to measure exactly what the appropriate result should be, as they often will want more. It can be addictive for some. A good rule of thumb could be measured by a 40 percent to 60 percent improvement. You will find that others are interested in a complete change, which may also include another procedure. Collagen will not help in the case of a sagging mandible or fat pads drooping in the buccal region, creating a hollowed lateral plane to the side of the face.

Indications   Collagen can be used as filler, as in the case of a deep acne scar or pitting, nasolabial folds, thin lips, or in feature restoration such as aging lips. All patients undergo pretesting for allergic reactions.

Contraindications

- herpetic breakout
- autoimmune diseases (lupus, arthritis, non-Hodgkin's lymphoma, where the body identifies its own cells as foreign bodies and attacks them)
- cancer
- diabetes
- bleeding disorders
- keloid or connective tissue problems
- Accutane use within 2–3 years
- allergies specific to materials used

Other Injectible Fillers

Other fillers are making a presence in the market. Hyaluronic acid has been used in many preps throughout the years. Swedish-born **Restylane**, an injectible filler for wrinkles, will be approved by the FDA and marketed in the United States. This filler promises to be longer lasting and low on the irritancy scale.

Artecoll is another injectible filler and tissue-augmentation product that has been undergoing trials in the United States and soon will meet FDA approval. **Polymethyl methacrylate** or **PMMA** is formulated into small beads, which are blended with **lidocaine** and collagen for use in tissue augmentation. This is a simultaneous, two-phase process. A hypodermic needle creates a tunnel into the dermis, and while the needle is being released, the Artecoll product is deposited. The indications and contraindications are the same as for other lip-enhancement products.

Lip Augmentation

In addition to using injectible fillers, lip implantation for augmentation continues to be popular, with varying degrees of success. **Gor-Tex, Softform, UltraSoft (polytetrafluoroethylene** or **ePTFE**), and **Facsian** (human cadaver material) are all used to enhance lips and are considered more permanent than some injectibles. These implants are threaded through the lip tissue through four incision sites located at the corner of the mouth, or interior to the nasolabial fold. Great precision must be taken to trim the implant and to secure a sterile field in the operating room to avoid infection. Strict home-care compliance is necessary to allow implant proper healing. No touching, moving, or picking the implant postoperatively.

When to Use

Indications   Implants are used in reconstructive surgery, cleft palette, deep nasolabial folds, uneven or imbalanced lips, and general lip restoration as in aging mouth.

Contraindications   As with many procedures there are those clients for whom lip augmentation should not be considered. They are as follows:

- herpetic breakout
- autoimmune diseases (lupus, arthritis, non-Hodgkin's lymphoma, where the body identifies its own cells as foreign bodies and attacks them)
- cancer
- other communicable diseases
- diabetes
- bleeding disorders
- keloid or connective tissue problems
- Accutane use within 2–3 years

Optimum Results with a Combination of Lip Enhancement Materials

The 1990s were full of over-augmented lips, which created an unrealistic and unattainable lip silhouette. Many patients were having implants removed as often as they were vying for position to have another implantation. With many new lip products available in the near future, we should see both more realism combined with more respect for the parameters of a given material. This especially presents in the implants that are being created for reconstructive surgery.

Lip augmentation works best when used in conjunction with other treatments and when the physician and the patient select both a natural and a feasible amount of augmentation. For example, the vermilion region may be slightly distended with one material, such as a very thin string of Gor-Tex, or superficially lifted with Artecoll, and then the more dense lip tissue may be injected with a lighter material such as collagen or hyaluronic acid. In addition, **micropigmentation** (cosmetic tattooing), can be applied for definition, once the lips have healed, along with lip-color enhancement (lip liner, gloss, or lipstick with pout highlight in center of bottom). It is difficult to suggest that one application or material can treat the whole lip, just as one procedure cannot rejuvenate the whole face.

Lasers and Laser Safety

Lasers and the use of lasers has often inadvertently landed in the lap of many an esthetician with no training, no interest in operating them, or—worst of all—none of the appropriate credentials to manage their use. For some estheticians, being locked up in the OR all day, running a laser hair clinic, may seem tedious and isolating; it can be illegal if you are in violation of your state's licensing regulations.

It is our responsibility to obtain appropriate credentialing and licensure to operate special equipment, or to acknowledge to our employer that we are not qualified to perform certain work. If you are in compliance with state requirements, appropriately credentialed, and interested in operating a laser, then obtain as much training, continuing education, and experience as possible before treating patients. In addition, it is recommended that we read the American National Standards Institute (ANSI) publications ANSI Z136.3-1996, American National Standard for the Safe Use of Lasers in Health Care Facilities and ANSI Z 136.1-1993 American National Standard for the Safe Use of Lasers.

The word **LASER** is really an acronym for **L**ight **A**mplification by **S**timulated **E**mission of **R**adiation. The difference between lasers and light from the sun or from a light-bulb is that lasers have one color (**monochromatic**); the light waves fall in phase or travel in one direction (**coherent**), and can be focused (**collimated**) to produce a very tiny spot. Sunlight, lightbulbs, or other types of light are more diffused and are incapable of creating this type of intense, directed, light.

Depending on the type and use of the laser, this pure form of light can be directed to remove hair, spider veins, and skin and tissue. It is important to observe extreme optical (ocular, eye) safety measures while operating the laser, or even while in the room during the treatment. The following precautions must be taken to avoid permanent damage:

- Laser wave–length approved safety glasses, with printed manufacturer label and side shields, must be worn by all in the treatment room during the operation of the laser.
- The physician should fit appropriate stainless steel eye shields into the eye of the patient if areas near the eye are being treated (i.e., eyebrows, widow's peak, temples, etc.).
- Avoid looking directly into the laser beam opening—with or without glasses.
- Cover all reflective surfaces, door windows, and regular windows, to avoid laser reflecting off these surfaces, and mark treatment rooms with laser warning signs.
- When not in use, apply *Standby* mode to laser to avoid accidental activation of the laser.
- Make certain in cleaning protective eyewear to not use solvents that may remove approved coating.

In addition, here are some guidelines for laser safety in general:

- Laser accoutrements such as foot pedals or continuous-flow hand pieces should be operated only by the clinician applying the treatment to avoid accidental injury.
- Appoint one person to check all phases of the operation of laser, and another to follow up on key elements such as calibration changes, patient compliance, record keeping in the mandatory journal, and protection eyewear placement.
- Apply the *Ready* or *Start* mode of laser only when the hand piece is over the area to be treated.
- Laser keys should be located in a separate location from laser to avoid vandalism or misconduct.

- Lasers can ignite flammable solutions such as alcohol or acetone; if using these preparations, allow them to dry prior to using laser.
- Water is used to extinguish fires involving lasers.
- Oxygen will accelerate fires, so watch the use of oxygen (O_2 facial machines) in the room while using a laser.

According to the American National Standards Institute, there are four classifications of lasers:

1. Class 1 lasers are laser printers and CD/DVD players for example; they emit very low to no radiation due to the hardware in which they are enclosed.
2. Class 2 lasers emit a visible beam; one example of this type would be a bar code reader in a store.
3. Class 3 (A and B) some lasers must be used with eye protection. A telescope is an example of this type of laser.
4. Class 4 lasers are definitely hazardous to eyes, skin, and other tissues—including other objects in the room. The lasers used in medical settings are considered Class 4. Eye protection is mandatory. They will start fires and can set off explosions (if targeted) with misuse or carelessness.

Photorejuvenation/Light Therapy

Photorejuvenation is a non ablative skin rejuvenation technique which uses high intensity pulsed light to reform pigmented lesions, vascular lesions, and fine wrinkles. It improves conditions such as rosacea, hyperpigmentation, and uneven skin texture by emitting light over many wavelengths (lasers produce a single wavelength), thus allowing light to penetrate all levels of skin, and reaching areas where sluggish cells and easily dilated vessels can be found.

It has become a favorite among clients and patients without time to recover from a more invasive or lengthy procedure as there is virtually no downtime. It is important to make certain that the expectations are realistic, however. It can be an excellent precursor to a facelift for preoperative conditioning, and can be used as maintenance between procedures.

Indications   Rosacea, photoaging, and hyperpigmentation.

Contraindications

- herpetic breakout
- autoimmune diseases (lupus, arthritis, non-Hodgkin's lymphoma, where the body identifies its own cells as foreign bodies and attacks them)
- Propionibacterium acnes (P. acnes)
- cancer
- skin cancer
- diabetes

- bleeding disorders
- keloid or connective tissue problems
- Accutane use within 2–3 years
- pacemaker/heart issues
- epilepsy

Telangiectases/Laser Spider Vein Treatments

The work on the newer vascular and hair reduction lasers is to be highly commended. Patients are sharing heartfelt stories and leaving our clinics in tears not because of the discomfort of a given treatment, but more because of the ease—and more importantly the results—they are achieving from their treatments. Clients speak of uncomfortable events with family, friends, and co-workers suspecting them of alcohol abuse, negligent hygiene, or other ill health issues; vascular laser has led to the improvement or near elimination of the rosaceous condition created by telangiectases.

Indications   Telangiectases, rosacea, small hemangiomas are all indications for use of vascular lasers.

Contraindications

- herpetic breakout
- autoimmune diseases (lupus, arthritis, non-Hodgkin's lymphoma, where the body identifies its own cells as foreign bodies and attacks them)
- cancer
- skin cancer
- communicable diseases
- rosacea flare
- diabetes
- bleeding disorders
- keloid or connective tissue problems
- Accutane use within 2–3 years
- pacemaker/heart issues
- epilepsy

Laser Hair Reduction

Just as vascular lasers have improved the lives of clients with rosacea and telangiectases, lasers for hair reduction have eliminated embarrassment for many women and men who are victims of excessive hair in unwanted places.

New technology promises to treat not only the darkest hair, but also light hair, and all skin types and colors. Many are anxiously awaiting the advent of these new machines. However, it may be prudent for us professionals to remember why it is that we have hair, and recall its role in the wound-healing process. Most patients who come in for treatment have discernable and legitimate complaints about unwanted hair, but let's responsibly guide those who may be hair-phobic. Some hair is necessary.

If you have your own machine and plenty of space, this treatment may be performed at any time by estheticians, medical assistants, and nurses. It may prove wise however, to lease a machine; that way you do not have to bear the expense of repair and obsolescence. Many marketing plans include messages such as "Make sure that your clinic owns the laser." Ownership may be unnecessary. When you consider that most machines are in the $100,000–$130,000 range, you realize that it takes thousands of procedures to pay for the laser before you are really making a profit, and by then there is new technology available.

It is best to have a well-orchestrated plan with specific dates when energy is put to good use. Employ the use of marketing, laser, product, and personnel. It is possible to treat between 25 and 30 people in a day set aside for hair reduction. The time spent with each client is dependent on the areas to be treated, so plan accordingly. Simply put, upper lip may take 5 minutes, but a full back will take a bigger chunk of your day. Fees are also based upon time and can be geographically determined. Market value is important here. A small rural community will not bear the fees that a large metropolitan area with suburbs adjoining will.

Indications   **Hirsutism**, dark wiry hair undesired by client or patient on areas of face, arms, legs, back or other areas, is a prime target. It may be necessary to refer the patient to a physician for an evaluation, as there may be an underlying condition promoting the hair—polycystic ovaries or a thyroid condition, for example.

Contraindications

- herpetic breakout
- autoimmune diseases (lupus, arthritis, non-Hodgkin's lymphoma, where the body identifies its own cells as foreign bodies and attacks them)
- cancer
- skin cancer
- communicable diseases
- rosacea flare
- diabetes
- bleeding disorders
- keloid or connective tissue problems
- Accutane use within 2–3 years
- Fitzpatrick skin type contraindication for your machine
- pacemaker/heart issues/circulatory problems
- epilepsy
- sunburn/tan

Summary

Looking at small procedures is good business. The esthetician's role may be primarily in the organization of these clinics or special events, or more directly involved in a hands-on fashion. Do keep in mind, however, if you get yourself locked into a schedule of full-day operating of a hair reduction clinic, for example, that is time you will not be able to use in building your practice or handling the retailing aspect of your business.

Often, what works most efficiently and effectively is that the esthetician works in partnership with the physician on the pretreatment consults (which incidentally can be worked into a skin-care consultation with product recommendations and purchases). Then the actual treatment is performed by the medical assistant, which keeps the overhead down for the physician as most estheticians make commission on treatments, and ultimately the client is sent back for follow-up with the esthetician (which in turn may result in further skin-care treatment plans, products, or subsequent surgical procedures).

Whatever you choose to do with regard to operating lasers, make certain that you are within the boundaries of your legal scope, that you continue to upgrade your training, and that you are compulsive about communicating any and all questionable issues regarding the treatment of a patient, client, or employee to the physician and medical personnel.

Frequently Asked Questions

1. **What does the esthetician do if she or he becomes too busy to handle the regular clientele while applying the laser for the hair reduction sessions?**

   This happens often in the clinic when there is a new treatment to perform. Everyone wants to jump on it. It is always beneficial to really look at all angles of who is best suited for applying treatments. Keep in mind what your goals are, and naturally, the physician's need at a given time. If there is no one currently available to help you with your load, consider bringing in an additional medical assistant or nurse for whom this type of work is an interest. Many nurses would like to have additional responsibilities and are interested in esthetics; some may have an occasional interest, in which case this could be an ideal match.

2. **To save a client a trip to the office, what are the rules to applying skin-care treatments on the days that clients have Botox or collagen injections?**

   This is common in medical spas, and we can perform many treatments without a problem. However, many clients will not be interested in having a peel or some other advanced treatment after having a small procedure such as collagen injections or lip augmentation. They are not without some discomfort, and if anesthesia was used, an additional treatment may not be possible.

   If a client insists on having a microdermabrasion, for example, at the clinic on the day of her **Botox** injection, speak with the physician about the sites that were injected, and avoid those areas. If it was just the forehead, no problem: do the remainder of the face. If, however, there were many sites injected with **Botox,** wait 2 weeks before applying microdermabrasion or other treatments that will stimulate circulation.

Individual Appearance Issues

CHAPTER 20

Camouflage Therapy and Cosmetic Support

- Introduction
- Basic Principles of Makeup Enhancement
- Individual Appearance Issues
- Short-Term Use of Camouflage Therapy
- Makeup Applications for Specific Cosmetic Procedures
- Long-Term Use of Camouflage Applications for Facial Disfigurement
- Summary
- Frequently Asked Questions

Introduction

The fine art and science of makeup application crosses all generations, gender, and times. Styles come and go; however, most of us in the industry have built our skill upon a foundation of basic science and artistic principles. Some estheticians have progressed beyond those fundamentals to use their acquired skills to help clients and patients build self-esteem and confidence.

Estheticians, stylists, personal shoppers, appearance counselors, therapists, physicians, cosmetologists, and dentists have all played important roles in the lives of individuals dealing with appearance issues. Clinical estheticians have become a significant adjunct in the medical field; we are specialized technicians with the training, time, sensitivity, and ability to help others with appearance transitions.

Whether makeup application is routine or camouflage, it is essential that it is *useful for the client*. Estheticians are educators, particularly in clinical work, as we are from the beginning demonstrating how clients can take the steps to apply the makeup themselves. This sets us apart from all other types of artistry.

Having patience and a kind demeanor is helpful while patients are learning something new. It rarely comes easily or second nature to people, and they may well be frustrated as they try to replicate the great job that they have experienced by the professional. You will need to give them as many opportunities as they need to master their own skill and style.

Basic Principles of Makeup Enhancement

In basic makeup application and in the crossover from routine to camouflage, the techniques are similar. We are using methods to enhance the appearance of some features while playing down others. Techniques known as shading and highlighting and blending are used in both genres.

Shading creates depth in areas that need sculpting, defining, and or form. *Highlighting* an area brings a subject forward. As with great watercolor techniques, *blending* is applied to soften the demarcation lines, so that you cannot see where the shading ends and the highlighting begins. In the case of shading, the darker the color, the more an object will recede, or go back into space. Conversely, the lighter a color is, the more the object will appear closer or move forward. Blending the two creates the illusion that the color becomes one, with accents/highlights and depth/contour. All other colors that you apply are just different values, or different levels of lightness and darkness.

Whether we are shading a face for more definition, applying color correction to a **hemangioma** (red birthmark), or toning down skin fresh from **abrasion**, we are working with the same basic principles in using lightness, darkness, and color amalgamation (combination) or blending.

Individual Appearance Issues

Camouflage suggests hiding, concealing, covering, veiling, or disguising something. Nature uses camouflage: birds, animals, and sea life all benefit from camouflage for their basic survival. This can be true for some people as well. Those with facial disfigurements experience problems arising from social interactions, and these can be devastating for them. Self-esteem issues run deep in those with disfigurements both congenital and acquired through an accident.

Disfigured individuals are as distressed by their self-perceptions as they are by those reflected back to them through the eyes of others. They may respond with a variety of behaviors—aggressive, passive, hostile, or receptive—to cosmetic support, depending on how they are approached, exposed, or intruded upon, and on how much time they have had to adjust to their situation.

For some, camouflage therapy is a temporary measure to employ while recovering from a surgical procedure, or to resolve a stage of adjustment in coping with a disfigurement. For others, it is a lifetime of searching and researching new products to deal with a congenital condition or the aftermath of an accident.

As in all clinical work, you may find camouflage therapy challenging. You may see some very difficult cases, and sometimes you will feel helpless. The following conditions will often prove to be the most emotionally challenging:

- **Accidents involving children and teenagers.**   Accidents both physically and mentally change children's perceptions, either permanently or transitionally, of who they are, and how they relate to others. Often teens will seek camouflage therapy in hope of covering scarring from the aftermath of an accident. Depending upon the severity of the wound, it may or may not work.
- **Burn survivors.**   Burn survivors have three sets of problems. Not only do they have scars, but also because of the mottling and morphing of the skin, makeup does not always hold. In addition, they may not be able to completely remove some of the heavier skin-care products, thus creating other problems with pore plugging and cystic type of acne.
- **Cancer survivors.**   Cancer patients who have lost a jaw or chin may seek camouflage therapy to cope with daily looks and stares from others—which are especially devastating as the individual is learning to cope. In addition, you may see clients coming in for cosmetic support while going through chemotherapy; they may have lost their hair.
- **Loss of eye.**   A client may come to you for makeup to add to the symmetry of a newly placed artificial eye. The prosthesis may be a type of large contact lens that is placed on the retina in the eye socket, or it may be a complete unit that takes the place of the original eye.
- **Self-abuse.**   An individual with a history of self-inflicted excoriations, razor blade scars, or in some cases self-surgical procedures, may come in for camouflage therapy. These are very difficult cases and require a team approach involving the physician and nursing personnel, and possibly a mental health specialist. It is important to have this individual fully evaluated prior to treatment, as you do not want to be a trigger for another self-abuse situation. This is a complex disease, not typically understood even by physicians or therapists.
- **Congenital disorders causing deformation.**   Individuals with childhood diseases and disorders may present for camouflage therapy. They may have had time to adjust to their unique problem and may just need support and skills for cosmetic enhancement.

Short-Term Use of Camouflage Therapy

Working with an individual for short-term camouflage therapy due to a cosmetic procedure will be quite different from treatment due to a lifetime condition, congenital birth defect, or traumatic accident. Often postoperative cosmetic patients are delighted about an appointment for makeup at this point, as they have felt exiled from their routine lives. They also may feel anxious about family and friends finding out about the surgery. Have the finest camouflage makeup available for purchase, as patients do not like to go to a department store during the postoperative phase. Make certain that it is easy to use. Have a schematic or face chart on which to indicate the colors that you use as you proceed with the instruction.

It is important to keep makeup sessions as simple as possible. Remember: you may be a fabulous artist, but your clients need to be able to perform the treatment on themselves. We should be able to apply the makeup and give them a lesson in about 20 to 30 minutes. If it takes you longer to apply this makeup, they may feel that they will never be able to acquire your skill.

If you do more than one session, it may be useful to apply the makeup to one side and then let the client do the other. However, on the first one, apply the full treatment to offer the gift of seeing a rejuvenated and sometimes restored face. This can be an emotional experience for some patients. It is important to have compassion and allow the feelings to come up, yet reassure them that they will be able to reproduce this new look at home.

Old habits are difficult to break, and at times, you may find that people will want to apply a treatment no longer appropriate to an area that has been positively altered by surgery. This happens particularly on the upper lid regions, where a heavy contouring shadow may have been used for a droopy eyelid. Again, with compassion and with an educational approach, show that individual why it is no longer necessary to apply dark shadow on the lid, and show them a fresh—and probably much easier—way to apply color.

Many clinical estheticians do not feel that their job description includes camouflage therapy, and that can be difficult for the patient or client requesting this type of private setting for cosmetic support. If you are adamant about not applying makeup, build an alliance with another practitioner who does.

Makeup Applications for Specific Cosmetic Procedures

Typically, camouflage therapy directed at postoperative conditions will be short-term. Once the affected areas have healed, the client will return to routine makeup and may use much less product or, in some cases, none. Each procedure will dictate the type and scope of camouflage therapy depending on the areas which require concealing and on the direct interest of the client. If a client has no interest in camouflage therapy or makeup in general, it is important to respect their wishes and make no judgments about their choice. Here are a few approaches to deciding when and how to apply camouflage makeup.

Laser Resurfacing/Chemical Peel

Each physician will determine when it is appropriate for the patient to begin using camouflage makeup therapy. When training, judgment, and trust have been established between the physician and the esthetician, the physician will defer to the esthetician for camouflage therapy.

When   Typically, this is done somewhere between 10 days to 2 weeks postlaser, depending on the home-care compliancy of patient, the specific healing pattern, or whether the skin has completely re-epithelialized (it has intact barrier as epidermis has grown back).

What   Today's high-tech, low-impact, sheer, inert mineral powders (such as titanium dioxide) work the best for postlaser camouflage. They can be lightly dusted or gently sponged on freshly ameliorated (laser resurfaced or peeled) skin to camouflage the redness created by the procedure. The redness (erythema) may last for 2 to 4 months depending on skin type and condition of the skin.

For this type of application, the days of using green color-correcting products have been all but eliminated by the use of mineral powders and foundations with "built-in" correcting measures. Yellow turns out to be a much better color-correction device in most preparations designed to camouflage redness, because it blends in with the natural skin tones of most ethnic origins. Green color correction must be covered with an additional product, and then powdered to set. Keep in mind that, as with all things, there are exceptions. You may have a client or patient for whom the green is necessary due to personal choice, or extreme erythema.

Mineral powders can also be fused with sunscreens, moisturizers, eye creams, and some gels, depending on the need of the patient at that point in his or her recovery. There are also liquid foundations containing titanium dioxide. Newer, lighter bases are excellent coverage, and these can be used in addition to the powders if a person prefers a liquid base.

How   When applying camouflage to a patient's skin postlaser, it is important to:

1. Always start with a fresh bottle or new powder.
2. Do not use a heavy makeup or powder because it may clog pores, which are more refined because of the surgery.
3. Use a quality, soft, powder brush or sponge.
4. Apply light layers of base, and gently pat in powder on areas of darker redness.
5. Make certain that the patient has an appropriate cleansing product that will not overstimulate the skin (use no performance agents), yet will collect camouflage product.

Face-Lift/Rhytidectomy

Camouflage treatment after rhytidectomy (face-lift) primarily targets bruising. We will often not be able to treat all of the bruising, but we can cover the various colors of yellow, green, plum, red, and dark purple, which are common following a face-lift.

The bruising may involve the face, neck, and chest, depending on the extensiveness of the surgery and the patient's skin type and color.

When   A full camouflage treatment may typically be performed at about day 10, after the sutures and staples are removed. It is important to avoid the immediate scar site with your therapy, until it is completely healed, to avoid irritation.

What   Once this area has completely healed, and you receive the go-ahead, you may apply base and/or powder directly on the scar to tone down the redness. Some scars will be slightly **hypertrophic**, or have a ridge; others will be flat and smooth. This will depend on the type of procedure and on the patient's ability to heal. Eventually most scars will lose color and blend in with the rest of the skin tone, and most will flatten. The patient will use products to conceal the scars for many months.

How   Use routine makeup applications for all areas that are not affected by bruising or incisions. In areas of bruising, use slightly more foundation and mineral powder. Pat or stipple makeup products on gently, these areas may be tender and may require several light application to cover. This applies to incision sites as well. Inform the client that it is advisable that they start with fresh makeup: their older products may contain bacteria.

Eyelift/Blepharoplasty

A blepharoplasty or eyelift will give an artist a rewarding challenge to meet. Nothing can change the look of a face like the rejuvenation of a crepey, baggy, tired eye. Albeit subtle, treatment of the eye area with a fresh application of shadow base to lighten and brighten the lid, which had hidden below droopy skin, is sometimes all these patients will want, particularly if they are older and are interested primarily in function.

When   Typically at about day 7 or 8 sutures will come out. However, the physician may want a day or two after removal before makeup such as shadow, mascara, or liner is applied. That said, many clients using quality mineral powders may choose to apply a light powder application to conceal bruising and erythema prior to suture removal.

What   Mineral powder as a base can typically wipe out redness or bruising, with a swipe of a shadow sponge. Using a slight yellow undertone to the powder can neutralize redness; this makes a great base for a light shadow color to adhere to. Mascara and liner can be used at about day 8 to 10 (depending upon healing and physician recommendations). Adding a darker shadow color on the incision in the crease may be appropriate at 3 weeks if substantial healing has taken place.

How   Covering the bruised area is often the first order of business, followed by applying the other eye therapy products on top. It is important that the patient have a gentle eye-makeup remover to remove this camouflage product. In addition, a cotton ball should be *patted* on the lid, not pulled across the new incision site. Instruct the patient to flush with water to make certain that the cleanser is off the eyelid.

Long-Term Use of Camouflage Applications for Facial Disfigurement

Often we all want to rush in to help a person who we consider in need of camouflage therapy due to an accident or a congenital birth defect. Susan Lindsey, a clinical esthetician and rehabilitation specialist from Edmonds, Washington, works with people seeking feature enhancement and restoration due to congenital disfigurements, cancer, burns, and accidents. She says, "The use of makeup is an option to ease the way back into an appearance-focused society. Not wearing makeup may be as important a choice as wearing it." Susan's wise statement is at the threshold of all camouflage therapy. For all of us working with appearance issues, it is important that we do not put our biases or judgments into the situation. We can guide, instruct, and demonstrate, but all decisions and choices about using camouflage therapy are up to the client.

Camouflage Therapy as a Choice

As a choice, camouflage therapy provides many with the opportunity to improve their quality of life through an increase in self-esteem and confidence. Here are a few guidelines in working with a client using long-term camouflage therapy:

- Do not assume that the client does not know how or what to use in camouflage makeup. They are more familiar with their faces than we are. They may be expert at applying makeup and are just looking for something new. Check it out.
- Maintain a private environment. Do not allow calls, interruptions, or other clients to view the session.
- Remain calm and relaxed.
- Keep full documentation.
- Attend camouflage therapy courses routinely. There are often new techniques and lighter products being introduced.
- Make certain to have the products available in samples for home trial and in regular stock ready for purchase.
- As with all clients, use care and active listening skills. Depending upon their physiological state and the length of time since the loss of a facial feature, they may not have come to terms with the changes. Pay attention here. Chances are that we may be able to improve the appearance of the disfigurement, but it is possible that we may not.
- Provide consistent results and be realistic.
- If the individual has not come to terms with an accident or postoperative feature-changing surgery, it may be best to just visit with the patient, with the physician in attendance.

When a Client Is Not Ready for Treatment

Depending on the type of accident or surgery, the severity of the injuries, and the coping abilities of the survivor, people are going to be traumatized to some degree by the changes in their appearance. Some accident survivors are angry and unhappy, or unsatisfied with anything you might suggest.

In addition, we never want to give false hope or the impression that we can take away the disfigurement. It may be that the survivor needs to just talk about the accident and slowly move toward acceptance. Allow the client to share feelings and concerns with you without making any judgments. Avoid statements like: "We will make you look better," or "We can cover this with makeup."

Once again, remember it is important that they feel that they are choosing their own method of recovery and coping, and that whatever they choose is the best for *them*, not for the challenge that it may present to us. We never want them to walk out feeling worse.

When the client *is* interested in trying some camouflage techniques, be patient, pleasant, consistent and ask:

1. What is your greatest area of concern?
2. What have you tried before? How does that work now?
3. What do you hope these sessions can do for you?
4. Take it at their pace. If they know what they want and are ready to move forward, go ahead. If they are hesitant, let them know that they can always come back another time when or if they are ready.

Do not assume that you know what the client is feeling, or know which areas they want treated. Always ask: What are your areas of concern? This goes for all cosmetic and esthetic support.

Summary

Many estheticians have become unsung heroes in their work, whether working with accident survivors, congenital facial disfigurements, restoring topical features, or directing short-term camouflage therapy. In assisting clients or patients to ease back into their routine lives feeling confident and rejuvenated, we have filled a major need. This is constantly demanded of professionals. Here are some Web sites that you may find helpful while working in camouflage therapy:

www.lookgoodfeelbetter.org
www.headcovers.com
www.bonsecourshamptonroads.com
www.letsfaceit.com
www.changingfaces.co.uk
www.victoriaraynor.com
www.cancer.com

Some agencies facilitate and assist clients or patients and volunteers in the process of recovery and beyond, while connecting the two groups. If you are interested in taking your experience and professionalism to another level, you may be interested in volunteering your time or gifts to them.

Frequently Asked Questions

1. **What does the esthetician do if the client can easily be helped, but just will not take the time required to apply the product?**

   Support the client in their decision, and realize that we do not know what is taking place inside of the client. They may be trying to come to terms with the scar or disfigurement—or other issues that may be taking precedence.

2. How does the esthetician cope with his or her own feelings of fear or repulsion when working with a severely disfigured person?

This can be a very frightening experience, particularly if you have not seen many people postoperatively, after an accident, or with a severe disfigurement. It is necessary for all of us to examine why we want to do this type of work, understand the level of our involvement, and to know our personal limitations and those in our work.

Reconstructive and plastic surgeons are always in front of people needing prostheses or restoration, and in general are coping with applying measures to reestablish symmetry. It is beneficial to consult with the physician about a client or patient, to understand what has happened and what the implications are for the specific condition. Often this is an inch-by-inch process. We never want to further impact the patient by presenting as fearful, repulsed, or shocked by the disfigurement. Preparation is the key.

It is not healthy for an esthetician to try to handle advanced cases without training and support. Many of us do take to this type of work very easily, however. The experienced professional will see the disfigurement in context and will address personal issues before entering into the situation. In addition, a clinical esthetician or rehabilitation specialist will understand the practical limitations, will know that the client will share their comfort level, and in time will lose any fear of the situation.

CHAPTER 21

Think Multiculturally and in Living Color, the Big Business of Makeup, Micropigmentation

- Introduction
- Build a Business Including All Skin Colors
- Products, Treatments, and Protocols Are Basically the Same for All Skin Shades
- The Business Side of Makeup
- Micropigmentation/Permanent Cosmetic Makeup
- Summary
- Frequently Asked Questions

Introduction

The term *multicultural* is not a word used to mark how dissimilar we are while living together in our politically correct world. Rather, it presents an opportunity to share how *similar* we are to one another beneath the surface. In esthetics, we view people from all cultures as having many things in common, and one of them is to enjoy the inherent beauty that lies within each person. We also see the beauty in diversity, because we are trained to use color and understand the importance of applying it to bring out natural features and enhance the existing characteristics of our clients. No two faces are the same, nor is the left side of a face exactly like the right side. We are equipped to embrace diversity and differences just by the nature of what we do.

Our world is demanding that we learn how to run our businesses to include people from all ethnic backgrounds and spiritual preferences and from both genders. We must have in place products, treatments, and the knowledge to use them on all types and colors of skin.

Build a Business Including All Skin Colors

Building an inclusive business rich in diversity is challenging, but it is also good business. We need to step out of our cubicles, to look at how we could be improving our practices to include people from ethnic and cultural backgrounds different from our own. It is easy to keep the status quo and remain comfortable with makeup color, skin-care products, and treatments that we are accustomed to using; it is exciting and growth promoting to evolve.

The greatest challenge that we face in doing this may be overcoming fear. That fear is generated by the lack of knowledge that we have about skin color that is darker or lighter than our own. If it is only a few shades lighter or darker, we seem to manage, but if it is completely different, to be honest, we are afraid that we might cause more harm than good.

Skin Color Myths

We are all "people of color." It is important that we begin to or continue to see ourselves in this way. We find different shades everywhere: within our ethnic group, within our own families, on our own bodies, on our own faces, and within our own eyes. There is a multitude of misunderstandings about skin color and the treatment of lighter, medium, or darker skin. Here are some of the myths about skin functions, conditions, and color:

- Darker skin has more melanocytes.
- Lighter skin is fragile and bleeds more easily than darker skin.
- African American skin contains more oil.
- Asian skin is less sensitive than white skin because it has more color.
- Native American, Hispanic, or East Indian skin does not burn.
- Light white skin never tans.
- The structure and function of darker skin is different from that of lighter skin.

Myth 1. Darker skin has more melanocytes.   Not true. The amount of melanin is the same; it appears darker because the melanocytes are larger, not because there are more of them (Thrower, 1999 p. 4). Cells in lighter skin break down more quickly as they move toward the surface than they do in darker skin. All skin is light just below the epidermis.

Myth 2. Lighter skin is more fragile and bleeds more easily than darker skin. Lighter skin has all of the complexities that darker skin has. True, it is more vulnerable to UV radiation, but some darker skin can be sensitive and fragile as well. Lighter skin is not as prone to inflammatory pigmentation as darker skin is, and it tolerates many acid peels without scarring (if proper applications are observed). Light skin can be resilient and durable.

Lighter skin does not bleed more easily. Bleeding disorders or a propensity to bleed crosses all skin colors. Lighter skin shows bruising, hematomas, or blood in an abrasion more easily because of the contrast in color.

Myth 3. African American skin has more oil.   Not true. African American skin has the same amount of oil as lighter skin; it just reflects more light from the oil in darker skin. (Thrower, 1999, p. 3). Darker skin may sweat more readily due to its absorption of the sun's UV rays, thus creating a heat-releasing system.

Myth 4. Asian skin is less sensitive than white skin because it often has more color.   Asian skin is typically the most sensitive of all skin types. It does not tolerate acid peels easily and is prone to hyperpigmentation. It will frost very easily during lower-level glycolic peels, and it should be considered a sensitive skin type subject to patch testing prior to using performance agents in home-care and in in-office peels. It responds well to products containing soothing agents such as **allantoin** or azulene and skin lighteners such as kojic and bearberry.

Myth 5. Native American, Hispanic, or East Indian skin does not burn.   This is false. These skin types, with a full range of colors, can and will burn subject to adequate exposure. In addition, with more exposure, they can hyperpigment, are at risk for hypopigmentation (in the darker shades), and, although rarely, can develop skin cancer.

Myth 6. Light skin never tans.   Again, this is a myth. Light skin can tan and retain a tan. Just as with all skin, light skin out of defense will produce the necessary melanin to rush to the surface to protect the skin from UVA/UVB radiation—hence the tan. It is, however, the most vulnerable of all of the skin colors to photoaging and skin cancer.

Myth 7. The structure and function of darker skin is different from that of lighter skin.   No. The structure and function of the skin are the same in all colors. The structure combines the three distinct layers: the epidermis, dermis, and the subcutaneous. The functions of protection, temperature, sensation, secretion, excretion, and absorption/metabolism are all necessary components of human skin.

Build Color Awareness

Dispelling myths about skin color encourages us to begin to look at our practices differently. When we go to trade shows, or look through journals and magazines, it is healthy for us to look for colors outside of our routine selections, and begin to increase our treatment plans to include masks, peels, protocols, and makeup tips that will help build a more complete color component to our practice.

Products, Treatments, and Protocols Are Basically the Same for All Skin Shades

Products and treatments for gold, brown, or darker skin are the same as for pink, creamy light, beige, or medium-light skin. However, due to pigment issues, the aggressiveness of a given product or treatment may vary. Obtain a full history prior to recommending a product or treatment for any client; you will want to know whether they are pregnant, on Accutane, or have allergies or sensitivities. There are products and treatments that create problems with all skin types and shades depending upon condition, age, health issues, environmental factors, and compliancy.

Special Considerations

It is best to really get to know a skin before you apply your favorite aggressive or antiaging treatment, and it is always good to test patch every client with a new treatment. Here are some special considerations for treating skin that is darker in pigment:

- **Do not assume that skin is oily.** The skin is not necessarily oily, and in fact may be dry or dehydrated. The skin may look oilier than it is, due to reflective quality of oil on darker skin.
- **Watch overtreating skin with machines such as brushes, microdermabrasion, or vacuum.** Be sure to not traumatize skin with abrasive actions which may increase potential for postinflammatory hyperpigmentation.
- **Be careful when performing extractions.** Extractions *always* should be done with care; however, be especially careful when treating dark skin due to its innate propensity to scar.
- **Use lighter concentrations of AHAs and BHAs.** Using less concentrated forms of glycolic, lactic, and or salicylic acid is indicated because higher levels may create pigmentary changes.
- **Use and sell sunscreen.** Darker skin will benefit from UVA/UVB protection and it will help to keep lesions with darker pigment from getting darker. Look for sunscreen without the minerals zinc oxide and titanium dioxide, which will look ashen and white on golden or brown skin.
- **Use natural skin lighteners, along with lower levels of hydroquinone for pigment issues.** Skin lighteners such as kojic, bearberry, arbutin, and licorice are used for lightening (albeit slowly) pigmented areas. The FDA has approved the use of hydroquinone in lower levels for darker skin (Thrower, 1999, p. 46). Studies show that higher levels in darker skin are not more helpful. Hydroquinone has been used for darker pigmented areas but has actually been removed from the shelves in other countries (Robinson, articles 2001). If overused, it can create a condition known as **exogenous ochronosis,** which is characterized by an extreme form of hyperpigmentation, and which can eventually create nodules and a permanent loss of pigment.

All clients will be especially appreciative of your taking the time to acquire the knowledge of product and process for serving them. In addition, having cosmetic support appropriate to their color range and undertone, when it may be different from yours, will keep a client loyal to you. It is important to understand some of the basics about color and its application based on undertone.

Understanding Undertones

The color of a person's undertone affects the outcome of applied color probably more than any other palette issue. We can select what we deem as the perfect shade for the individual, but if it does not possess the same color undertone as the client, it will not match regardless of what you try to do.

All color comes with a predominant base. The bases either are warm in tone (the autumn or spring shades of gold, orange, or bronze) or cool-toned (pink, rose, or blue, often the colors of summer or winter). Taking this one step further, there can be some browns with cooler undertone such as taupe, and some blues with a warm undertone such as teal. Even though some companies will call products neutral shades, you will see the colors favoring a warm or a cool base.

This concept works for house paint, dyes for clothing or paper, and in nature in general. Everything we see will have predominant undertone. Some leaves on plants will have a cool green undertone with a hint of blue, while other green plants will have a warmer undertone and contain a hint of yellow. There are ranges and overlaps in warm and cool colors; nonetheless, there will be a primary proclivity toward one or the other.

This phenomenon exists in skin color. A Fitzpatrick Skin Type I, blond with blue eyes, will often have a cool, pink/blue undertone, and so may a Fitzpatrick Skin Type V. A Fitzpatrick Skin Type III may have a warm undertone, but another client in the same color classification may have a cooler undertone, thus making a warm/gold foundation look orange on her skin. This is where paying attention to undertone makes a big difference.

A foundation or powder with a cool undertone (pinkish-bluish) will look ashy on a person whose skin has a warmer undertone. Conversely, a client with a cool undertone to the skin will look yellow or orange if a warmer product is applied. The best way to test is to use four stripes of foundation in each color key near the shade of the client and see which one disappears. The one that vanishes or looks the least noticeable is the correct one.

Keep in mind that many people with darker skin may have several shades on the face. You may need to apply two different shades: the forehead and chin may be darker than the cheeks, for example. Most clients will be pleased that you have this capability and will not mind buying an extra product to even out skin tone. Fair-skinned clients typically will have two or three shades that are rotated throughout the seasons, depending on sun exposure.

The Business Side of Makeup

Makeup is annually a billion-dollar business. We all take the industry for granted and often assume that we can leave it to the department stores or salons to sell makeup. This is a mistake. You can increase your business by 20 percent just by offering makeup. Trends come and go, but typically women who come into a physician's office for products and treatments are often those with considerable self-knowledge. They are not looking for the latest in lip gloss. They are more interested in having makeup that suits their skin condition, color key, age, image, and lifestyle. Not to mention the fact that they appreciate being able to walk out after a treatment all ready for a lunch date. A woman at a luncheon with other women, or back at work, will be flattered by friends and co-workers complimenting her on her apparently refreshed appearance. Another benefit to you and to your client.

1. Determine whether client is warm or cool undertone.	1. Need a range of warm and cool shades.
2. Apply foundation and concealer to properly prepped face with sponge.	2. Need sponge to apply makeup and concealer.
3. Apply powder with powder brush.	3. Need powders in warm and cool ranges and brush.
4. Apply blush with blush brush.	4. Need blush shades in warm and cool tones, along with brush.
5. Apply shadow light-medium range.	5. Need shadows in warm and cool tones with light and medium tones.
6. Apply eye liner, mascara.	6. Need liners in light-medium and dark colors.
7. Apply lip liner and lipstick.	7. Need lip liners and lipsticks.

Regarding makeup application and sales, the basic question is: "What do you need to serve makeup requirements?" Walking through a simple makeup application may prove useful in determining how to integrate this service:

Granted, this is oversimplified, but one does not really need a major expenditure to set up a makeup business in the office. Look for makeup that is of excellent quality, as you cannot put a poor quality makeup on freshly ameliorated skin (laser resurfacing) or on skin with allergies or other sensitivities. Make sure that it is oil-free and low in fatty additives, which can be pore clogging. Dryer skin type clients can always use slightly more moisturizer, but they of course will benefit from not having skin clogged as well.

Consider that with every treatment that you perform, you have an opportunity to sell the skin-care products you are using. Foundation, a powder, a blush, liners, lipstick, mascara, and a brush or two will benefit you threefold.

Micropigmentation/Permanent Cosmetic Makeup

Tattooing, permanent makeup, dermagraphics, intradermal pigmentation, and micropigmentation are all names for **permanent cosmetic makeup.** Decorating the skin by applying colored dye into the dermis has been in existence for millennia. Dating back to the ancient Egyptians as early as 2000 B.C., tattooing has developed as a popular form of beautifying the body. Both ancient and current tribes use forms of tattooing to distinguish one another and in rites of passage ceremonies. Cultural expressions have been realized by skin markings, whether through color implantation or scar creation (slashing the skin to produce a certain marking).

Medical Applications

Modern uses for permanent makeup are vast, and serve as a blessing for those who have undergone reconstructive surgery due to cancer or accidents, or those born with disfigurements. For people with cleft palate, or for breast reconstruction after mastectomy, permanent cosmetic color can be used to improve the appearance of a restoration when the limits of surgery have been reached. Skin pigmentation in burn survivors can become more even, and keloids may relax after the treatment. For those patients who have lost hair due to cancer, **alopecia** (hair loss), or trauma, brows can be simulated and eyes lined to give definition to the face, and to help boost self-esteem. It is also useful for people with physical disabilities such as arthritis, Parkinson's disease, multiple sclerosis, and visual impairments. For others just wanting to spend less time applying makeup, for contact lens wearers, for those allergic to makeup ingredients, or for those wanting to define features on an aging face, this can be an easy solution.

Typical uses for permanent cosmetic makeup   Routine uses include eyes (eyebrows, eye liner) and lips (lip liner, full lip color).

Medical applications and feature restoration   These include:

- lip or cleft palate: vermilion restoration/asymmetry
- breast: areola (nipple)
- hair simulation: eyebrow (loss of hair)
- pigment loss: vitiligo
- scar camouflage (burns, accidents)
- aging feature

The Treatment

Practitioners recommend a series of visits. First, an artist will test patch to prove that the client is not allergic to the product. If well tolerated, color is gradually applied in a pointillist manner (small strokes or dots) or with hair-like strokes into the dermis.

Advancements in topical anesthetics have made it more comfortable for the client, and these are preferred to injected anesthesia, which is associated with swelling that renders the treatment less feasible. Using newer modalities such as light therapy can minimize swelling and postoperative healing time.

After the treatment, the client is told to follow strict home-care instructions to allow pigmentation to heal. If the affected area is manipulated by pulling or picking the pigmented areas, color may be lost. An ointment is applied for approximately 72 hours.

Education/Training

If properly trained, the clinical esthetician with an aptitude for graphic art, good color awareness and acuity, and a background in general cosmetic principles is in an excellent position to perform permanent makeup. *Strict protocols and standards must be followed for performing this treatment*. This is not something learned via a correspondence course. One should find a program fully accredited with extensive hands-on training. From there, specialists recommend that you work as an apprentice. The Society for Permanent Cosmetic Professionals and the American Academy of Micropigmentation are organizations with membership available to support industry standards, offer continuing education, and provide mentorship. Both associations require 40-hour minimum basic training courses and recommend apprenticeships.

Summary

The world of color is fascinating, true, and natural. Where would we be if we lived a monochromatic existence? It would be uninspiring. Many estheticians have an inherent interest in science, art, and commerce, thus it is a productive way to support and bring together people from all ethnic backgrounds. Building a skin-care practice that includes a variety of people, ages, and health conditions makes for a lucrative business in the twenty-first century. Unfortunately, many do not take advantage of the wonderful opportunities that we have before us now. For those brave few, however, the rewards will be great.

Frequently Asked Questions

1. **How does an esthetician get started working with a more ethnically diverse clientele?**

   Start slowly. Attend workshops, seminars, and conferences that offer programs in areas where you have no training. Work at building your knowledge bank to include skin care for a variety of skin colors and undertones. Consciously increase your friendship base to include people from cultures other than your own. We need to allow people from various ethnic groups to teach us about their views on beauty whether or not we agree or have the same ideas.

2. **Will the esthetician lose makeup business if the client decides to have permanent makeup or micropigmentation?**

   No. Most of us will continue to purchase shadows, mascara, liner, lipstick, foundation, blush, brushes, and concealer right along with the season changes. Most women who wear makeup like change and use the permanent makeup only as a base.

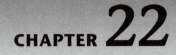

CHAPTER 22

Scientific Methodology and Case Studies

- ■ Introduction
- ■ Use the Scientific Method
- ■ Case Studies
- ■ Acne Profiles
- ■ Laser Hair-Reduction Profile
- ■ Dyschromias/Hyperpigmentation Profile
- ■ Summary
- ■ Frequently Asked Questions

Introduction

Providing case studies in your practice can accelerate learning for all estheticians. Being prepared to offer a special rate or exchange program to a client willing to participate in a case study may bring about an opportunity to provide a necessary service that an individual may otherwise be unable to pursue.

Use the Scientific Method

Whether we are aware of the **scientific method,** or just following the manufacturer's instructions on a given treatment, we are using an accepted method. The scientific method has been used by scientists dating as far back as Galileo, a seventeenth-century astronomer. It is based on five basic steps of observation, research, hypothesis, experimentation, and conclusion, to solve a problem. In very simple terms, we have a method to follow. In context the five steps are as follows:

1. **Observe.** State the problem. Make an unbiased observation about what you see. This is the same principle that we apply in chart SOAP note writing (see Chapter 13).

For example, you are visited by a woman in her early forties who states that she is interested in smoothing her dry, parched skin and softening the furrows in her forehead. In observing, you note she is a Skin Type II, has some photodamage, and is experiencing some cystic acne.

2. **Do research.**   Ask yourself, "What is known about solving this condition or set of issues?" Look for answers that have worked in the past. That may include home-care programs, in-office treatments, and possibly a consultation with the physician.

3. **Form a hypothesis.**   Form a treatment plan as a possible solution to these problems. It may be necessary to take one problem at a time. The plan will be based upon a client's health condition, lifestyle, compliance, and level of interest in solving his or her skin problems. In this case, you may look at the various peels and hydrating masks in your repertoire, AHA/BHA home-care products including a skin lightener, and possibly at setting up an appointment with the doctor for Botox.

4. **Experiment.**   Apply your hypothesis. Work the plan that you have created with the client. Try the peels and have her start the home-care regimen. The doctor applies the injection of Botox. Begin with the simplest of programs first. Then continue to experiment until results are notable.

5. **Conclude.**   If your experimentation was successful, you are on the way to solving the issues. Document these findings through writings, computer or digital images, and measurements if necessary. If not, the hypothesis may be incorrect, and you may need to go back to the original fact-finding stage and try some different products or treatments, based on the new information that you have from your experiments. Test the new hypothesis, and repeat until the condition resolves. If it does not lead to good results, refer to the physician.

As we all know, skin issues may take several cycles to resolve and may involve hormones or deeper subclinical conditions. Moreover, the client will need to make appropriate lifestyle changes and maintain constant home-care compliance.

Case Studies

The following case studies utilize a scientific approach, and have been applied with full in-office and home-care compliance. The cases address acne (various levels), dyschromias, and hair reduction. The appropriate informed consent forms have been signed.

All clients were given respective protocols, sun protection UVA, UVB, and diet/nutritional and lifestyle/behavioral instruction. Clients with acne were advised to monitor foods such as dairy, caffeine, and sugar that may indirectly affect stress levels. The client with dyschromias was instructed to use high-performing sunscreens containing zinc oxide and titanium oxide and to watch sun or light exposure. In addition, it was advised that the client use home-care products containing skin lighteners with lower level AHAs and in-office treatments that do not create inflammatory pigmentation due to the increased amount of melanin in Skin Type IV. The client presenting with hirsutisim was advised to consult a physician for evaluation.

Acne Profiles

Clients struggling with acne often feel desperate about their condition. They will be some of the strongest, most optimistic, and tenacious partners the clinical esthetician will serve. For most, having an opportunity to become part of an ongoing clinical study will give them the reassurance that they need to feel that research is being done on their behalf. In addition, it gives them hope and a dream that, one day, having better-behaving skin is within their reach.

Client A Profile (Images Located in Color Insert)

The client in this study is a 22-year-old woman with Eastern European ancestry. She is a Skin Type II, presents with normal to slightly oily orientation. In addition, she has Grade II acne, some roughness, uneven texture and pore size, acne scarring, and slight erythema to some lesions (*observation*). She was generally dissatisfied with the appearance of her skin: she was training to become a nurse and wanted to appear healthy.

Her hope was to clear up her skin and to be able to manage it easily with a few products and in-office treatments, as she is a busy student. She had tried various OTC skin-care products and has found them to be drying, ineffective, and inconsistent; she did not try prescription medications. She was willing to participate in the study, and she has a friend who may also be a candidate with a similar profile.

Esthetician's Treatment Plan

To start, this client was put on a consistent home-care program involving a cleanser, toner, a light hydrating gel and a sunscreen. In addition, she received in-office peels, masks, and microdermabrasion treatments. (*hypothesis*)

Home care

A.M.

1. foaming cleanser: gel with 12% AHAs and 1.5% BHAs (3.5 pH) for deep pore cleansing
2. toner: light water-based fluid with 2% salicylic acid to fight bacteria
3. hydrating gel: hydrator containing hyaluronic acid for moisture
4. sunscreen: a light moisturizing environmental protector with 3% micronized zinc oxide to prevent further pigment changes and photoaging
5. Mineral powder replaces client's existing cosmetic product.

P.M.

1. Repeat foaming cleanser.
2. Repeat toner.
3. Apply lotion containing AHAs, BHAs and retinol.

Weekly in-office treatment   The in-office treatments were given every 8 to 10 days. The plan included a combination of glycolic, modified Jessner's, and microdermabrasion peels, along with extractions, cryogenic, and copper-hydrating therapies. Standard protocols for each treatment were used, followed by the use of copper peptide hydrating gel and sunscreen appropriate to skin type. The client was advised to avoid AHAs, BHAs, retinol, and retinoic acid for 2 days after treatment, and she was given alternative products to use, such as a gentle cleanser and a non-AHA, BHA hydrating product. (*experiment*)

Treatments 1–6	*Treatments 7–12*	*Treatments 13–present*
Glycolic Peel	**Modified Jessner's Peel**	**Microdermabrasion**
(1) Glycolic Acid 3.2pH, buffered in 70% solution —1 layer	14% glycolic buffered, 14% lactic, Resorcinol —1 layer	Two passes nonparticle, medium stainless wand and modified Jessner's Peel as
(2) Extractions		needed—1 layer

Conclusion

Client A tolerated home-care and in-office treatments well. She was compliant and enthusiastic about her new program. Results appear to be incremental and are notable. The program has been successful by all accounts. *(conclude)*

Breakdown by Weeks

Weeks 1–6
Upon using her home-care products, Client A began to observe that her acne was drying up along the mandible, yet skin felt too dry in other areas such as in the zygomatic region. She commented that she had avoided using the moisturizer, because she was concerned that it might create more acne. She was given instructions to use the hydrator as it would help to improve the barrier, cut down on localized dryness, and keep the sebaceous glands from surging. She also noted that after the fourth peel her skin seemed to start to look smoother.

Weeks 7–12
An indication of slowed improvement marks a need for a change in treatment and peels. Modified Jessner's has replaced the glycolic peel. Improvement in acne scarring and texture smoothness had increased. There was light reflecting off the skin, and the gray color was improving. It began to look pink.

Weeks 13–18
Client still had an occasional cystic lesion, but in general skin had improved. Infection resolved, and texture continues to improve. Client was concerned with a few residual scars from the original acneic condition, and her interests remained in maintaining current excellent condition. Changed treatments to once every 2 to 3 weeks and move to microdermabrasion in combination with modified Jessner's for new acne as needed.

Weeks 19–24
Client A continued to improve. Her home-care program continued to be beneficial and she remains compliant. Microdermabrasion is used approximately every 3 weeks to continue improvement on scarring and acne management. She became ecstatic about her skin

and appeared to have more self-confidence and greater self-esteem. She recently turned 23 years, and she is nearly finished with her nursing degree while holding down a full-time job.

Client's Story

I have had acne and scars on my face, and I hated my skin. I tried OTC products containing benzoyl peroxide and salicylic acid, but not medication. When I first started my program at the clinic, I was experiencing some clearing of the breakouts, sometimes it was dry, but it really made it clearer. After about 3–4 peels, I began to see a difference.

Now I use the cleanser and moisturizer, which work much better and faster than products that I had used in the past, and the microdermabrasion is working the best. My skin has almost cleared up. I am glad that I was able to try this program because it worked for me. I used to hate my skin, and now I can handle it, and I am hoping that it will completely clear up.

Client B Profile (Images Located in Color Insert)

Client B is a 24 year-old woman with sensitive, oily, Grade III acne, exhibiting many open and closed comedones, many pustules and papules, several cystic lesions, pigment changes, inflamed skin, and some signs of **erythema** in general. Fitzpatrick II skin type, some sensitivity, with no known allergies (she suspected an allergy to yeast, but no diagnosis) or other health problems or conditions. (*observation*)

She was interested in treatment, and had tried many remedies on her own with OTC drugs, to no avail. This client would benefit from a comprehensive program of proper home-care products, in-office treatments, and medical intervention. However, she was not interested in ABs (antibiotics) at the time. (*hypothesis*)

Esthetician's Treatment Plan

To begin, we addressed the sensitivity issues that the oily sensitive skin type had with Grade III acne. The very products that may dry up her acne may also create secondary problems that we did not want to develop. She was placed on skin care for sensitive, intolerant skin including a moisturizer, which the client said she did not use. By not using a moisturizer on her sensitive, oily skin she was inadvertently allowing potential irritants to increase her susceptibility. In addition, in-office treatments consisted of a combination of acids peels, enzymes, hydrating and soothing masks, packs, **cryotherapy** (liquid nitrogen), microdermabrasion, and ultimately, a consult with the physician for oral and topical medication. (*experiment*)

Home care

A.M.

1. cleanser containing glycolic 8% free acid, salicylic 3% and glycolic 8% toner
2. hydrating gel with vitamins A and E

3. sunscreen lotion with antioxidants such as pycnogenol (pine), (bioflavonoids), and zinc oxide
4. mineral powder makeup

P.M.

1. cleanser/toner-gel or light lotion based with a light sulfur base (anti-inflammatory, antibiotic), or lower-level AHA with a high pH (not as irritating) at 3.5–3.8
2. hydrating lotion: allantoin, hyaluronic acid, and lower-level AHA with high pH, alternating with an azulene hydrator

Weekly in-office treatment   The in-office treatments were given every 8 to 10 days, and the plan included a combination of glycolic, sulfur mask, papaya enzyme therapy, modified Jessner's and microdermabrasion peels, along with extractions, cryogenic, and copper-hydrating therapies. Using standard protocols for each treatment, the client was advised to avoid AHAs, BHAs, retinol, and retinoic acid for 2 days posttreatment. Client was given alternative products to use, including a gentle cleanser and a non-AHA, BHA hydrating product. (*experiment*)

Treatments 1–6	*Treatments 16–21*
Glycolic (1) 70% buffered glycolic peel (2) Extractions	**Acne Clear-Up Peel** (1) Acne clear-up peel containing 2% azelaic, 2% salicylic, 14% lactic and 14% glycolic (2) 2–3 layers (3) Extractions
Treatments 7–12	*Treatments 22–24*

Modified Jessner's Peel
(1) 14% glycolic buffered, 14% lactic acid,
      Resorcinol
      1 layer
(2) Extractions
	Papain Peel and Microdermabrasion
	(1) Papaya mask
	(2) Microdermabrasion
	(3) Extractions

Treatments 13–15	*Treatments 25–present*

Microdermabrasion
(1) Two passes nonparticle, medium
      stainless wand and modified Jessner's
      Peel as needed—1 layer
(2) Extractions
	Microdermabrasion
	(1) Microderm—2 passes, nonparticle
	(2) Modified Jessner's—lesions only, or acne
	      clear-up peel—only on few remaining lesions
	(3) Extractions

Conclusion

Client B continued to be a challenge. She cleared up, and then created new cystic acne. In general, the skin health improved, and she appeared optimistic. She often veers from her home care and tries her own home remedies. In this effort, she feels determined to seek products that work best for her. With time, trust in the process, and experience in working together, Client B became more compliant. Medical intervention was introduced rather early on in the form of oral antibiotics (doxycycline 100g, b.i.d. for 60 days).

Client B is affected by her diet and stress greatly, and she does well when she improves these areas by eating well and exercising regularly. We continued to help and revise our work together accordingly. Ultimately this client could benefit from Accutane therapy. However, costs and logistics were prohibitive for her at the time.

Breakdown by Week

Weeks 1–6
Client B was given glycolic peels every week to condition her very sensitive skin to the stronger agents that we would be using. She responded almost immediately, and skin began to look more luminous and appeared cleaner. Some lesions began to dry up and others were less inflamed. There was a 10% improvement within the first 5 weeks. Wanting more of an improvement, she elected to try oral antibiotics. The physician was consulted, made the diagnosis (dx) and prescribed the medication as per usual.

Weeks 7–12
The treatments were reevaluated at 7 weeks, and we felt that we had hit a plateau. The treatment plan changed to include a modified Jessner's, extractions, and an azulene soothing mask. In addition, we added retinoic acid to the home-care regimen every other night and added mineral skin-care makeup, in powder, blush, and shadow. The Jessner's was successful for six treatments.

Weeks 13–15
Client was introduced to a light therapy session during this period, which ended in a major step back in our progress. The acne flared and took 2 subsequent weeks to calm. The light therapy consisted of two 90-second treatments on each side, as client was draped and prepped according to manufacturer's specifications. Did not try again, so cannot judge efficacy of this therapy.

During this time, we added a benzoyl peroxide 10% cleanser and tea tree oil (as an antiseptic), as client felt that skin was not feeling clean with original cleanser. Had severe reaction to BP cleanser, recovered by going to a basic lotion cleanser without performance or active agents. Client B began to alternate light, inactive cleanser with original cleanser containing glycolic and salicylic acids, along with leave-on solution containing the same. This works well for her when she is in acne flare. In-office treatments returned to tried-and-true modified Jessner's peel, with excellent results.

Weeks 16–21
Client became slightly resistant to modified Jessner's; moved to an acne peel containing 2% azelaic, 2% salicylic, 14% lactic and 14% glycolic. This peel increased smoothing of the acne scarring, and virtually dried up the cystic acne she had been developing. Home-care compliancy generally good, however admitted to not cleansing face at night on occasion. Client retained regimen of alternating nonactive soothing products with glycolic-salicylic cleanser and toner/solution.

Weeks 22–24

Client became interested in scar management as cystic acne became more cyclical with menses, and she had days free of lesions. Microdermabrasion returned as method of treatment along with a papaya enzyme peel. New oil-controlling hydrator was introduced and well tolerated. Occasional cystic acne along buccal region was noted and treated with two layers of acne peel containing azelaic acid, and this proved beneficial.

Weeks 25–Present

Client B continued to have outbreaks typically at buccal and lower zygomatic regions; however, this seemed to be connected to three issues: not cleansing properly, monthly cycle, and stress. Microdermabrasion was the method of treating this client along with supplemental acid peels as indicated. The treatments were well tolerated, her home care was easy to apply, and she is happier, in general, with the improvements and condition of her skin. However, we did not consider victory yet, and continued with weekly visits until more improvement was apparent.

Client's Story

When I first started this program my skin was very oily, and sensitive, with lots of acne. The more treatments and products that I bought and used (OTC), the more irritated and itchy my skin became. I did not like the way that I looked; I avoided looking into mirrors, and did not want anyone to take my picture. About a month after washing with the face wash, and using the lotion and having the treatments, I began to see a difference. The light cleanser and lotion have worked the best. Benzoyl peroxide did not work.

Five minutes in the morning and in the evening, I can keep my skin looking better. I don't have to hassle with going to the stores and reading all of the labels to try to figure out what may help. Now, if I get occasional acne (one or two), I can cover it with coverup, and my skin looks great. I like the way I look when I see myself in the mirror; also, I take pictures and do not worry about how they will turn out.

Client C Profile (Images Located in Color Insert)

Client C was a pre-teen male with Grade IV level acne who had seen a dermatologist, as well as tried oral and topical antibiotics, OTC drugs and preparations, over several months. According to Client C none of these remedies had been helpful, and he says, "Nothing is working." He was clearly a candidate for Accutane at first glance, but parents and physician had chosen not to use the therapy at the time.

Client has not been diligently using program detailed by dermatologist, and he appeared generally not interested in helping himself. Client was counseled and told that he would need to participate to improve his condition, and that it would be important to follow the plan, otherwise we would all be wasting our time. He became agreeable and we proceeded. The following details were given as his skin-health plan:

1. Client would use cleansers, solutions, and topicals as directed. He purchased a cleanser and toner containing glycolic and salicylic acids to be used 2–3 times a day.

2. It was recommended that he keep using all preparations prescribed for him by his dermatologist, and to consult his physician about possible allergies (environmental and foods), stress level, and other potential personal issues that could be affecting him.

3. It was recommended that he keep a daily journal that included thoughts, ideas, and the practical aspects of caring for his skin. He would write information such as when he cleansed, when he noticed more breakout, if he began to clear up, and general information about his skin care to report to the esthetician.

4. He was to buy new hair supplies from a professional cosmetologist, as the OTC leave-on product appeared to be heavy and could be contributing to his problem near the hairline.

Esthetician's Treatment Plan

The treatment plan consisted of requiring consistent home-care compliance, in-office treatments, and skin-care counseling. Knowing that his acne had developed into a potentially disfiguring disease, we worked in complete partnership with his dermatologist.

We started with a glycolic and salicylic acid–based cleanser and toner program; this slightly improved condition. Then skin became resistant, and we changed to benzoyl peroxide program as indicated.

Home care

A.M.

1. benzoyl peroxide cleanser
2. benzoyl peroxide topical gel and sulfur (leave on)
3. sunscreen lotion with antioxidants and zinc oxide

Midday Cleansing

Repeat steps 1 and 2.

P.M.

1. Repeat A.M.
2. Repeat P.M.
3. Write in journal.

Three times a week at night: alternate sulfur- or clay-based mask (to draw out infection, and using anti-inflammatory benefit of sulfur) with retinoic acid .05% as prescribed by physician.

In-office treatments
Client did not tolerate acid peels. For treatment, used enzymes papaya, citrus/clay masks (no steam, too much erythema), and microdermabrasion only on areas without cysts or pustules (blackheads on nose). In addition, extraction therapy (cotton swab evacuation) was used in brief, and without lancet or needle as he had no tolerance to any of these procedures.

Treatments 1–2

Slight improvement from home care

1. modified Jessner's applied for 5 minutes, slight discomfort, but otherwise tolerated
2. extractions—low level of tolerance

Treatments 3–7

Client described discomfort with acid peel and says "it was too hot," asks for another type of treatment.

1. papaya enzyme peel 10–20 minutes—well tolerated
2. extractions—well tolerated

Treatments 8–12

Client arrives with a haircut which allows more air to the skin at hairline, and reveals a marked improvement in general skin health in the frontal region.

1. papaya peel 20 minutes
2. microdermabrasion—nose
3. extractions

Conclusion

Client C has received minimal results, and it has been slow. Since he is young, and extremely sensitive to procedures, this may not be the best form of treatment for him. The client, with support of his parents, decided to try Accutane. The outcome of Accutane therapy is successful, as noted in color insert.

Client D Profile (Images Located in Color Insert)

Client D is a college student with Grade III acne. She came to the clinic via Web site, for cosmetic support and for help in clearing up her acne with microdermabrasion. As a college student, the client is under stress and her response to it did affect her acne. A discussion took place between the client, parent, and the esthetician, in which the esthetician shared that the microdermabrasion would be one facet of the treatment plan, to be supplemented by other applications such as peels and home-care products and compliance. In addition, it was determined that the client had no known allergies or general health problems, and that she had tried a variety of finer skin-care products, drugs, and OTC preparations to no avail. The treatment plan was laid out, and was agreeable to all. The client visits the clinic weekly for multilayer/purpose treatments and skin health-care counseling.

Esthetician's Treatment Plan

The first step in setting a skin-care treatment plan for the client was to move her from seven products that she had been using that were formulated for an older, dryer, skin type.

Home care

A.M.

1. cleanser containing benzoyl peroxide 10% and tea tree oil
2. acne gel with benzoyl peroxide 5%, antioxidants, and kojic acid (for acne scar lightening)
3. sunscreen: light lotion with micronized zinc oxide
4. mineral makeup powders

P.M.

1. Repeat A.M.
2. Repeat A.M., or, if feeling dry, alternate with lipid replacement product containing phospholipids and glycosphingolipids.

In-office treatments

Treatments consisted of chemical peels, microdermabrasion, extractions, azulene masks, and lipid replacement applications. Client was given nonactive cleanser and hydrator to use 2 days after peel.

Treatments 1–6

Home-care pretreatment phase improves condition by small percentage. In-office treatments start as follows:

1. Patch testing was performed to left frontal region near hairline. Well tolerated after 5 minutes.
2. 20% salicylic acid peels were applied in three layers in 1-minute intervals. Slight frosting was achieved, thus drying acneic lesions.
3. Microdermabrasion (nonparticle) was then applied to all areas, avoiding cystic lesions.
4. Extractions were performed on all lesions that were in a treatable phase (surface pustule).
5. Soothing azulene mask or lipid replacement mask was applied.
6. copper gel for hydrating
7. sunscreen with antioxidants and zinc oxide

Treatments 7–12

Skin health improves by 50 percent. Change in program is warranted as most of the infection has resolved. At treatment 10, physician added oral antibiotic b.i.d. for 60 days.

1. microdermabrasion—2 passes
2. Modified Jessner's to areas with acne only
3. extractions
4. cryotherapy
5. copper gel
6. sunscreen with antioxidants and zinc oxide

Treatments 13–Present

Client has continued to improve. Treatments currently addressing a few new or active lesions, but in general health had been restored. Scar management is being visited.

1. microdermabrasion
2. Modified Jessner's on lesions only
3. extractions
4. cryotherapy
5. copper gel
6. sunscreen with antioxidants and zinc oxide

Conclusion

Treatments and home-care program have been successful. Due to client compliance and willingness to receive treatment, she is observing a positive change in her skin health and appearance. She will need to continue her clinical skin-care program, and may want laser therapy later to address scarring.

Laser Hair-Reduction Profile

Laser hair reduction is being continuously improved. It has brought solace to those suffering the painful, embarrassing experience of heavy, dark hair growing in areas where people do not want hair.

The clinic program in this case is a combined effort of the physician and two other personnel, the CMA (Certified Medical Assistant) and the LE (Licensed Esthetician). The esthetician typically does the laser hair consultations, which involves presenting the treatment to the client or patient, determining the skin type (for the laser calibration), sharing risks, patient selection, patient education, and essentially selling the service package. Once the client is scheduled for treatment, the CMA is responsible for obtaining the signature for the consent form, the condition and calibration of the laser, the treatment, and the immediate care after treatment. The two share responsibilities in collecting fees and in making the subsequent appointments.

If there are any special cases, health issues, or contraindications, the physician is then notified and brought into the consultation; the appointment may need to be rescheduled so that the patient may meet with the doctor prior to receiving any treatments.

Client E Profile (Images Located in Color Insert)

Client is a female in her early forties, with hirsutisim, primarily about the mandible, zygomatic, and mental regions. The hair is dark and coarse on her Fitzpatrick III skin type. She had tried various methods of hair reduction including laser, electrolysis, waxing, tweezing, and shaving, to no avail. She was quite emotional about this hair and its apparent tenacity.

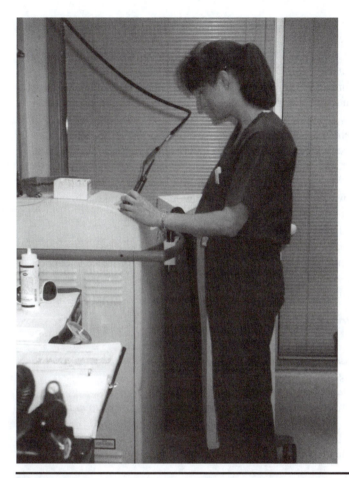

Figure 22–1   Certified Medical Assistant calibrating laser

Esthetician's Treatment Plan

The client needed 4–6 treatments, did not appear to be at risk for hyperpigmentation, and was not tan. She has no known serious health problems or disorders. She has experienced laser hair treatments 5 years ago at another location, with an earlier model system.

Treatment application   Katy Denooyer, CMA, of Bellingham Ear Nose and Throat and Facial Plastic Surgery, describes the standard laser hair-reduction protocol that was used as follows:

1. Patient was checked in. Collected payment, made next appointment, signed consent form.

2. Rechecked laser. Made appropriate setting/calibration adjustments prior to patient entering room; made sure that all supplies were organized, as this helps treatment flow more smoothly.

3. Took patient back to laser room. Discussed results of laser treatment, looked to see how area was responding to treatment, and made sure that the area had been prepped or shaved for optimum comfort and efficacy. Asked if patient had a music preference. Started CD.

4. Applied gel to treatment area.

5. Put on approved laser safety glasses, both CMA and patient's.

6. Applied the treatment. During the procedure encouraged breathing to the patient. Used statements like, "You are doing great!" and "Almost there . . . " At points, noticed that the patient was struggling, asked if she would like to take a break. Also, offered a squeeze ball to the patient to hold during the treatment.

7. Post-treatment. Offered ice pack or liquid nitrogen to cool.

8. Applied copper gel and sunscreen.

9. Patient was reminded not to use retinoids, AHAs, or other performance agents for at least 3 days.

10. Walked patient back out, and said goodbye.

Supplies that make a difference:

- *4 × 4s*
- *post-laser hydrating gel such as copper peptide*
- *ice packs or liquid nitrogen*
- *squeeze ball or toy for hand during treatment*
- *topical anesthetic for next treatment (pt can put on up to an hour prior to next visit)*

After Treatment 1

Patient has lost 30%–35% hair.

After Treatment 2

Patient is encouraged by more hair loss.

After Treatment 3

Patient has lost 85% of hair. Patient was doing well with results thus far, and did not come back for a fourth treatment.

Conclusion

Treatment was successful. Patient satisfied with results after three visits, has not needed subsequent treatments.

Dyschromias/Hyperpigmentation Profile

The appearance of pigment changes can change the topographical appearance of skin. In some cases, due to the shading as in hyperpigmentation, this can actually make the skin look as if it has an indentation at the site. By lifting the color—using skin lighteners,

AHAs, and sunscreens—we can increase the blending of skin tones and decrease the uneven appearance to the texture of the skin.

Client F Profile (Images Located in Color Insert)

Woman in her mid-thirties presents with multiple skin-care concerns, one being the pigmented area in her buccal region on her left side. Her Fitzpatrick IV skin type and dark hair in that region makes it appear deeper than it is; she was not using a sunscreen daily. A cautionary measure needed to be observed as we can create more pigment in the region by overstimulating the melanocytes by aggressively treating it with chemicals that may generate heat, or using the microdermabrader, for example.

Esthetician's Treatment Plan

To start, we decided to improve and guide her home-care regimen to include products that addressed some light acne, slightly oily skin, along with hyperpigmentation. An in-office treatment plan was created to support her home-care efforts and help boost the program along.

Home care

A.M.

1. cleansing gel containing 6% glycolic acid and 2% salicylic acid
2. toner containing 6% glycolic acid and 2% salicylic acid
3. skin lightener with 4% (to start) hydroquinone with physician support
4. sunscreen with antioxidants and zinc oxide and titanium dioxide (will need to blend well as this will initially show up on her darker skin)
5. oil-free makeup and light powder

P.M.

1. Repeat steps 1–3.
2. Add hydrator, light facial fluid if dry.

In-office treatments   Treatments will consist of bimonthly applications of Jessner's, microdermabrasion, and lightening preparations postpeel.

Treatments 1–6

Jessner's—14% glycolic, 14% lactic, 14% salicylic peel applied for 5 minutes, slowly building to 10 minutes over time. These were well tolerated. By the third treatment and with compliant home care, we began to see a lift in the pigmented area.

Treatments 7–12

Client came in for treatment, and happily shares that she is pregnant. We took her off all AHAs, BHAs, and skin lighteners. We switch to nonactive home-care treatment products for home care including clay- and sulfur-based cleansers, along with kojic and bearberry, for skin lightener. She continued her sunscreen applications along with her treatments, which consisted of:

- microdermabrasion
- extractions
- clay and papaya masks along with steam and light brushing
- combination microdermabrasion and sulfur, hydrating and soothing masks, along with hand and arm treatments
- full makeup after treatments

Conclusion

We were beginning to see the pigmented area lightened from the dark color, but will put off all aggressive attempts until the client had completed breast-feeding. Her skin looked healthier and she is radiant.

Summary

Case studies require patience, dedication, a willingness to try different experiments, and to acknowledge what you observe. As much as we want a new product or treatment that we have invested in to work, we must admit the shortcomings and limitations of preparations when they do not work, and move on. We must communicate to our client the potential risks and failings of treatments or products, and many clinical trials are performed at a discounted rate. Documentation is key to running a case study. Keep your notes organized and separate from the patient's chart, as it is easy to fill up several pages on just observation. Keep in mind the SOAP model (see Chapter 13) for the ease of writing and to provide a context for your work.

Frequently Asked Questions

1. **What does the esthetician do if they spent countless hours working with a client, and one day they just do not show up for a treatment in a study phase?**

   Call and let them know that they have missed their appointment; maybe they forgot and are embarrassed. This will let them know that you are still interested in working with them. Let them know in a pleasant way that you hope that they can continue, and that they can call or e-mail you any time they need to change their scheduled appointment.

   Sometimes when people are receiving discounted or free services, they do not value them or they begin to take advantage. You need to let go if they are no longer reliable or have received the help that they wanted.

2. **What if I have never done a study? Who would want to read mine?**

   You will be pleasantly surprised at how few studies are available—even just the simple case studies like these (not true clinical trials) that have been shown here. In addition, we can learn so much about our work by keeping a journal, and reviewing it periodically.

Handling Challenging Situations and Issues

CHAPTER 23

Handling Challenging People and Safety in the Workplace

- Introduction
- Self-Abuse
- Signs of Trouble—Distress and Rudeness
- Drug Addiction and Untreated Mental Illnesses
- Disgruntled or Unhappy Patients
- Safety in the Workplace
- Sexual Harassment
- Domestic Violence
- Summary
- Frequently Asked Questions

Introduction

On occasion we find ourselves in a room with someone with a mental imbalance that may not be evident at the onset of the consultation—or even after a few visits. It may take stress in a person's life to reveal paranoia or a developing psychosis. Working in plastic surgery in particular, we may see such cases on a more regular basis than might a professional in another setting. Image issues can be high impact for people.

A mentally healthy person is one who possesses knowledge of themselves; meets his or her basic needs, assumes responsibility for actions and behaviors; has learned to integrate thoughts, feelings, and actions; can successfully resolve conflicts and maintain relationships; communicates directly with others; respects others; and adapts to change (White, 2001, p. 1175). Conversely, a mentally unhealthy person is characterized as one having an impairment of normal intellectual and social functioning. The condition may range from mild anxiety to the need for hospitalization, and various disorders in the middle (Keir, Wise, & Krebs, 1998, p. 747).

From the beginning of your work with a client or patient it is important to note and report all comments made by that person describing depression, sadness, or unhappiness. Clear mention of an interest in suicide or attempts made must be reported. Patients may reveal an attempt at suicide at an earlier point in their lives, and the doctor will need to make a full evaluation before you treat them. This goes for an individual with a tendency toward self-abuse.

Self-Abuse

This disorder can present from the very lightest of afflictions such as "skin picking" or scratching to people who actually perform surgeries on themselves. For those with compulsive behavioral patterns of picking at acne, scabs, or lesions, you may be able to help them by showing them what actually happens in this process, which ultimately creates the scar. Showing them that their picking, squeezing, and subsequent ripping off the scab may create a rupture in the dermis and hence create a breeding ground for a whole new pustule—not to mention one right next door on the surface, as it becomes impossible to remove all of the bacteria.

Sometimes this client will come in showing good skin health, and other times you will see them complaining apologetically that they have been on a rampage; they may have six or eight lesions on their face. It comes and goes, depending upon how much stress they are under, and how conscious they have been of their behavior. Most of the time, the clients are unaware that they are creating damage to themselves. The key to helping here is to try to get the clients to keep up with regular treatments to clean up lesions, which are triggers to their picking.

Other clients may come into the office in hope of receiving help for scarring that they had sustained over years of abusing their skin with various implements. These individuals will need a full evaluation by the doctor prior to your treating them. It is good practice management to share with them that you are concerned about treating them. You can explain that your main goal is to look out for the health of their skin and that you want to do what is best for them. They will typically understand, and if they are in recovery they will agree to a physician's analysis. Otherwise, do not perform a treatment: you may create a trigger for their compulsion.

If a client or patient comes in for self-treatment items such as professional peels that they want to perform at home, wants to buy implements, wants samples of medications and seems to have been injecting, cutting, or performing any other type of self-procedure, decline to participate. Refer them to the physician for the help that they need. This can be a progressive disorder and they may change dramatically each time that you see them. It is very difficult to understand, and even more difficult to deal with this situation. You will not be able to help such individuals. They need psychiatric help, medication, supervision, and possibly hospitalization.

Signs of Trouble—Distress and Rudeness

Signs of mental distress can be as simple as a client or patient not following instructions, and/or becoming argumentative about the protocol, treatment, or products that you are recommending. It is important that you share this with the doctor as soon as possible. This could alert the staff that this person may need more direction, or could be a problem further down the road. Try to have as much patience as you can with such people; often they are under stress and just need someone to coach them. Go back over the protocol, using numbered sentences and A.M. and P.M. instructions. Reiterate the importance of using the recommended method and give them a more direct reason for the use of the protocol. Remind them the outcome of their surgery depends on their willingness to follow these instructions. Document your experience with the patient in their chart, and the fact that you are reviewing protocols for the second, third, fourth, or fifth time.

Further along on the continuum, you may find a patient who is rude or condescending to the staff. They may use statements like "You told me not to . . ." when you know this would not have been part of your instructions. This is a very good reason to document in detail your instructions to patients, and to make a copy of the instructions that you have given them for their file. Again, tell the doctor and an experienced supervising nurse about the incident. If this person gets out of hand in subsequent visits, you may need help. In addition, sometimes we need to relinquish our job to another staff member; there may be a personal issue that the patient has with you, or a more a clinical problem that you may never be able to figure out. Do not take this personally. Move on. Most people are balanced, confident, and easy to work with, and will listen to most of what you say when they learn that the outcome of their surgery is dependent on their diligence.

Drug Addiction and Untreated Mental Illnesses

The most difficult patient may be one with a drug addiction or a mental illness that is not being treated. These individuals can become belligerent, hysterical, and sometimes violent. If at any time you sense that you are in danger emotionally or physically, it is important to get up and leave the room to get help. By then, it may be difficult for you to effectively deal with the patient. If they have become violent, have someone call the police or 911, alert the clinic administrator, and the physician. The patient may need medical intervention. It is important to not excite or make verbal judgments about their behavior. To defuse potentially volatile behavior:

- Remain calm at all times, and encourage the person to talk while you wait for help.
- Acknowledge the person's feelings without taking sides.
- Move to another location such as near the entrance or outside.
- Do not make sudden moves or invade the person's space.
- Do not criticize, threaten, or belittle the individual.
- Whether standing or sitting, position yourself to the side instead of directly in front of the individual.

Turn the situation over to the authorities when help arrives. This incident must be documented; an incident report must be filed and a copy placed in the chart of the individual. Be aware of this person's subsequent attempts to visit the clinic and report it to the administrator.

Disgruntled or Unhappy Patients

Most difficult situations can be avoided by applying appropriate risk management techniques. However, in rare cases problems—real or imagined—do arise with surgeries, and we must deal with them. The physician will deal with the patient who is dissatisfied with surgery results. You as the esthetician may also be brought into the situation if there are revisions or subsequent surgeries: it may be part of your job description to set up protocols, prepatory treatments, or dispense products or education. It is at this time that you observe the following:

- Do not say anything disparaging about the physician, procedure, or outcome. It is possible that the patient is trying to create a case against the doctor. Always watch your words. They may show up on a tape recording.
- Do not agree with the patient or exacerbate their level of anger or pain.
- Refer all questions and comments back to the doctor.
- Be compassionate and let the patient know that you are available to help where you can.
- Remind the patient that you are the skin-care practitioner.

Support in the Practice

It is sad but true that in surgery there is always a risk, and in a rare case a procedure may not turn out as planned. There may be an underlying condition, which creates an unforeseen or unfortunate outcome. Most problems can be rectified. Occasionally they cannot. It is important for the staff to hold a meeting and talk about the situation. This is not only a good business practice, but it will stop the rumor mill from circulating erroneous information, and clear the path to healing for everyone.

It is important for physicians to get the support they need. Physicians need compassion and understanding from a network of colleagues who can serve as counsel when needed. They perform under a tremendous amount of pressure and responsibility; although they are the ones that everyone looks to for all of the answers, they are people first.

Extreme Measures to Be Employed with an Imbalanced, Dissatisfied Patient

The patient may need the help of a mental health counselor as well as follow-up care given by the physician. Depending on the nature of the problem, and on the personality, support, and family situation of the patient, the patient may become revengeful. This can range from a slight mention of dissatisfaction, to firm, clear demands to remedy the situation, to threatening with a lawsuit, to the patient threatening the doctor. It is imperative that the physician is monitored and observed with the patient, as a desperate patient may attempt to harm the doctor. Such cases have been documented, often occurring in the early morning before office hours, or late at night when the doctor had forgotten to lock the office doors. Having good lock-up procedures as well as efficient patient monitoring is essential to a healthy practice. Remain aware of the comings and goings of others at all times. Tag-team each other when leaving the facility.

Safety in the Workplace

We do not like to imagine that harm may come to any of us at work, but the realities are quite to the contrary. Crime in health-care facilities is on the rise due to long health-care delivery systems (even though most cosmetic procedures are cash up-front and typically are performed in upscale areas), high staff turnover, the accessibility of handguns, drugs and the presence of money in our facilities, and staff members not trained to recognize or manage potentially hostile or violent situations.

OSHA Standard for Violence Prevention

OSHA (Occupational Safety and Health Administration) has standards for safety and violence prevention guidelines. They date back to 1970 under the General Duty Clause. It is necessary to have these guidelines in place, so that upon inspection an office could be cited if there was a potential hazard and precautions were not taken. Here are seven steps as recommended by OSHA in establishing your violence prevention program (www.osha.gov):

1. **Management commitment.**   It is important to commit to spend the money on necessary changes that need to be made in the workplace—be it lighting, alarms, locks, restricted areas, or overall security.
2. **Employee involvement.**   Employees should be encouraged to make suggestions about making the workplace safer. Valuable input comes from those who are faced directly with the situations routinely. Employees should also be recognized for making good suggestions and carrying out policies.
3. **Work-site analysis.**   Have a work-site analysis performed to help identify risk factors in the facility. The team will evaluate and note security hazards such as:
   • hidden doors, closets, halls, driveways
   • isolated work areas
   • unrestricted areas
   • blocked escape routes
   • lack of comfortable, nonthreatening environment
   • potential for violence based on locations and demographics
4. **Written program.**   A written program with clear policies and procedures helps to show how the program relates to each employee, to reinforce management responsibility and support, and to clearly detail what has been done to improve the work site. The written program will:

- emphasize a zero-tolerance toward any workplace violence, including both verbal and nonverbal threats. It will encourage employees to report incidents and suggest means for elimination or reduction of hazards.
- protect employees who participate in reporting and suggesting changes
- outline the facility's security measures and assign responsibilities
- include employee support, especially for any employees who are facing termination or other personal hardships

5. **Administrative controls.** These are the policies and procedures that are developed and supported to reinforce the program such as:
   - provide sensitive and timely information to patients
   - respond promptly to complaints
   - control access to other clinic areas
   - provide security escorts after hours
   - reinforce excellence in customer service and provide the training to back it up

6. **Engineering controls.** These are adjustments in the physical structure or layout of the office such as:
   - alarms, cell phones, panic buttons
   - waiting rooms that maximize comfort and privacy, and minimize stress
   - furniture arrangements that prevent entrapment
   - staff rest rooms that can be locked and secure
   - bright lighting

7. **Incident follow-up.** Pay attention to all incidents that occur, regardless of size or significance. If changes are necessary, implement them. Training is to be provided yearly for all employees.

A Violence Incident Report form should be filed with the clinic administrator in the case of a threatening remark or act of physical violence against an employee or property of the facility. The police are to be notified and a formal complaint filed.

Having a Crime Prevention Speaker

Invite a police officer to visit and speak at your staff meeting. He or she can give you tremendous insights regarding the issues that are specific to your community, as well as general information that you could take anywhere in your travels. Some general guidelines are as follows:

- The most difficult times for personal safety are in coming and going to the office, particularly in the dark.
- Wear a fanny belt pack, leaving the hands free, instead of toting a purse or handbag, backpack, books, papers or other materials.
- Do not carry more than your license, cell phone, keys, and a credit card in your fanny pack.
- If you must carry materials with you, put them on a rolling suitcase that you can easily drop if necessary.

- Lock your car as soon as you get in. Leave the area. Do not sit and refresh lipstick or make a call. Go.

As health-care professionals, we must serve as stewards to protect those we work with as well as ourselves. Having these policies and procedures in place makes one so much more confident and aware of potential situations that may arise. It is not meant to create unease at work but will help you identify something going wrong—and will give you an opportunity to change it.

Sexual Harassment

Sexual harassment does exist in the twenty-first century. Most claims can be avoided by taking reasonable care to prevent sexual harassment in the workplace. By reviewing office policy and keeping abreast of new information through memos, meetings, and workshops, we can become more aware of what constitutes sexual harassment.

Title VII of the Civil Rights Act of 1964

Cultural, familial, and personality differences can create ambiguities. Something that may seem offensive to one person may not be noticed by another. However, there are some guidelines that can be followed by the esthetician—and anyone in the office for that matter; everyone has a right to be free from sexual harassment. Title VII of the Civil Rights Act of 1964 defines sexual harassment as:

> Unwelcome sexual advances, requests for sexual favors, and other verbal or physical conduct of a sexual nature when submission or rejection of this conduct explicitly or implicitly affects an individual's employment, unreasonably interferes with an individual's work performance or creates an intimidating, hostile or offensive work environment.

Other more specific forms of sexual harassment may consist of:

- derogatory or vulgar statements regarding a person's sexuality or gender
- unnecessary touching; unwanted sexual compliments, innuendos, jokes, or rumors about a person's sex life
- sexually suggestive materials such as magazines, posters; remarks about a person's anatomy
- leering, whistles, or catcalls
- sexually graphic or lewd e-mails
- repeated unwelcome pressure for dates or sex

What You Can Do

If an esthetician feels that she or he is being harassed by a co-worker, physician, administrator, visiting physician, or some other person, it is important to tell the offender that the behavior is unacceptable and that they must stop at once. This often will stop the harasser.

If it does not stop the behavior, or if you do not feel comfortable expressing disdain for the behavior to the harasser, it may require an informal meeting with your office manager, the clinical administrator, or the physician in the office. If the behavior continues, it may become important to file a formal complaint. The formal complaint may involve an investigation by obtaining a statement from the harassed individual, the alleged sexual harasser, and/or witnesses who may have important information to share.

It is definitely unwise to use sexual harassment in either a malicious or a frivolous manner. All accusations are taken seriously, and offenders are subject to disciplinary action and potentially, termination.

Domestic Violence

Domestic violence occurs in relationships where conflict is the continuous result of power inequality between partners (White, 2001, pp. 1204–1206). It may be expressed in a variety of ways and may be a combination of actual or threatened physical injury, sexual assault, psychological abuse, economic control, and/or progressive isolation. Most survivors are dependent on the abuser for basic security needs such as home or shelter and finances.

The Esthetician's Role While Working with Survivors of Domestic Violence

As estheticians, we may be brought into contact with domestic abuse survivors, as many cosmetic surgeons, dermatologists, and other physicians will be seeing these patients or clients for reconstructive surgery. Your role may be one of patient educator or you may assist in pre- and postoperative care and camouflage.

It is important to report all information regarding abuse to the physician. We do not want to ask questions about how they sustained their injuries, or pose other personal questions about the assault, but if the client or patient voluntarily shares information with you, it is necessary to tell the doctor. If it also involved the survivor's children, this needs to be reported as well. *You may be saving lives.* Guidelines for working with survivors of domestic violence are as follows:

- **Do not probe into their personal lives.** This individual will need intensive therapy, and we are not adequately trained for this type of counseling. We do not have the necessary credentials to be practicing mental health.
- **Refer all questions to the doctor.** The physician is better equipped to handle the forthcoming questions regarding the surgery, potential outcomes, or results. This person may become especially anxious and frightened, and may become confused about the surgery. Have them work primarily with the doctor.
- **Do not try to save them from their problems.** Keep the codependency issue here in mind. This individual will benefit the most by having a team of trained professionals helping them with their issues. Again, *do not counsel them.* Specifically, do not tell them to stay away from their spouse or abuser, suggest that they see someone else who

might be better for them, or mention any other escape methods. This problem runs very deep, and it will require more than you can do for them alone, unless you are a qualified, credentialed therapist.

- **Stick to skin care and the basics.**   If you find the survivor returning to discussions of their problems, remind them that you can help them with skin care, pre- and post-operative care, and makeup and appearance concerns, but that you are not qualified to help them with the other issues. Have on hand cards, brochures, and other informational material regarding domestic violence, and refer them to someone who is well trained and qualified to help them through this difficult time in their lives. This is not turning your back on them or shutting them out. Stay within your scope. They will thank you for it later.

Your Own Domestic Violence Problem

Many fine and intelligent practitioners have found themselves in abusive situations—whether cumulative, slowly getting worse, or happening all at once, with a partner or spouse—due to stress or alcohol/drugs—just snapping one night. It is important to not go into denial. If you perceive an incident as abusive, it probably is. If you feel that you are in an abusive relationship, call a trusted friend and remove yourself from the abuser. Do not go back into the situation alone. You need to develop a coalition of supporters. Some of the health-care professionals may include:

- mental health therapist
- life coach with degree in social work or counseling
- domestic violence victim support and advocacy
- criminal intervention

Recognize that you probably have been slowly programmed to believe that you are not able to exist on your own. This is not true. If you have children, it is vitally important to remove them from the abuser to prevent further trauma. Most children will recover if they are dealt with honestly and openly, and if you take control of the situation and not subject them to further abuse.

It is important for you to develop a safety plan for yourself and your children. In addition, this type of dynamic in a relationship can affect co-workers and others trying to help you. You will not want the abuser coming to the workplace. Here are a few tips for creating a safety plan:

- Change locks and install a security system.
- Move to a new location.
- Create a buddy system with friends and survivor advocates.
- Have important phone numbers and a buddy system available in an emergency.
- Tell neighbors about what has taken place, and ask them to call the police if they hear or see suspicious activities around the house.
- Have copies made of all important documents, and keep them in a safe place such as a deposit box.

- Tell children what to do if an abuser attacks—such as immediately running to a prearranged location and calling 911.
- Have extra money, clothes, and keys in another location.
- Get a restraining order against the abuser.

If you *are* the abuser, it is vitally important that you get help. Life has a way of making us all pay for harm that we have perpetrated on others. There are ways to end the cycle in which you find yourself.

If you need to be "right" or correct about everything and want complete control of others, co-workers, friends and family members; if you make threats or emotionally hurt others by constantly putting them down by "making fun"; or if you hold back money from loved ones or use children against a partner, these are all forms of abusive behavior. This may be the onset of more devastating behavior to follow, such as pushing, shoving, or throwing objects at others. This can then escalate to even more dire conditions for those around you. Talk to a trusted friend about your feelings, and be open about receiving information or interventions attempted by loved ones.

Take time out from your relationships to get professional help from a trained therapist or mental heath counselor and begin the healing that you need. It may be that you have a chemical dependency, need a lifestyle change, or need to de-program a learned behavior that has been carried through generations in your family. Whatever the cause, it is better to admit that you are struggling with this problem, so that you may start to become healthier, and create a more nurturing environment for you, your family, friends, and co-workers.

Summary

Keep in mind that the bottom line is: always keep yourself clear about what you can offer and what you cannot. Every day will present tremendous opportunities for personal growth and great lessons if you are willing to learn about helping others while not becoming caught up in their own life-path work.

Many talented, gifted people have survived and have become victorious in the face of abuse at all levels. It knows no economic, social, gender, or age boundaries. Keep your health and the welfare of your family as priorities. Whether at home or at work, recognize the signals of needing help, and find it. Know that with a little work, you can be healthy, happy, and free.

Frequently Asked Questions

1. **What does the esthetician do, if a client discloses that she has been beaten by her husband?**

   Unfortunately, this happens. Ask the client if she is safe at home currently, and tell her that she needs to file a police report. If someone in the office has training (many physicians do) in dealing with domestic violence, tell your client that you have a person for them to speak with, and that they will help in the next step. Typically, the children are moved to another location such as the home of a family member or friend. However, if the survivor has nowhere to go, they will be directed to an undisclosed facility.

The family will require professional counseling and support, and the client may feel embarrassed or humiliated about the disclosure, so it is important to remain nonjudgmental, and allow them to take the lead in conversation. If she continues as your client, and has a need to tell you her problems, gently let her know that you care about her, and want to assist her in getting the help that she needs by referring her to an appropriate support group. These groups meet regularly in communities and are often facilitated by survivors and health-care providers who specialize in issues of domestic violence. Two helpful Web sites are: www.ncadv.org and www.ndvh.org

2. How does the esthetician deal with the unwanted advances of a physician in the office?

Just be honest. Tell them that you are involved with someone, or that you are not looking for a relationship. It does not need to be a formal complaint. If the doctor does not take your words seriously, it may be difficult to work for him or her. You may need to make a change, as it may become difficult to work through the individual's lack of perception.

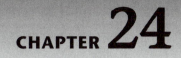

CHAPTER 24

Meeting the Challenges Within

- ■ Introduction
- ■ Types of Situations that You May Encounter
- ■ Codependence
- ■ Interdependence
- ■ Dealing with the Death of a Client
- ■ Dealing with the Death of a Co-worker
- ■ Stages of Dying and Death
- ■ Summary
- ■ Frequently Asked Questions

Introduction

You will find that your innate ability to adapt and to cope with challenging situations and people will serve as the bedrock of your career as an esthetician practicing in a medical office. One may be a fine esthetician and be adroit at performing treatments and product orientations, but these two key elements in your repertoire of personality characteristics are needed to round out your career and your profession. One may *learn* to adapt, and one can be *trained* to handle difficult people and situations, but this work may still prove to be stressful for you and your co-workers if they are not natural characteristics.

Types of Situations that You May Encounter

While working as an esthetician in a doctor's office you will come in contact with the typical situations that you will encounter in any esthetic setting, but there will also be plenty of special situations. You will be asked to use your common sense, professionalism, clinical proficiency, and intuition—as guideposts along the way through sometimes uncharted territories. Here are a few of the unusual situations that may present in the clinic:

- A client or co-worker becomes extremely clingy and dependent and leaves an inappropriate amount of messages for you or other co-workers.

- You begin to feel alone and that no one other than you understands or can help your client/patient.
- A client or co-worker becomes abusive, either to themselves, to you, or another co-worker.
- A co-worker becomes distant and seems to be unusually burdened by patients or the workload.
- The death of a client or co-worker.

Scenarios such as these may affect the team as a whole and the health of the practice. Some estheticians may find they have unknowingly entered into a relationship with a client that may create undue stress and bring about dependencies with others, which can be unhealthy or detrimental for the clients and themselves.

The Esthetician's Caregiving Tendencies

The goal of the clinical esthetician is often to provide help and service to all people including staff members, clients, and patients in the clinic. Initially, one will feel rewarded for attempting this: being able to genuinely help others is a powerful experience. However, we may find ourselves attempting to help when it is inappropriate to do so. When caregiving (or dispensing) becomes caretaking (or receiving) we need to examine our motives and make some changes.

Caretaking vs. Caregiving

What is the difference between caretaking and caregiving in our work setting? In *caregiving*, we are providing needed care in a healthy, team-approached manner, where we feel supported and balanced in the duties and tasks of doing our work. We recognize that we are being paid a salary for our work, and we do not feel taken advantage of or inappropriately used. In addition, we are able to recognize—and turn over—issues that are beyond our scope, and we become empowered and more effective as a result.

In the case of *caretaking*, we are *using the care that we are giving* to fill unmet needs of our own. Often this translates as a need to be needed, to be in charge, and thus to be in control. We do not feel empowered by helping; instead we have ulterior motives of receiving from our giving—thus, the caretaking. We ultimately feel resentful that we can never do enough, become enough, or help enough, because that is how we feel about ourselves to begin with—depleted. In this situation, we often feel isolated, and unfortunately we become unnecessarily burdened. It is easy to believe that others need you. On the other hand, is it that you need them? Watch out. This notion of being able to help all is suspect and later leads to burnout. It may, furthermore, reveal some deeper personal issues.

Be Clear about Your Role

Although some patients may not be clear about your role in the office, you need to be. If you have a nurturing personality, a constant need to be in control, or like to do everything on your own, you may need to work on perspective and boundaries. If not, you will in short order find yourself feeling the weight of the world on your shoulders, and you may worry about clients and patients even when it is inappropriate to do so. Here are some signs that you may be heading into trouble, and solutions to redirect you and get the support that you may need:

- **If it seems as if you are giving constantly and not receiving anything in return.** It may be that you are overextended, and you may need a visit with a trained co-worker or possibly the clinic administrator to create a healthier work plan for yourself. It is important to find out why you feel that no one appreciates you. Are you giving of yourself appropriately? Examine your motives for wanting something in return and ask yourself, "What would be a fair trade of my giving in this situation?" Then go about asking for it.
- **If you cannot stop thinking about a patient, a client, or co-worker, and all of their problems seem to continue to play in your mind.** Why are you thinking about this person? Do their issues represent some problems that *you* are having, or your own unresolved issues? Do you feel the need to tell them how to handle their problems? If so, you need to know that you are crossing the boundaries and a code of ethics as an esthetician. Clients need to work out their own issues with an appropriate health-care professional.
- **If you truly believe that you do not have any real issues.** If you truly believe that you have no issues of your own, you are in denial. We all have issues, and we need to work out our own. If you are able to let go of other people's problems and let them work on their own, you will be free to see that you have plenty of work to do on your problems.
- **If you always feel misunderstood or as if you are all alone.** This can be a red flag, a very unhealthy place to stay. We are not ever alone while working with doctors, medical assistants, RNs, LPNs, or administrators; there is always someone to help. Additionally, you could find someone outside of your workplace to help you sort out your feelings. Good communication is essential to a healthy work environment.

Codependence

If you find that some of the issues mentioned are ones that you are routinely struggling with, you may be codependent. Codependency is a learned pattern of feeling and behaving in a negative manner, which creates problems in relationships (White, 2001, pp. 1231–1232). It is characterized by a low self-esteem, by being out of touch with one's own feelings, by feeling shame and never feeling good enough, and by trying harder to fulfilling the needs of others. Such individuals hope others will feel good about them and are "people pleasers"; yet they *demand* attention and love from others and will try to manipulate and control the lives of those around them.

The Codependent Professional

In codependent practitioners, there is a sense of *only I* can perform this task, or *I really know* this patient better than anyone else does. They may actually keep information from the rest of the team, to protect their sense of control. Poor communication patterns and family-of-origin dysfunctions can emerge when codependent personalities are stressed.

This can also create occupational stress on the entire team. Professional rivalry grows, and staff members form allegiances, trust breaks down, and—the first thing you know—you have a major conflict on hand. On the surface it may only look as though you have an over-achiever on staff. Be aware of this problem. If it is you, a few sessions with a licensed therapist may help to relieve some of this burden for you. If it is a co-worker, bring it to the attention of your administrator or physician, because it may eventually erode the integrity of the patient-physician relationship.

When the Client Is Codependent

You will find that most people will have a clear sense of what they want or need from you, and they will view you as a resource for skin-care products and treatments, and a link to the doctor should they become interested in Botox, collagen injections, or a procedure. However, there will be clients who are not so clear about their objectives and may really want a friend to listen to all of their problems (and at a moment's notice they will be trying to help you with yours). If you encourage this type of situation and become a sounding board for this person, you may find yourself facilitating a codependent relationship. It is insidious and sometimes complex. These people can be great shoppers and loyal clients, so often the tendency is to hear them out, because you know that they will buy something. Watch your part in this relationship, however. You may need to let go and refer them to another professional.

One way to gracefully handle this referral is by building a library of Web sites, calling cards, brochures, books, articles, and phone numbers to give to the client or patient to redirect the conversation. The individual can see that you have taken the time to research the matter, and yet at the same time you are letting them know that you are not able to pursue their request or interest further with them. You remain *pro-them*, so to speak.

Interdependence

In healthy relationships, there is *interdependence*. This is an even flow of helping, giving and receiving, sharing with others, and mutual respect. The real key difference between codependence and interdependence is that there is no real investment in the outcome or in the results of the giving and sharing.

This is necessary in the clinic for both the health and integrity of the team working together, but it also benefits the client and patient. We need to keep in mind that we are being paid to do a job—and to be a reliable, observant, objective, attendant to the physician. This is a healthy way to develop a full repertoire of skills and abilities necessary to work in the helping, the healing, and the art and science of health care.

Dealing with the Death of a Client

It is inevitable: at some time we will be dealing with the death of a favorite client, patient, or co-worker. Just as we experience loss of loved ones within our families and friends, the loss of someone we have come to know in our work life can be devastating. Whether death suddenly comes by accident, or is drawn out over time through a terminal illness, we can never really prepare for its coming and finality. We will deal with denial, suffering, and pain when we lose a person who has become part of our work life, be it a client visiting the clinic monthly for services; or a co-worker coming to work each day. Once they are gone, it is incomprehensible and overwhelming to accept the fact that they will not be returning to the office.

There is never a way to prepare for a death even if we know that a client or patient has a terminal illness. The stages of grieving may be more or less intense depending on the nature of your relationship with the deceased; your cultural beliefs, spirituality, and faith; and the amount of support you may have. It is important to take care of your feelings while grieving the loss. Here are some ideas for coping with the loss of a client:

1. Allow yourself to cry and feel the pain of the loss of your friend.
2. Share your pain with others, both those who knew the person and those who may not have.
3. Pray or meditate about the delivery of your friend to a better place.
4. Continue to work and keep your scheduled plans.
5. Make time to share good times and laugh with friends and family members.
6. Attend services if you feel comfortable doing so, or create a special ritual in which you say good-bye to your special friend.

Dealing with the Death of a Co-worker

It is important to share your thoughts and feelings with other staff members, and to express how you felt about your co-worker. Peer support groups are essential at a time of death or loss. Having a special day for remembering your friend, where you invite in their family members for lunch to share thoughts and feelings is helpful for both co-workers and family members. Often family members will not even be aware of how much their loved one impacted the lives of clients, patients, and co-workers. You may get together as a group and purchase a beautiful painting or sculpture to give to the family or to put in the office in memory of your co-worker. Check with the family from time to time to see how they are doing, or send a nice "thinking of you" type of card, to let them know that you care.

If you are struggling to get through each day, join a bereavement group, where you will find mental and spiritual support in your grieving process. Your presence will bring hope and comfort to the others in the group, as every person will be in a different stage of the grieving process. If you are uncomfortable in groups, you may want to see a therapist who deals primarily with death and dying issues. You may also visit your local hospice for information and to explore your experiences. Hospice is a comprehensive system of care in which terminally ill patients and their families can find relief from the issues around dying and the death of a loved one.

Stages of Dying and Death

Swiss-American psychiatrist Elisabeth Kübler-Ross states in her book titled *Death and Dying* (1969) that there are five grief stages of grief. They can be experienced by both the dying and those caring for the dying, or after a death. They are as follows:

1. **Denial.**   The patient may say, "This is not really happening to me." The family member or friend may say, "This doctor is wrong, we'll find someone else who knows what they are doing."

2. **Anger.**   Anger toward caregivers or loved ones is not uncommon while the patient is thinking, "It's not fair, I do not deserve this." The family member or friend may say, "Why do these horrible things happen to you?" They may even become angry with their ill loved one for becoming sick.

3. **Bargaining.**   The patient may begin to try to pray or negotiate a time frame as in "Let me live long enough to see the holidays." The family member or friend may say, "Please stay around long enough to see your grandchild come into the world."

4. **Depression.**   The patient begins to lose interest in worldly issues, and begins to face the inevitable. The caregiver, family member, or friend begins to see that the reality of loss is inevitable, and they begin to lose hope that the loved one will recover; hence they begin to accept that death is inevitable.

5. **Acceptance.**   This is the final chapter in the stage of dying. The patient begins to get affairs in order by changing or creating a will. He or she wants to see friends and family members and is at peace with the fact that death is approaching. Once the patient has seen those they are the closest to, and that their affairs are in order, he or she begins to rest and sleep most of the time. Sometimes a dying patient will wait until loved ones coming to visit extend permission to die or utter the words "It is safe for you to go." Family members are sad but know that their loved one is dying. They may begin to see the physical changes and accept the fact that their ill loved one cannot go on in this state. They, too, begin to accept the final stages.

All stages are transitory, but each of them will generally be experienced by the dying, the caregivers, family members, and friends. It is an unknown factor as to how long terminal patients will stay in the final stage before they die. However, they may speak of having seeing relatives who have passed over, or dream about a journey they are taking as if they are currently traveling. This can be disconcerting to those around them, but it is advisable to let it go. Do not try to explain what they think they see, or what you feel is reality.

Summary

As we travel through the challenges of dealing with ourselves, the personalities of co-workers, and the needs of clients and patients, it is healthy to maintain objectivity about our work and the impact that it has on others.

A healthy, balanced approach and outlook can be beneficial to clients, patients, and co-workers—as well as to the esthetician. With the help of co-workers and the guidance of mentors or those more experienced in the office, there is support for almost any type of issue that arises. One can reap so many rewards through the giving of help and through the experiences learned in any of these situations. Not to mention the appreciative cards, letters, flowers, cookies, articles, books, and a myriad of other nontangible gifts such as love, respect, faith, strength, and hope that we receive as practitioners.

Here are a few ideas to keep a healthy flow going in your dealings:

- Keep others abreast of the work you are doing with a client so that at any given time you may be able to receive the help you may need from the doctor or nurse.
- Do not keep secrets about the care of a patient, client, or staff member. Be aboveboard.
- Do not be come possessive about a person, whether they are a staff member or client.
- Remember that you cannot *save* people; they need to do their own work.
- Be a team player. Rely on the talents and expertise of those around you at all times.

Hospice and **palliative care** workers are helpful in learning about the process of dying and death itself. We do not have full understanding about this natural occurring stage in our lives. In our culture, we are often removed from the death itself. Health-care workers often perform all of the immediate duties for our loved ones who are passing, or have passed.

People will deal with their feelings around the dying differently, and in some cases they may choose *not* to deal with it directly. Being of support to another during a death changes one's perspective on life forever, and quite possibly on death as well.

I WILL MISS YOU

I will miss you—
My friend
My confidant
My mentor

I will miss you—
Your caring thoughts
Your honest, ready smile
Your glowing optimism

I will miss you—
The hope in your eyes
The truthful words when you spoke
The wisdom and inspiration that lives on in your work

I will just miss you—

Frequently Asked Questions

1. What is the best thing to say to a person who has lost a close family member?

If you know the family well and have stories to share, share them. It is helpful for everyone to work through their grief in their own way. If you feel like speaking about the person, it would be fine to do so. It is best not to say that you understand how they feel if you do not, but let your heart guide your words. People can always feel kindness and thoughtfulness.

2. How does the esthetician handle the profile or intake form of a deceased client?

For some, dealing with these documents may be very difficult. All patient charts are kept with the medical records department where they are processed. The esthetician's profile or intake sheets may be given to the clinic administrator or medical records clerk, for archiving. This can be a difficult task and depending on how close the relationship was between the client and the esthetician it may require support and/or time.

3. One of the nurses in our facility is always discussing her problems with another co-worker. She spends an inordinate amount of time trying to help this person, and then feels upset and disappointed when the advice she has given is not used. What should she do?

This type of situation occurs in all settings, but it is especially pervasive in health-care settings. Sometimes people are just releasing tension, and are not that concerned about others; they rather like to blow off steam. However, in some cases, a person may seem unusually compulsive about the habits of another, and it may be worth exploring the issue.

Some people feel powerless and will use helping others as a guise for not dealing with their own problems. It may be helpful to suggest that the staff member seems unduly concerned about the other co-worker, and recommend getting a professional opinion.

4. How does the esthetician deal with a client or patient who is overly demanding?

We all have experienced a self-oriented client. This requires recognizing the signs, drawing strong boundaries, and resisting the impulse to be overly accommodating. When we are asked by an individual to come in on a day off, or stay late repeatedly; or when a client does not pick up on cues such as your opening a door and picking up their coat, you may have a client who knows no boundaries. Be clear about what you will and can do for them—and conversely what you are not going to do for them. You should not feel that you have to constantly cater to one individual to the detriment of another, or to yourself.

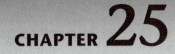

CHAPTER 25

Self-Care for the Clinical Esthetician: Mind, Body, and Spirit

- Introduction
- The Mind-Body-Spirit Connection
- Applying Mental, Physical, and Spiritual Care
- Summary

Introduction

It is difficult to discuss self-care without looking at the aspects of self, and of what self-care means. For some, self-care may suggest carving out a few minutes in a busy day for a quiet lunch. For others, it means adding an exercise or workout program that reduces stress. We need to create a *comprehensive* program of self-care and its applications because the mind, body, and spirit are connected.

The Mind-Body-Spirit Connection

As difficult as it may be to believe, it has not been long since scientists thought that the body, mind, and spirit were individual and separate. Today we know that the mind can affect the body, the spirit can affect the mind, and the body can affect both. The definitions of these three aspects, for our purposes, are:

- **Mind:** the brain, intellect, and the psyche
- **Body:** the physical manifestation of the being
- **Spirit:** an inner strength, peace, and/or possible belief in a higher power

The Mental/Emotional Connection

Research has shown that the mind can alter physiology. In an emerging field of study known as psychoneuroimmunology (PNI), scientists study the way that the brain transmits signals along the nerves to stimulate the body's normal immune system (White, 2001, p. 225). Once this communication takes place, there is a direct relationship between brain cells and other cells in the body; hence, cells can be directly affected by emotions and other functions within the scope of the being.

Biofeedback can clearly measure the body-mind connection. It has been used for decades to assist people in learning to change or modify conditioned responses to stressful situations, phobias, and illness. By connecting them to a device which then monitors their bodily responses such as body temperature, muscle tone, brain waves, and breathing, the individual is able to recognize, mentally, the physiological responses to the stressors; they are then able to change their involuntary responses. Neurofeedback or neurotherapy is a newer therapy, which is being used for attention deficient disorder, epilepsy, and severe migraine headaches.

The Body Connection

The body creates and receives countless messages every minute from its various systems and structures. The nervous, skeletal, muscular, respiratory, circulatory, immune, digestive, endocrine, reproductive, and **integumentary** (skin) systems are working in synchronicity. When we consider the vastness of the body's coding system alone, we can imagine that should a system or structure become stressed or overwrought with tension, it ultimately can lead to mental disorders and physical disease.

The immune system is the body's gateway to health. In order to perform at optimal condition, the systems must work together harmoniously. Maintaining the body's immune system is vital for the health of all systems because, officially part of the circulatory system, it acts as our environmental protector against all invaders. When the immune system is compromised, so goes the body's defense mechanism. Thus we see breakdowns in other structures through transmission of a **pathogen** (potentially a disease-producing microorganism or substance).

We have all heard of the importance of building the immune system, and safeguarding one's immune system, but what does it really mean? Keeping the immune system up or high means to create and cultivate a defense system using rest, proper nutrition, exercise, mental and emotional wellness, and spiritual connection.

The Spiritual Connection

The spirit is connected to the body and mind. We see its expression through faith, courage, will, strength, and fortitude. It is in our humanness that our spirit is present. By honoring spiritual expression ourselves and in others, we derive love, peace, conviction, hope, and endurance. These all contribute to a healthy body and mind.

Applying Mental, Physical, and Spiritual Care

The challenge in applying self-care is assessing our needs. Full-blown symptoms are typically required before some of us address our self-care issues. It suffices to say that *planning* may create a healthier life; we can work to avoid having experiences that require emergencies, crises, or recovery care.

Mental/Emotional Care

Self-care for the mental/emotional aspects of our being comes from a variety of methods. Some are intuitive, and others pragmatic—intended and dutiful. Creativity serves as the watershed for much of our mental and emotional lives, yet we often do not consciously see it this way. Teaching and learning are also vital expressions of mental health and self-care. By learning something new, we push beyond our limited thoughts, and thus create more room for personal growth, cognitive development, and understanding. Features of caring for our mental beings are:

- creativity
- education
- mentorship
- meaningful relationships
- coaching/therapy
- vacation

Creativity   We are all born with creativity. It need not be measured by societal standards such as the presentations of creativity that we seen in magazines, television programs, or paintings that we see in a museum, but rather *our own particular signature* or stamp that we place on the way we do things.

Creativity comes in many forms. It can be the way that we relate to another person, colors and scents that we choose to apply both therapeutically and strategically, methods that we develop in business or performing treatments, arranging flowers, cooking, or our own particular version of art. When we are in a state of creating we are connected to our intuition and spirituality, to mental and emotional processes, and, of course, to our physical beings.

We need not look far for creativity as healing agent. Most breast cancer survivors will share stories of the creative expressions that helped them through the process from diagnosis to recovery. Many create art for breast survivors' exhibitions. Some write books, sing songs, and share stories while dealing with their therapy. Others creatively try to help their families and friends cope with their illness through humor, kindness, and leadership. Estée Lauder can be credited for creative expression and support in the pink ribbon vehicle used to raise awareness and funding for breast cancer research.

Creativity is necessary for our mental and emotional health. By unlocking our creative energy, we allow flexibility, ingenuity, and adaptation into lives that may otherwise be rigid, lackluster, and vacuous. Problem-solving ability is fueled by creative expression just by the inherent nature of creating; we are always more open-minded when in a state of creating. When we allow creativity to flourish we are less apt to feel that the success of any one task determines our worth. While we are engaged in creating, matters resolve naturally, in an ebb and flow, like a cycle or season.

Education   Education is a fundamental aspect of caring for our mental health. If we think in terms of comprehensive education, we need to look at the entire picture, not just a few accents that will take us through the next season, or create a flurry of activity to our practices.

In addition, we need to think of adding the necessary components to our knowledge that will bring our awareness to the next level by increasing the *value* of what we know. So often we are not aware of the positive impact our empirical research, for example, has made to our milieu in the helping arts. We need to be able to use the results of our study in a manner that is academically sound and well respected.

When we look at developing our awareness, an interdisciplinary approach is more helpful than looking at one guru, or known personality who seems to have all of the answers. It is also important to acknowledge our own intelligence in the process of learning. We so often feel that someone else knows better. We need to remember that we bring an entire package including cultural/tribal background, gender, socioeconomic demographics, empirical research, business experience, and individual history to our educational experiences, not to mention our biases. It may be beneficial to take courses in accounting, sculpting, ancient Greek mythology, cultural studies, or the environment. Work on building up your academic acuity by starting college, or slowly obtaining your AA, BA, BS, MA, MS, or Ph.D.

Mentorship   We all need mentors. We often feel that we need to handle everything alone, or the hard way, but the truth is, until we are properly mentored, we do not have a sense of connectedness to a world larger than that of our own self-interest. Self-interest will only carry us so far and may be fraught with anxiety and self-doubt. Ultimately we need to view others and ourselves as connected and serving with intention and purpose for the greater good. This is found in both the receiving and giving of mentorship.

Meaningful relationships   Meaningful relationships are the conduits to healthy living. The speed and busyness of the environment in which we live and work today often leads to a void where caring, meaningful relationships are concerned. Because we feel isolated in our busyness and work lives, our own world—and all of its apparent problems— takes on more importance than it's due. With good, meaningful relationships, our issues are easier to keep into perspective, and create less frustration and angst.

Therapy/life skills coaching/support groups   At certain points in our lives, we may feel the need for the help of a mental-health professional. Whether it is due to a crisis, such as death or divorce, or other life changes, we may feel overwhelmed, confused, and in general unable to cope with our particular situation. It is at this point—when the problem is still reasonably manageable—that we should seek help. We should not wait until everything is out of control, and we become unable to function, or ill.

Therapy

Therapy is useful when trying to gain perspective on life, in part or as a whole. It may seem as if every attempt at working through an issue or a problem is ineffective. Some underlying issues may need to be resolved prior to moving forward. A trained therapist or counselor may be able to assist in the discovery of roadblocks. Often the commitment to a few sessions can resolve most problems; issues that are more complex may take longer.

Life-Skills Coach

Life coaches have become a blessing in the lives of those needing support and direction in careers or encountering impasses in perspective, and those who have found traditional therapy not an option. For some, disappointments and unrealized goals may be just a matter of focus and outlook. This is where a trained life coach may prove useful. Some life-skills coaches are also licensed mental-health specialists, so this can be a great union. Coaches work as paid mentors for the client in routine meetings; others work by phone, or via e-mail.

Support Group

Support groups are the best choice for people who may feel that a one-on-one relationship may be too direct, or intensely personal. Groups show us how we see ourselves, how others perceive us, and ultimately how we might increase our effectiveness in life. We can improve our interpersonal skills by listening and supporting others while they are sharing, and then in turn, we feel supported. The American Group Psychotherapy Association (AGPA) is a resource; their Web site is www.agpa.org.

Vacation   Vacations are necessary. Take one. That means time away from work, school, home details, everything. We do not always need an expensive getaway, but surely we need time for refreshment and recharging. By not taking time away from routine doldrums, we increase our burnout factor. In addition, when we do not take time out away from our overprocessed and overmanaged lives, we become detached and thus less effective. Being less effective leaves a breeding ground for contempt for anyone doing well, and this can stir nonproductive competitive feelings toward others at work. Petty grievances begin to rule as coping strategies, we become unable to take in anything new, and our brains feel overloaded and nonfunctioning. A vacation will neutralize these self-sabotaging thoughts and behaviors, and breathe fresh air into our lives. We should not wait until danger signals show up. It is far better to plan to get away on a regular basis.

Physical Care

Of the three aspects of self-care, the physical may be the easiest to recognize; physical needs are the easiest to assess. Most of us in our industry are acutely aware of, and concerned about, age and weight management. While these issues may seem obvious to us, we are not as apt to recognize the effects of other influences on our bodies such as stress, inadequate nutrition, and lack of proper rest. We can describe the effects and counsel clients easily enough in these areas yet have trouble applying what we know to ourselves. The features of taking care of and maintaining our physical beings are:

- rest/sleep
- stress reduction
- nutrition/diet/vitamins/minerals
- exercise
- checkups
- body work/massage, facials other

Rest/sleep   In our overall health and fitness plan, it is essential to bring about restful sleep. Stress reduction, diet, exercise, and meditation are all good examples of triggering a positive resting experience. *Rest* refers to a state of relaxation, calmness, and an altered consciousness which affects both the mental and the physical (White, 2001, p. 375). We have always heard that the body needs at least 8 hours of sleep for adequate restoration and rejuvenation. Depending on individual need in terms of age, hormonal stage, and physical and mental condition, we require a consistent amount of time each night in the state of repose and tranquility. Sleep brings about a slowing of the physiological being, and hence its systems.

Stress reduction and management   Stress and its management are certainly the focus of every seminar, training program, and conference in most industries today; however, we wonder how much is truly being managed. There are two types of stress. *Eustress* is a type of stress that culminates with a positive result, while *distress* is stress gone awry. Eustress is necessary and often short-lived; it is the type of stress that we experience while preparing to give a presentation or asking an employer for a raise. Distress is the type of stress that often becomes categorized or generalized as *stress*, which has a negative and often cumulative effect. It can stem from not getting enough sleep, having to work longer hours, in addition to not getting enough exercise and overeating or drinking. Distress, when compounded by other issues such as divorce, death of a friend or family member, or job loss, and left unchecked, will ultimately result in disease and decay of body, mind, and spirit.

Physical Benefits of Being Calm

Studies show that when we are in a calm, relaxed state we can accomplish more, our body systems function properly, we have more creative energy, we are more resilient, and we have a better sense of well-being (Wilson, 2000, p. 30). We are finding that meditation, visualization, and methods using the martial arts are being included as therapy in progressive cancer and disease centers. So it should not be surprising to us when these programs are recommended for lesser-compromised health issues.

Simple Stress Reduction and Management Applications

Stress-management programs work by consistent application, and follow-through. Many simple measures can be easily implemented as stress-management tools, which will have a positive result on the body's ability to thrive. The following are vehicles for calming:

- **Good communication.**   Approach every opportunity to communicate as if it really matters. Ask for a consensus, and determine that the information you have given has been received correctly, and that it is understood. Often misunderstandings are at the root of stress.
- **Think before you speak.**   Slowing down and giving yourself time to speak gives the other person permission to do so. In the big picture, what difference does it make if we take a couple more minutes to give people a more accurate account of a perspective or situation?
- **Look at the big picture.**   Ask yourself how much really matters. Do not get caught up in details that are not important to the whole.
- **People first.**   Always put people first, then money, then things (Orman, 2002, p. 45).
- **Think of yourself as a change agent.**   Be flexible and learn to adapt. If you open up to new possibilities, you may find less stress and more calm in a new way of approaching your life, your work, your *being*.
- **Take care of your whole being.**   Get adequate rest, exercise, and nutrition; use spiritual guidance/intuition.
- **Know yourself.**   Learn as much as you can about you. This can alleviate many stressful moments throughout the day. The more that you understand about why and what you are reacting to, the more opportunity you may have to resolve the specific stress and thus relieve your body of its negative effects.

Nutrition/diet/vitamins/minerals   Nutritionists suggest that proper diet is at the helm of good health. We know that our body functions according to its intake, or lack thereof. In 1992, the U.S. Department of Health and Human Services developed a system to help with the selection of a healthy diet. Called the *Dietary Guidelines for Americans* (Roth & Townsend, 2003, p. 21), it offers the following general suggestions and goals:

- Aim for a healthy weight.
- Be physically active each day.
- Choose whole grains first and then a variety of grains daily.
- Choose a variety of fruits and vegetables daily.
- Keep food safe to eat.
- Choose a diet that is low in saturated fat and cholesterol, and moderate in total fat.
- Moderate your intake of sugars, caffeine, and alcohol.
- Use less salt.

This seems reasonable, yet many of us are suffering from information overload regarding why it is suggested that we eat certain foods.

Confusion about What to Eat Today

It is no wonder that we are confused about what to eat these days; there are so many conflicting reports. Depending upon geographic location, body type, physical issues, cultural and spiritual beliefs, and access to health information, we are, unfortunately, subject to various trends with respect to nutrition. One year a food product is in favor; the next, something else becomes in vogue. We are bombarded by information not only gathered from magazines, but put out by our government agencies, physicians, and research scientists.

Sensible Eating

It is helpful to look at a simplistic approach to eating and acquiring the nutrition that our bodies need to function at optimum levels. A sensible eating plan consists of three main nutrients. They are:

1. **Fats** are necessary to the healthy immune system in delivering energy, distributing hormones, equalizing blood sugar levels, and hunger management. In this context, we will briefly discuss the four main types of fats: saturated, polyunsaturated, monounsaturated, and hydrogenated. Saturated fats are solid at room temperature and found in butter, meat, eggs, and cheese. Polyunsaturated fats are liquid, such as cooking oils (soybean oil, sunflower, safflower, or corn oil); fish or fish oils; and oily substances. Within the polyunsaturated fats are two key essential fatty acids:
   - Omega-3 (v-3) found in flaxseed, leafy vegetables, soybeans, fish, and fish oils
   - Omega-6, (v-6), found in oils from flax seed, corn and soy, and vegetables such as kale, greens, and Swiss chard

   Both essential fatty acids have been associated with lowering the risk of cholesterol and therefore heart disease (Gittleman, 1998, p. 25). Monounsaturated fats are olive oil, canola oil, avocado, and nuts. Hydrogenated fats are polyunsaturated fats to which hydrogen (gas processed) has been added, making them a saturated fat such as margarine.

2. **Carbohydrates** are necessary to drive our energy, by administering proper sugar uptake into the bloodstream. There are three types of carbohydrates: monosaccharides, disaccharides, and polysaccharides; all are a form of sugar. Depending upon the glycemic index, which is a measurement of how quickly sugar is absorbed into the bloodstream, they are classified as:
   - **Monosaccharides** are the simplest form of sugar, and absorb directly into the bloodstream. Berries, carrots, corn, honey, and sodas are examples.
   - **Disaccharides** are combinations of monosaccharides and require hydrolysis (refinement by adding water) before they can change into simple carbohydrates. Examples are sugar cane, syrups, candy, jams, and milk (Roth & Townsend, 2003, pp. 72–73).
   - **Polysaccharides** are complex carbohydrates, the slowest acting sugars. They consist of grains, potatoes, starchy foods such as rice and pasta, and some fruits with fiber such as oranges and apples.

   As we know, sugars give us energy, and if we have a lack of sugar in our bloodstream, energy levels drop and cravings go up. The key is to offset the amount of sugar that is directly being distributed into the bloodstream, by selecting the carbohydrate, or combination of carbohydrates, that best fits the need.

   The polysaccharides are slow to break down, thus limiting the amount of a surge in the bloodstream. This will determine the amount of insulin (also a fat-storing hormone) that is produced in the pancreas. Insulin is the distribution center for the sugar being stored, and its administration to the cells as nutrients. Simple carbohydrates, monosaccharides, have a higher glycemic index, so they enter the bloodstream much faster. The insulin can take on only so much, so it begins to store the excess. Whether the sugar is stored or used is determined by how well the hormones **glucagon** (which stores energy in the muscles and liver) and insulin have been balanced (Gittleman, 1998, p. 104). By controlling the glucagon and insulin, through eating carbohydrates from the lower glycemic index and through having fiber in the diet, we are more apt to burn fat, fuel energy, and store less.

3. **Proteins** are essential to repair and build cells, and to bank usable fuel for the body. Proteins make new cells and rebuild tissue and organs. In the average adult body protein content reaches 18 percent of the total body weight (Roth & Townsend, 2003, p. 103). There are two types of proteins: complete and incomplete. The *complete* proteins supply us with nine essential amino acids, which are vital to normal growth and development. *Incomplete* proteins are proteins that lack one or more of the essential amino acids. In order for incomplete proteins to be beneficial, they must be combined with other proteins. The food sources of complete proteins are: meat, eggs, fish, cheese, and poultry. The incomplete proteins are nuts, soybeans, dried beans, and grains.

   If we do not have adequate protein in our diet, our immune system become compromised, we lose muscle mass, and the body begins to create enzymes which will in turn cannibalize its own muscles and organs. Conversely, if we have too much protein, we will suffer from liver and colon ailments and from high cholesterol, which may lead to heart disease.

Putting It All Together

By mindfully selecting the amount of protein, carbohydrates, and fats that you take in, you can control:

- the amount of insulin that is produced to store fat
- the amount of glucagon, the hormone which moves fat
- the amount of energy that you store and use
- the amount of food you desire

Simply put, high-glycemic carbohydrates will produce high levels of insulin, which will make you gain weight. By eating complex carbohydrates, you will slow down the amount of insulin that is being made, thus not storing it as fat. By taking in more protein, you will stimulate the hormone glucagon to use fat in your body as fuel; and by eating healthful fats such as Omega 3s and Omega 6s, you will lower levels of cholesterol, increase your immune system for protection, stabilize hormones, and aid in hunger management. It is always advisable to seek professional nutritional counseling. If you have specific health needs, follow the advice of your health-care provider.

Drugs/Supplements/Vitamins/Minerals

Drugs and dietary supplements create a multibillion-dollar business worldwide. Moreover, just as in diet fads, skin-care products, and small plastic surgery procedures, we see trends come and go. When considering using any type of supplement, our first comment should be: "This is going into my body." Then the question should be: "What is the cost/benefit ratio?"

We really need to know whether a product is appropriate for our particular needs. It is vital that we learn as much as we can about taking any supplements internally, or recommending them to others. Have your health-care provider show and tell you why a drug, herb, vitamin, or other supplement is being recommended, and ask about a *viable method for measurement* for its use in your body.

Exercise   The American Heart Association recommends 30 minutes of exercise, 6 days a week. It need not be strenuous, but aerobic. This covers all forms of movement from walking, running, hiking, swimming, skating, snowboarding, skiing, golf, weight lifting, dancing, tennis, handball, and racquetball. In addition, albeit more slow-moving, Pilates, yoga, and Tai Chi have been added to the index of viable, if not essential, forms of exercise because of the meditative value inherent in performing them. They provide a reduction in injury and a deliberate approach to movement, which combines the body, mind, and spiritual connection.

Body Awareness

The topic of body awareness is not as esoteric as it sounds. We must become consciously aware of our body's ability to move—and, conversely its limitations. Not all bodies are meant for all activities, at all ages. Movement strengthens the skeletal, musculature, integumentary (skin), and immune systems—in addition to supporting a sense of well-being at the mental/emotional level. By increasing stamina, it reduces tension and anxiety, which in turn, increases the ability to rest and sleep. The key is to determine which program of movement suits your particular fitness needs, factoring in your body awareness, condition, age, and requirements. Here are some ideas for developing a fitness schedule:

- **Hire a professional personal trainer with knowledge of nutrition, lifestyle, and physical parameters.**   Work closely with someone you trust—and who is highly trained.
- **Start slow and build steadily.**   Do not start in the middle or at the advanced level; give your body time to adjust to the new exercise.
- **Listen to your body.**   If a movement or exercise hurts, do not do it.
- **Do not try to keep up with others who may have a different fitness level.**   Well-meaning friends may be at a different level of competency than you. Go at your own pace.
- **If you stop your program for a week or more, start back slowly (not where you left off).**   This is where many injuries occur. Always start over if you have been off for an extended period of time.
- **Have fun with your program.**   If it is boring or something that you do not like, you will not stick to it; find something more fun.
- **Apply a calm, relaxing form of movement to the end of every session.**   Slowly stretch after all exercises so that muscles have a chance to restore.

- **Breathe.**   Always breathe through your movement or fitness program, and focus on breathing through your nose (your body's natural filtration system), while exercising.

Routine checkups   Having routine physical examinations with a qualified health-care professional is not only necessary, but makes excellent business sense. If we become ill, our livelihood is likely to become compromised.

A routine health examination should begin even before you get to your health-care provider's office. Take a half hour or more, and sit down at the computer, or with a pen and paper, and begin to write down questions and concerns that you may have. Then organize them in order of priority, making certain this information is concise and easy to read. If you have a specific issue, give a brief history; describe in a sentence or two what is going on now, and what you have been trying to eradicate the problem. Print two copies, one for you, and one for the provider.

This is always appreciated by the provider and can be placed in your file. It gives a personal account (subjective), which is not as easily misinterpreted as a verbal explanation. Once we get into the doctor's office, we often forget some of the less pressing concerns, as we are being prepared for the physical exams. We can expect from our health-care partners their time, good communication, and compassion.

Physical exams should be performed as follows:

- 20–35 years of age: every 1–3 years
- 35–50: every 1–2 years
- Every year for those over 50

Pap tests

According to Christiane Northrup, M.D., Pap smears (Papanicolaou test—a smear of exfoliative cells) have decreased deaths of cervical cancer by 70 percent. They should be performed every 2–3 years after the beginning of sexual activity, annually for those over 40, and possibly more often if a positive or abnormal test has been detected. A manual breast and rectal exam should be performed at the time of the Pap smear for all ages.

Mammograms

Mammograms are recommended every year for women over 40 years of age. Studies continue to show that early detection of breast cancer results in more curable disease and greater survival.

Male exams

Men should have a testicular exam with every physical exam and rectal exams to check the prostate yearly after the age of 40.

Dental exams

Dental exams should include both an internal exam and an external exam of the zygomatic region, the mandible, and the throat and neck. Every 2 to 3 years a set of X rays should be taken. Under the age of 40, yearly cleansing should be performed by a dental professional, and biyearly after.

Bodywork, spa treatments, facials   The value that we extend to our client is related to the care that we give to ourselves. If we are not walking our talk, it can be felt, if not seen. Factors of money, time, and convenience should not keep us from receiving what we are advocating for others. Routine bodywork could be considered maintenance for the health-care professional. In addition to spa treatments or facials (which may leave us feeling like we are still at work), regular bodywork may include the following:

- **Reiki:** A gentle Japanese technique used for stress and pain relief
- **acupuncture:** Ancient Chinese method of health care that utilizes needles applied to meridians or zones of the body believed to be in distress or congestion
- **Rolfing:** A deep massage which helps to soften connective tissue, hence making it more easily manipulated to ultimately restore health in an area of the body
- **craniosacral therapy:** Works to release tensions in the body through a gentle head massage, which increases or decreases the amount of spinal fluid held by stress, trauma, or injury
- **Trager:** A gentle, nonmanipulative movement that releases stress from tension and negative thought patterns. Its use includes bringing about a sense of well-being.
- **neuromuscular therapy:** Utilizes advanced techniques to break the stress, tension, and pain cycle. The goal is to relax the muscle, thus increase circulation and restore health to the area.
- **Pfrimmer deep muscle therapy:** A deep-tissue manipulation, which stimulates circulation, and lymphatic movement, thus promotes purification of the body's circulatory system

The Spiritual Care

Caring for our spiritual beings in this context will be interpreted as developing a relationship with oneself in order to find meaning in all aspects of life—including death—with hope, faith, strength, courage, and peace. Whether this includes intuition, religion, or a connection to a higher power, the meaning is open to individual interpretation and celebration.

Our spiritual being needs to be fed and nourished; it cannot be separated from our physical and mental/emotional needs. Considering the intangible concept of spirituality brings up a variety of meanings. For some, spiritual care is met on a hike in the woods, viewing the landscape from the top of a mountain, or strolling along the seaside. For others it is being a parishioner at a place of worship; and for still others, it does not necessarily mean believing in an entity, but believing in a personal connection to something larger than our present awareness. Ways of caring for our spiritual beings are found through:

- affiliations with spiritual groups
- unconditional love
- meditation/prayer/self-hypnosis
- music/dance

- communing with nature
- volunteerism/giving back
- tithing

Affiliations with spiritual groups   Many feel most connected to their spirituality while attending services at a church, synagogue, mosque, or temple. Religion provides a context for their beliefs in a higher being. It gives hope and peace to its followers through an organized sharing of values and beliefs.

Unconditional love   Love is considered unconditional when it is given freely, without expectation. When giving or receiving unconditional love we experience the intrinsic nature of light, warmth, and spirit. When we allow expressions of unconditional love through kindness, good intention, faith, hope and strength, we feel a connectedness, which moves beyond our immediate needs and worldly values.

Meditation and prayer   Meditation is a vehicle for opening our hearts and minds to quiet and renewal. We are blasted daily with so much information creating a sensory overload and a false sense of reality. We often begin to believe, through our daily dose of exposure to worldly doings, that we are not complete enough as human beings. Because we feel depleted, we think that we need more things; yet, when we get into a state of relaxation or meditation, we find that the opposite is true.

Prayer

Prayer has been used by groups and individuals as far back as time records for the purposes of communicating with God or a Higher Power. There is a belief that by praying the Supreme Being will hear, affect, or answer prayers and chants. Studies have shown that patients in critical-care units have fewer complications when prayer has been introduced (Byrd & Sherrill, 1995, pp. 21–23).

Gratitude

There are countless examples of prayer being offered as a way of giving gratitude for what we have been given in our lives. Being grateful for another day, peace of mind, beauty in the world, and the kindness of others, is at the base of finding one's way through the trials of life. A belief that we come and go from this world in a purposeful way gives meaning to our lives, although we may not understand at the time the conditions of our parting. It is with prayer and meditation that we may find peace and solace, and thus meaning to our living.

Music   Music is a universal language. It acts as a vessel, which can affect our moods, physiology, and consciousness. The use of chanting, drumming, singing, and playing instruments, dates back to ancient times. In ancient mythology, it was believed that through music the gods would be called, crops would grow, the sick would be healed, game would be brought closer for hunting, and the evil would be put to death (Pinkola Estes, 1992, p. 160).

Music can bring peace and a sense of well-being to the listener. It affects biochemistry in the body as it can calm, soothe, or energize an individual depending upon the type of music that is used. "The song, like the drum creates a nonordinary consciousness, a trance state, a prayer state (Pinkola Estes, 1992, p. 160)." Sounds affect both humans and animals, and we respond accordingly.

Communing with nature   Naturalist Aldo Leopold said, "There are two spiritual dangers in not living on a farm. One is the danger of believing that breakfast comes from a grocery store, and the other that the heat comes from the furnace (Leopold, 1966, p. 6)." These points are well understood. Watching the natural cycles of life can bring about a greater understanding of its process, and enhance one's spirituality.

Volunteerism/tithing   We come full circle when thoughts of volunteerism are considered self-care. The most satisfying form of volunteerism is anonymous. Giving from one's heart without expectation or acknowledgement breathes fresh new energy into the life of the giver. A conscious, deliberate expression of unconditional love generates a cleared mind, tenderness toward others, hope, and a demonstration of peace and goodwill.

Giving of one's earnings in a consistent, small amount shows good faith and gratitude for the money that one receives for labor, and it demonstrates a belief in abundance. Whether we consistently tithe at a place of worship, or give to benefit endangered species, the environment, or children's groups, we are not only benefiting the recipient of our tithing, but we are making room for the next level of growth in our own lives.

Summary

We are very complex beings with needs that are not always met. We must learn as much as we can about our minds, our bodies, and our spirits so that we can begin to meet our needs in healthy and productive ways. Once we have met our needs, we are better equipped to handle the needs of others; and in many cases to allow them to meet their own.

Concluding Thoughts

We have entered into a very exciting time for estheticians and for the skin-care industry. Technology and training have long surpassed the state requirements for licensing estheticians. This is bittersweet as we have the tools to apply new treatments or procedures, however current state licensure may not allow us to practice, hone, and develop our emerging skills.

Time has come for us to institute a separate designation for the clinical esthetician, perhaps as a subspecialty of dermatology or plastic surgery. In the meantime, we need to follow current guideline and licensing regulations so that as we develop our profession within the medical milieu we are in compliance.

As clinical or medical estheticians we have what it takes to be successful. We can make a tremendous difference in the lives of our clients, patients, and coworkers. The greatest gift that we can offer to those we serve is the recognition of value that we bring with us. Revealing the strength, passion and enthusiasm that we each hold deep in our hearts for the work that we do is inspiring in and of itself.

Believe in yourself and your abilities and you will be honored with a wonderful, successful career in medical esthetics.

Many blessings,

Sallie Deitz, clinical esthetician, patient educator

Glossary

ABCD—A system of checks for skin cancer, it stands for Asymmetry, Border, Color, Diameter.

abrasion—A removal of skin by friction.

Accutane—An oral medication also known as Isotretinoin (vitamin A) used for advanced cases of acne and extreme cases of rosacea.

actinic keratosis—Solar keratosis, sunspots; they can be dry, flaky and red. In addition, can be precancerous.

AHAs—Alpha-hydroxy acids—generally fruit acids—used to exfoliate and hydrate the skin.

allantoin—A product of the comfrey root, used to sooth and promote tissue growth.

alopecia—Loss of hair.

alpha lipoic acid—An antioxidant.

ancillary profit center—Separate department within the medical office that generates a profit, such as a skin-care center.

anthralin—An anticancer drug often used for the control and management of psoriasis and alopecia.

antioxidant—A chemical or ingredient which is used to block or neutralize effects of free radicals, a group of reactive atoms which encourage cancer.

arnica—An herb used to reduce swelling.

Artecoll—A filler for wrinkles and tissue augmentation, and acne scarring.

atopic dermatitis—Also known as eczema, a rash with crustiness and oozing.

avobenzone—(parsol 1789) A UVA absorbing ingredient used in sunscreen products.

azulene—(German chamomile) An ingredient used in products for calming and soothing

balance sheet—A balance sheet is a document that shows how much cash, accounts receivable and accounts payable, inventory, and debt that you have at a given time.

benzophenone-3—(oxybenzone) A sunscreen chemical with UVA and UVB absorbing properties.

beta carotene—An antioxidant, found in dark green and yellow vegetables.

beta-hydroxy (BHA)—A peel compound made from salicylic acid

blepharoplasty—Eyelift—could be upper or lower.

blepharospasm—Uncontrollable blinking.

bloodborne pathogens—Pathogenic organisms that are present in human blood and can cause disease in humans. These pathogens include but are not limited to HBV and HIV.

Bloodborne Pathogens Standard—OSHA issued the Bloodborne Pathogens Standard (29 CFR 1910.1030) in 1991 to prevent needle sticks and other exposures to blood and other body fluids that contain blood at work.

body-kinesthetic intelligence—Excellence in, tendency to respond positively to physical movement

Botox—A bacterium known as Botulinum toxin type A. It is injected to suppress muscle overactivity.

botulinum toxin type B—Myobloc, an injectible bacterium used to treat contracting muscles that are pain inducing such as **cervical dystonia**.

break-even point—A figure, which is determined by knowing how many products and services that you need to sell each month to cover all of your expenses.

bromelin—(pineapple) Enzyme used to dissolve keratosis.

business plan—A formal written plan which serves as a road map for a business to meet goals with appropriate financial and staffing support.

cash flow statement—A financial statement of the amount of cash that moves through the business in the form of receipts, expenses, and capital expenditures (decrease in cash).

cellulitis—A form of staphylococcus; its origin can be from a streptococcal bacterium. Cellulitis is characterized by swelling, warm-to-hot-feeling skin, and may appear blistered or bumpy.

ceramide—Substance to strengthen the skin's barrier by creating a barrier to reduce the skin's own moisture, thus increases hydration. It can be animal or plant derived.

cervical dystonia—A condition in which the muscles in the neck contract abnormally.

charting—Recording of information about a patient; there are various types, such as narrative, problem oriented, source oriented, computerized

chief complaint (cc)—Used as cc, charting shorthand to record the patient's main concern.

client profile form—The esthetician's form for recording information about the client or patient, separate from the form that goes into the physician's patient chart.

coherent pattern—One travelling in one direction.

collagen—A protein serving to connect tissue.

collimated—Parallel; light can be specifically directed because light rays are parallel to one another.

comedones—Blackheads, primary lesions of acne.

copper peptide—A substance to increase collagen formation.

cosmeceuticals—Professional clinical skin-health products that contain more aggressive ingredients than commercial varieties.

cost of goods sold—(cogs) In financial planning, the price that you paid for products.

cost of sales—Products, wages, and overhead requirements must be developed and transferred into cost data for each product or treatment/service.

cryotherapy—Liquid nitrogen or dry ice used briskly over affected area, as treatment for cooling or soothing the skin after a chemical peel or at the culmination of a treatment to calm and relax stimulated skin.

delta hepatitis—A liver disease caused by the hepatitis D virus. Symptoms are similar to hepatitis B and may include fever, lack of energy, nausea, vomiting, abdominal discomfort, and jaundice.

demographics—Data on populations such as in income levels, ages, births, deaths.

dermatitis—General term for inflammation of the skin, characterized by an itchy rash; various specific types exist, many in reaction to specific or temporary stimuli or allergens.

differential advantage—The reason that someone would come to you for products and service over someone else.

differentiation aspects—The features that make you different from the competition.

dimethicone—Hybrid form of silicone used in products to protect against moisture loss. It also acts as ingredient to aid in ease of application of product.

dyschromias—Discoloration; pigmented lesions.

ecthyma—An advanced, ulcerated form of *impetigo*, which can be from a strep or staph origin.

eczema—Also known as atopic dematitis, it is characterized by severe itching and oozing blisters; may be chronic.

emotional intelligence—Another name for *interpersonal intelligence.*

endermology—A body treatment given before and after liposuction as it helps stimulate the reduction of adipose tissue (fat) in areas such as the buttocks, thighs, and calves.

ephelides—Freckles, macules.

erysipelas—An inflamed, painful rash caused by streptococcal bacteria.

erythema—Redness of skin, an inflammatory skin reaction; the cause is often difficult to determine; may be due to infection.

evening primrose oil—Contains essential fatty acids, which are necessary for skin's hydration and thus improve proper barrier functions.

executive summary—The summary is a condensed version of a business plan which serves to summarize and emphasize the key elements, points and features of a business plan.

exogenous ochronosis—Blue-black patches that develop primarily on darker pigmented skin through the use of hydroquinone or lighteners.

expanded polytetrafluoro-ethylene (ePTFE)—Material used in lip augmentation and for wrinkles and soft tissue defects

facial bra—Replacement for bandages following lift surgery; used to enhance healing of newly placed skin.

Facsian—Human cadaver material used for wrinkles, depressions, and lip augmentation and in reconstructive surgery.

Fitzpatrick's Skin Typing—An instrument created by T. B. Fitzpatrick, M.D., to classify skin types by its tendency to sunburn or tan.

folliculitis—Infection of hair follicles.

free radicals—Atoms or molecules that are unstable due to an arrant electron. If left uncorrected, the damage created by this chemical process can affect all components of the body systems. Antioxidants counteract this process.

furnicle—A large boil.

galvanic current treatment—A method of deincrustation. Using electrodes through which a current passes to create a chemical reaction that transforms sebum of the skin to soap. Used primarily on oily skins or areas.

Glogau Photodamage Classification—A classification of photodamage as theorized by R. Glogau, M.D.

glucagon—A hormone produced in the pancreas that increases blood sugar.

glycolic acid—An alpha-hydroxy acid used for exfoliation and hydration.

Gor-Tex—Expanded polytetrafluoro-ethylene (or ePTFE); material used for lip augmentation, and soft tissue defects.

hemangioma—A red birthmark also known as port wine stain, caused by benign tumor of blood vessels.

hemophilia—A bleeding disorder in which the blood fails to clot properly.

hepatitis A, B, C—(HAV, HBV, HCV) Hepatitis means "inflammation of the liver." It is usually caused by one of three viruses: Hepatitis A, B, or C. The effects of each virus are different, but in some cases viral hepatitis can lead to cirrhosis of the liver, eventually causing serious, life-threatening disease, and even liver cancer. Hepatitis A is spread through swallowing contaminated food or water that has been infected feces. Hepatitis B (HBV) is caused by a virus found in blood, semen, vaginal fluids, breast milk, and saliva. It is spread by needle sticks, sharing syringes, and through body fluids. Hepatitis C (HCV) is another virus found in blood and mostly transmitted through blood-to-blood contact. *See also* delta hepatitis.

herpes simplex Type I—(HSV-1) Cold sores, fever blisters caused by herpes virus.

herpes simplex Type II—(HSV-2) Genital lesions caused by herpes virus.

Hippocrates—A Greek physician of the 5th century.

Hippocratic Oath—A pledge taken by those beginning to practice medicine; and, a promise made to observe a professional code of ethics, honor, and behavior.

hirsutism—Overgrowth or excessive hair growth.

HIV/AIDS—HIV is the virus that causes AIDS. As blood cells CD4 T lymphocyte, or T cells die off, the body becomes more and more vulnerable to other diseases. AIDS is short for acquired immune deficiency syndrome. AIDS is a disease that slowly destroys the body's immune system. Without these important defenses, a person with AIDS can't fight off germs and cancers.

home-care compliance—The client or patient using products at home in a manner consistent with plan created by esthetician and physician.

hospice—A hospital or program where a comprehensive system of care is offered to terminally ill patients and their family members.

HPIP—acronym for the chart writing method: History, Physical Exam, Impression, Plan.

hydroquinone—Melanocyte-suppressant skin lightener.

hyperhidrosis—Excessive sweating.

hyperpigmentation—Dark pigmented lesions.

hypertrophic—Raised or extended, such as in a hypertrophic scar.

hypopigmentation—Void or loss of pigment.

impetigo—Another form of strep (can also be caused by staph), and is characterized by weepy, crusty lesions that grow in clusters. Children often experience impetigo, and spread it amongst themselves due to a lack of hand washing with soap.

informed consent—A signed agreement by both the practitioner and client, to agree to treatment or procedure, with risks disclosed; it typically releases the esthetician or physician of liability.

integumentary—The skin system.

interferon—A type of chemotherapy.

interpersonal intelligence—Talent for dealing with people; higher than usual amount of compassion and emotional depth.

intrapersonal intelligence—Great self-knowledge and self-awareness.

isotretinoin—A medication also known as Accutane (Vitamin A), used for a advanced cases of acne and extreme cases of rosacea.

keloids—Raised, wormlike scars. Aka hypertropic scars.

kinesthetic intelligence—*See* **body-kinesthetic intelligence.**

Kligman's Classification—A classification of levels of acne as theorized by Alfred Kligman, M.D.

ladies' thistle—A natural wound healer.

laser—Light Amplification by Stimulated Emission of Radiation

laser resurfacing—A cosmetic surgical procedure that uses lasers to vaporize layers of skin.

lecithin—A phopholipid found in animals and plants having antioxidant qualities; attracts water and is a natural hydrator.

lentigines—Freckles.

Let's Face It—A nonprofit support group for people with facial differences.

lidocaine—Topical anesthesia.

light therapy—(not a laser) known under various names, it in theory is supposed to bypass the epidermis and stimulate collagen in the dermis.

linguistic intelligence—Excellence in the use of words and verbal communication.

linoleic acid—(vitamin F) Essential fatty acid that helps to improve barrier functions, and acts as an emulsifier, which binds ingredients together.

logical-mathematical analytical intelligence—Exceptional ability with numbers and logic; comfort with using statistics, graphs, etc.

loss leader—Product offered at a special price to encourage purchase of other items.

lupus—(Systemic Lupus Erythematosus) (SLE) is an autoimmune disease, which means the body's immune system attacks its own healthy cells.

malaria—A serious, sometimes fatal, disease caused by a parasite, which is transmitted through the bite of a malaria-infected mosquito.

malpractice or professional liability insurance—A separate insurance policy that the physician or practitioner purchases to protect against a malpractice lawsuit filed by a client or patient.

market trends—The market's growth potential and movement toward a target.

market value—What the market will pay for an item.

marketing strategy—Method of identifying and finding potential clients.

marketing vehicle—A medium used for delivering a marketing message such as television, radio, or print ads.

markup—Amount of increase on cost of product to sell for retail.

mathematical intelligence—*See* **logical-mathematical analytical intelligence.**

medical documentation—Legal binding information written in a patient's chart.

melanocytes—Pigment cells that determine the color of skin and hair.

melanin—Pigment found in skin and hair.

melanoma—Malignant lesion, frequently metastisizing.

melasma—Pregnancy "mask"; darkened hyperpigmented skin, generally about the periorbital and perioral regions. Hormonally driven by melanocytes often located in the upper layers of the dermis.

merchandising—Displaying products for optimum presentation and sales.

metastasize—Spread, as in cancer.

methotrexate—An anticancer drug often used for the control and management of psoriasis.

microdermabrasion—A mechanical exfoliation that aids in the elimination of surface build-up and stimulation of circulation.

micropigmentation—Cosmetic tattooing.

milia—Small encapsulated sebum or fat beads just under the skin.

Mohs surgery—Microscopically controlled removal of skin cancers where clean margins around the cancer can be detected through careful monitoring during the surgery.

monochromatic—One color.

Multiple Intelligences—A theory created by renowned psychologist Howard Gardner, Ph.D., that delineates a concept of eight different types of intelligence that people may possess. *See* specific types.

musical intelligence—Above-average ability in music; response to rhythm and sound.

Myobloc—Botulinum toxin type B.

naturalist intelligence—Strong ability to interact with the natural world.

nevus (nevi, plural)—A mole.

octyl methoxycinnimate—A UVB chemical-absorbing ingredient used in sunscreens.

operating expenses—All expenses including cost of goods, sales expenses including marketing and distribution costs, sales, salaries, commissions, promotion, education and advertising.

OPIM—Other Potentially Infectious Materials.

OSHA—Occupational Safety and Health Administration; sets standards for safety in the workplace.

palliative care—Care given to the dying for their comfort such as medication, touching, holding, along with support to the family members.

papain—(papaya) Enzyme to dissolve keratin.

papules—raised lesions that are usually red.

parsol 1789—(Avobenzone) A UVA chemical-absorbing ingredient used in sunscreens. Stability in sun is in question.

pathogen—A potentially disease producing microorganism or substance.

patient education—Formal term for informing and teaching patients about products, treatments, procedures.

patient consultation form—Formal, legal, medical, document filled out by patient in medical office.

patient selection—Physician evaluation of patient candidacy.

phospholipids—Lipids often combined and used in moisturizers due to compatibility with skin's own natural lipids.

photorejuvenation—(or light therapy; not a laser) known under various names; in theory it is supposed to bypass the epidermis and stimulate collagen in the dermis, treat vascular redness and hyperpigmentation with little down time.

polymethyl methacrylate (PMMA)—Microspheric beads contained in Artecoll filler for wrinkles and tissue augmentation.

population—Group connected by common characteristic.

profit and loss forecast—Forecasted sales and losses instrument to determine cash flow, capital, and equity you will need until the practice generates a positive cash flow.

profit margin—The difference between the cost of the product and the price that it was sold.

profit—The difference between the cost of the product, the cost of doing business, or all expenses subtracted such as cost of product, shipping, commission/wages, versus what is left over.

projected cash flow statements—A document that shows your projected or targeted cash flow, an educated guess about money with which you can do business.

Propionibacterium acnes—(P. acnes) A bacterium that normally lives on the skin that will multiply quickly when trapped in sebum-rich environments, creating inflammation and thus nodules and cystic types of acne lesions.

psoriasis—A condition where skin cells that multiply faster than normal on hands, scalp, and knees creating a silver whitish scale that itches; can be painful.

pulse method—Intermittent application.

re-epithelialized—Skin has intact barrier; epidermis has grown back.

Restylane—Hyaluronic acid injectible filler for wrinkles.

retinoic acid—*See* **tretinoin**.

rhinophima—Bulbous nose, resulting from a severe form of acne Rosacea.

rhytidectomy—Face-lift.

rhytides—Wrinkles.

risk management—Measures put in place to avoid potential risks of malpractice Lawsuits.

Rubin Classification—Instrument used to classify photodamage as created by renowned dermatologist, author, Mark Rubin, M.D.

Safety Bill of Rights—The original name of OSHA.

sage—An anti-inflammatory substance.

scientific method—A method using five steps: observe, hypothesize, experiment, and conclude to solve a problem.

seborrheic keratosis—A thickening of the epidermal cells. Looks like a scab, usually light brown, can itch and flake.

sebum—Oily substance that lubricates the surface of the skin.

selenium—Antioxidant found in whole grains, meats and fish.

sharps—All needles, lancets, syringes, and other sharp nonreusable equipment.

Silon dressing—Semipermeable wound care dressing used for laser resurfacing made of silicone and polytetrafluoro-thylene (PTFE)

skin tags—Small flesh-toned skin drops that are loose and often are found on the neck, chest, and underarms.

SOAP—Acronym for Subjective, Objective, Assessment, and Plan used in problem-oriented charting.

SOAPIE—SOAP plus Implementation and Evaluation.

SOAPIER—SOAPIE plus Revision.

Softform—Expanded polytetrafluoro-ethylene (or ePTFE); material used for lip augmentation, wrinkles and soft tissue defects.

spatial-visual intelligence—Orientation towards arrangment in space and ability to move images around in space; tendency to visual a process.

SPF—Sun protection factor.

spontaneous granulation—Wound heals by itself.

staphylococcus—aureus (or staph) is a bacterium that can exist on skin or on other surfaces such as in the nose or mouth without symptoms. The symptoms can range from pain and swelling around a lesion, small milia like bumps, or general inflammation in the lymph nodes at any point in the body. It must be treated with antibiotics.

strabismus—Eyes that are misaligned or lazy eye.

streptococcal—Bacteria found within the body and on the skin. Cellulitis a common form of strep infection and presents as an area on the skin that is erythemic (red), inflamed, sensitive, warm or "hot" to the host, and may appear blistered.

subclinical condition—Undetected to naked eye.

syphilis—A sexually transmitted disease, which is caused by a spiral-shaped bacterium called Treponema pallidum, which can enter the body through minor cuts or abrasions in the skin or through mucous membrane. The disease is curable and progression is preventable if syphilis is caught early and treated. It was more common in the nineteenth and early twentieth century.

SWOT—Acronym for Strengths, Weaknesses, Opportunities, Threats; the elements you need to determine effective marketing strategy.

target audience—A group that has been identified for marketing purposes as potential clients.

TCA—Trichloracetic acid used in chemical peels.

telangiectases—Spider veins.

The Centers for Disease Control—A federal agency acting to protect the health and safety of people.

tinea—General term for fungal infection.

tinea versicolor—White patches where production of melanin has been compromised.

transconjunctival blepharoplasty—Fat pads are removed through an incision made inside lower lid.

tretinoin/retinoic acid—(Retin-A, Renova, Activa) a vitamin A derivative that stimulates growth of fibroblasts, which are tiny spindle-shaped cells present in connective tissue from which collagen and elastic fibers are formed. It is also used for exfoliation on the upper layer of the stratum corneum.

UltraSoft—Expanded polytetrafluoroethylene (or ePTFE); material used for lip augmentation, wrinkles and soft tissue defects.

Universal and Standard Precautions—A government regulation standard created by the Occupational Safety and Health Administration (OSHA) to treat all body fluids as if they are infectious, and assume all tissue as being hazardous. Frequent hand washing and wearing gloves and appropriate body protection devices during treatments, and clean up are essentials to following this rule.

vehicle—Method used to send an advertising or promotional message.

vitamin C—An antioxidant found especially in citrus fruits. Ascorbic acid and its derivatives are also found in skincare products

vitamin E—An antioxidant found especially in seed germ oils and leaves.

vitiligo—Extreme loss of pigment.

von Willebrand's disease (vWD)—A combined bleeding disorder of platelet function and mild to severe deficiency of factor VII. Can be both male or female and is genetically transmitted.

xanthalasmas—Whitish or yellow-toned fatty deposits usually found around the eye area.

xerosis—A condition of extremely dry skin.

Bibliography and Recommended Reading

Acello, R. (2000). *Advanced skills for health care providers*. Clifton Park, NY: Delmar Publishers/Thomson Learning.

American National Standards Institute (ANSI). (1988). *Standard for the safe use of lasers in health care facilities.* ANSI Z136.3-1988.

Byrd, R. C., & Sherrill, J. (1995). The therapeutic effects of intercessory prayer. *Journal of Christian Nursing, 12* (1), 21–23, 28. Retrieved from http://www.stkate.edu/library/guides/spiritbib.html

Chopra, D. (1994). *The seven spiritual laws of success, A practical guide to the fulfillment of your dreams.* San Rafael, CA: Amber-Allen Publishing.

Collier, P.F., & Son. (1910). *The Hippocratic Oath*. From Harvard Classics Volume 38, text placed in public domain June 1993. [Electronic version.] http://members.tripod.com/nktiuro/hippocra.htm

D'Angelo et al. (2003). *Milady's standard comprehensive training for estheticians.* Clifton Park, NY: Delmar Publishers/Thomson Learning.

Estes Pinkola, C. (1992). *Women who run with the wolves, Myths and stories of the wild woman archetype.* New York: Ballantine Books.

Fitzpatrick, T. B. (1988). The validity and practicality of sun-reactive skin types I through VI. *Archives of Dermatology 124* (6) 869–871.

Furman, R. (2000). *Drugs & cosmetics, Combinations that can kill you.* Studio City, CA: CRF Publications.

Furman, R. (2002). *Cancer & cosmetics, Combinations that can hurt you.* Studio City, CA: CRF Publications.

Gittleman, L. (1998). *Before the change, Taking charge of your menopause.* New York: Harper Collins Publishers.

Grogan, F. J. (2001). *Pharmacy simplified: A glossary of terms.* Clifton Park, NY: Delmar Publishers/Thomson Learning.

Johnson, E. A. (1985). *As someone dies, A handbook for the living.* Santa Monica, CA: Hay House.

Kaiser, Shirley E. (1998). *What is healing music?* [Electronic version.] www.shirleykaiser.com/healing/articles/healing.html

Keir, L., Wise, B. A., & Krebs, C. A. (1998). *Medical assisting, Administrative and clinical competencies* (4th ed.). Clifton Park, NY: Delmar Publishers/Thomson Learning.

Lees, M. (2001). *Skin care: Beyond the basics.* Clifton Park, NY: Milady/Thomson Learning.

Leopold, A. (1966). *A sand country almanac.* New York: Ballantine Books.

Maister, D. H., Green, C. H., & Galford, R. M. (2001). *The trusted advisor.* New York: Touchstone, Simon & Schuster.

Martin, L., & Jung, P. (2002). *Taking charge of the change, A holistic approach to the three phases of menopause.* Clifton Park, NY: Delmar Publishers/Thomson Learning.

Mazlow, A. (1954). *Motivation & personality.* New York: Harper & Row.

McCutcheon, M. (2002). *Where have my eyebrows gone? One woman's personal experiences with chemotherapy.* Clifton Park, NY: Delmar Publishers/Thomson Learning.

Michalun, N., & Varinia, M. (2001). *Milady's skin care & cosmetic ingredients dictionary* (2nd ed.). Clifton Park, NY: Milady/Delmar Thomson Learning.

Moore, T. (1992). *Care of the soul.* New York: HarperCollins.

Northrup, C. (2001). *The wisdom of menopause: Creating physical and emotional health and healing during the change.* New York: Bantam.

Olson, M. (2001). *Healing the dying* (2nd ed.). Clifton Park, NY: Delmar Publishers/Thomson Learning.

Orman, S. (1997). *The 9 steps to financial freedom, Practical & spiritual steps so you can stop worrying.* New York, NY: Crown Publishers, Inc.

Propionibacterium spp. Retrieved May 6, 2002, from http://www.geocities.com/ mtmccue2000/propionobacterium.html

Propionibacterium. Retrieved March 28, 2001 from http://medic.med.uth.edu/ path/0001503.htm.

Provost, Thomas T., M.D. 1995. Lupus and skin care. *The Lupus Lighthouse 17* (4) (Winter). Vancouver, B.C., Canada.

Puchalski, C. M. (1999). Spiritual Life *Touching the spirit: The essence of healing.* Retrieved from http://www.spiritual-life.org/id30_m.htm

Reardon, K. K. (2000). *The secret handshake.* New York: Doubleday, Random House, Inc.

Robinson, S. (2001). *Color blindness.* Timeeurope.com: Africa. Retrieved from www.time.com/time/europe/af/magazine/o,9868,170111,00.html

Roth, R. A., & Townsend, C. E. (2003). *Nutrition & diet therapy* (8th ed.). Clifton Park, NY: Delmar Publishers/Thomson Learning.

Rothfield, Naomi, M.D. (1995). Lupus and skin care. *The Lupus Lighthouse 22* (2) (Summer).Vancouver, B.C., Canada (newsletter).

Rubin, M. (1995). *Manual of chemical peels, Superficial and medium depth.* Philadelphia, PA: J.B. Lippincott Company.

Silverman, H. M. (2000). *The pill book* (9th ed.). New York, NY: Bantam Books.

Thrower, A. P. (1999). *Black skin care for the practicing professional.* Milady SalonOvations Publishing, Clifton Park, NY: Delmar Publishers/Thompson Learning.

White, L. (2001). *Foundations of nursing, Caring for the whole person,* Clifton Park, NY: Delmar Publishers/Thomson Learning.

Wilson, P. (2001). *Calm for life.* New York: Dorset Press.

Index

Note: the letter *t* denotes a table